125.00

369 0240475

This

AUTOPHAGY

CANCER, OTHER PATHOLOGIES, INFLAMMATION, IMMUNITY, INFECTION, AND AGING

VOLUME 1

Edited by

M. A. HAYAT

Distinguished Professor
Department of Biological Sciences
Kean University
Union, New Jersey

AMSTERDAM • BOSTON • HEIDELBERG • LONDON
NEW YORK • OXFORD • PARIS • SAN DIEGO
SAN FRANCISCO • SINGAPORE • SYDNEY • TOKYO

Academic Press is an imprint of Elsevier

ALISTAIR MACKENZIE LIBRARY
Barcode: 3640 240475
Class no: QU 375 HAY

Academic Press is an imprint of Elsevier
525 B Street, Suite 1900, San Diego, CA 92101-4495, USA
32 Jamestown Road, London NW1 7BY, UK
225 Wyman Street, Waltham, MA 02451, USA

Copyright © 2014 Elsevier Inc. All rights reserved

No part of this publication may be reproduced, stored in a retrieval system, or transmitted in any
form or by any means electronic, mechanical, photocopying, recording or otherwise without the prior
written permission of the publisher.

Permissions may be sought directly from Elsevier's Science & Technology Rights, Department in
Oxford, UK: phone (+44) (0) 1865 843830; fax (+44) (0) 1865 853333; email: permissions@elsevier.com.
Alternatively, visit the Science and Technology Books website at www.elsevierdirect.com/rights for
further information.

Notice
No responsibility is assumed by the publisher for any injury and/or damage to persons, or property
as a matter of products liability, negligence or otherwise, or from any use or, operation of any
methods, products, instructions or ideas contained in the material herein. Because of rapid advances
in the medical sciences, in particular, independent verification of diagnoses and drug dosages should
be made.

British Library Cataloguing-in-Publication Data
A catalogue record for this book is available from the British Library

Library of Congress Cataloging-in-Publication Data
A catalog record for this book is available from the Library of Congress

ISBN: 978-0-12-405530-8

For information on all Academic Press publications
visit our website at elsevierdirect.com

Typeset by MPS Limited, Chennai, India
www.adi-mps.com

Printed and bound in the United States of America

14 15 16 17   10 9 8 7 6 5 4 3 2 1

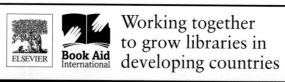

Working together
to grow libraries in
developing countries

ELSEVIER   Book Aid
International

www.elsevier.com • www.bookaid.org

Dedication

To

Patrice Codogno, Ana Maria Cuervo, Guido R.Y. De Meyer, Vojo Deretic, Fred J. Dice, William A. Dunn Jr., Eeva-Lisa Eskelinen, Sharon Gorski, Daniel J. Klionsky, Guido Kroemer, Beth Levine, Noboru Mizushima, Yoshinori Ohsumi, Brinda Ravikumar, David Rubinsztein, Isei Tanida, Sharon A. Tooze, Herbert W. Virgin, Eileen White, Tamotsu Yoshimori, and others:

The men and women involved in the odyssey of deciphering the molecular mechanisms underlying the complexity of the autophagy process that governs our lives.

Life in the Balance, Longevity the Goal
Self-eating, recycling, cash-for-your clunkers:
Trade up to the mitochondrial equivalent Prius.
The road to rejuvenation is paved with destruction
For clearing the rubble precedes reconstruction
But remember that life's circular dance
Depends on opposite forces in balance
Excess destruction, too much biogenesis,
Brings heart failure, cancer or neurodegeneries

Roberta A. Gottlieb

Contents

II

CANCER

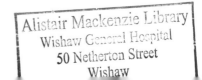
Alistair Mackenzie Library
Wishaw General Hospital
50 Netherton Street
Wishaw

III

TUMORS

Preface

The ultimate goal of research in this field is to decipher the molecular mechanisms underlying the exceedingly complex autophagic process and use them for the development of effective therapy against diseases. This goal becomes urgent considering that presently available treatments (chemotherapy, radiation, surgery, and hormone therapy) for major diseases such as cancer are only modestly successful.

During the past two decades, an astonishing advance has been made in the understanding of the molecular mechanisms involved in the degradation of intracellular protein in yeast vacuoles and the lysosomal compartment in mammalian cells. Advances in genome-scale approaches and computational tools have presented opportunities to explore the broader context in which autophagy is regulated at the systems level.

This is Volume 1, *Autophagy: Cancer, Other Pathologies, Inflammation, Immunity, Infection, and Aging*, of a four-volume series that will discuss almost all aspects of the autophagy process. The text is divided into three subheadings (General Diseases, Cancer, and Tumors) for the convenience of readers. The Introduction to *Autophagy* contains brief summaries of the large number of autophagic functions, including their roles in disease and health, especially with regard to both oncogenic and tumor suppressive roles during tumor and cancer development. Autophagy protects us not only from cancer but also against the development of other diseases. The role of autophagy in cellular defense against inflammation is also included.

The role of autophagy in the suppression of tumors and in tumor survival is discussed. Induction of autophagic cell death by anticancer agents is presented. On the other hand, some anticancer drugs induce autophagy that protects cells, while autophagy inhibitors sensitize cells to chemotherapy, which then becomes more effective. The importance of autophagy, stem cells, and dormancy in health and disease is also explained. That death-associated protein kinase 1 suppresses tumor growth and metastasis via autophagy and apoptosis is included in this volume. The role of autophagy in the treatment of diabetic cardiomyopathy is explained.

By bringing together a large number of experts (oncologists, neurosurgeons, physicians, research scientists, and pathologists) in the field of autophagy, it is my hope that substantial progress will be made against terrible diseases inflicting humans. It is difficult for a single author to discuss, effectively and comprehensively, various aspects of an exceedingly complex process such as autophagy. Another advantage of involving more than one author is to present different points of view on specific controversial aspects of the role of autophagy in health and disease. I hope these goals will be fulfilled in this and other volumes of the series.

This volume was written by 56 contributors representing 11 countries. I am grateful to them for their promptness in accepting my suggestions. Their practical experience highlights the very high quality of their writings, which should build and further the endeavors of the readers in this important medical field. I respect and appreciate the hard work and exceptional insight into the autophagy machinery provided by these contributors.

It is my hope that subsequent volumes of the series will join this volume in assisting in the more complete understanding of the complex process of autophagy, and eventually in the development of therapeutic applications. There exists a tremendous urgent demand by the public and the scientific community to address the treatment of major diseases. In the light of existing disease calamities, government funding must give priority to eradicating deadly malignancies over global military superiority.

I am grateful to Dr Dawood Farahi and Mr Philip Connelly for recognizing the importance of medical research and publishing through an institution of higher education. I am thankful to my students for their contribution to the preparation of this volume.

M.A. Hayat
March 2013

Contributors

Patrizia Agostinis   Cell Death Research and Therapy Laboratory, Department of Cellular & Molecular Medicine, Faculty of Medicine, Campus Gasthuisberg, K.U. Leuven, Herestraat 49, Bus 901, B3000 Leuven, Belgium

Macarena Alanís Sánchez   Pathophysiology Group Cell in Development and Disease, Lab 210, Andalusian Centre for Developmental Biology – CSIC UPO, Carretera de Utrera Km 1, 41013 Sevilla, Spain

Gizem Ayna   Department of Biochemistry and Molecular Biology, Stem Cells, Apoptosis and Genomics Research Group of the Hungarian Academy of Sciences, University of Debrecen, H-4010 Egyetem Tér 1, Debrecen, Hungary

Mario D. Cordero   Pathophysiology Group Cell in Development and Disease, Lab 210, Andalusian Centre for Developmental Biology – CSIC UPO, Carretera de Utrera Km 1, 41013 Sevilla, Spain

David Cotán   Pathophysiology Group Cell in Development and Disease, Lab 210, Andalusian Centre for Developmental Biology – CSIC UPO, Carretera de Utrera Km 1, 41013 Sevilla, Spain

Ana Delgado Pavón   Pathophysiology Group Cell in Development and Disease, Lab 210, Andalusian Centre for Developmental Biology – CSIC UPO, Carretera de Utrera Km 1, 41013 Sevilla, Spain

Mario de la Mata   Pathophysiology Group Cell in Development and Disease, Lab 210, Andalusian Centre for Developmental Biology – CSIC UPO, Carretera de Utrera Km 1, 41013 Sevilla, Spain

Luisa De Martino   Department of Pathology and Animal Health, University of Naples Federico II, Via Delpino, 1, 80137 – Naples, Italy

Guido R.Y. De Meyer   University of Antwerp – Campus Drie Eiken, Laboratory of Physiopharmacology, Universiteitsplein 1, B-2610 Antwerpen, Belgium

Karin Eberhart   Sabanci University, Faculty of Engineering and Natural Sciences, Orhanli-Tuzla 34956, Istanbul, Turkey

Alejandro Fernández-Vega   Pathophysiology Group Cell in Development and Disease, Lab 210, Andalusian Centre for Developmental Biology – CSIC UPO, Carretera de Utrera Km 1, 41013 Sevilla, Spain

László Fésüs   Department of Biochemistry and Molecular Biology, Stem Cells, Apoptosis and Genomics Research Group of the Hungarian Academy of Sciences, University of Debrecen, H-4010 Egyetem Tér 1, Debrecen, Hungary

Filomena Fiorito   Department of Pathology and Animal Health, University of Naples Federico II, Via Delpino, 1, 80137 – Naples, Italy

Yuuki Fujiwara   Department of Degenerative Neurological Diseases, National Institute of Neuroscience, National Center of Neurology and Psychiatry, 4-1-1 Ogawahigashi, Kodaira, Tokyo, 187-8502, Japan

Padmaja Gade   HH 333B, 660W Redwood Street, University of Maryland, Baltimore, Maryland 21201, USA

Juan Garrido Maraver   Pathophysiology Group Cell in Development and Disease, Lab 210, Andalusian Centre for Developmental Biology – CSIC UPO, Carretera de Utrera Km 1, 41013 Sevilla, Spain

David A. Gewirtz   Department of Pharmacology and Toxicology, Massey Cancer Center, Virginia Commonwealth University, Richmond, Virginia, USA

Madan M. Godbole   Dr Brian Herman's Lab, University of Texas Health Science Center at

San Antonio, South Texas Research Park, 8403 Floyd Curl Dr., San Antonio, Texas 78229-3904, USA

Devrim Gozuacik   Sabanci University, Faculty of Engineering and Natural Sciences, Orhanli-Tuzla 34956, Istanbul, Turkey

Rafael Guerrero-Preston   Johns Hopkins University School of Medicine, CRB-II, Room 2M05, 1550 Orleans Street, Baltimore, Maryland 21231, USA

M.A. Hayat   Department of Biological Sciences, Kean University, 1000 Morris Ave, Union, NJ 07083, USA

Eun-Kyeong Jo   Infection Signaling Network Research Center, Department of Microbiology, Chungnam National University School of Medicine, 6 Munhwa-dong, Jungku, Daejeon 301-747, S. Korea

José A. Sánchez Alcázar   Pathophysiology Group Cell in Development and Disease, Lab 210, Andalusian Centre for Developmental Biology – CSIC UPO, Carretera de Utrera Km 1, 41013 Sevilla, Spain

Tomohiro Kabuta   Department of Degenerative Neurological Diseases, National Institute of Neuroscience, National Center of Neurology and Psychiatry, 4-1-1 Ogawahigashi, Kodaira, Tokyo, 187-8502, Japan

Dhan V. Kalvakolanu   HH 333B, 660W Redwood Street, University of Maryland, Baltimore, Maryland 21201, USA

Jin-A. Lee   Department of Biotechnology, College of Life Science and Nanotechnology, Hannam University, Dajeon 305-811, Korea

Jiankang Liu   Institute of Mitochondrial Biology and Medicine, School of Life Science and Technology, Xi'an Jiaotong University, Xi'an 710049, China

Jiangang Long   Institute of Mitochondrial Biology and Medicine, School of Life Science and Technology, Xi'an Jiaotong University, Xi'an 710049, China

Wim Martinet   University of Antwerp – Campus Drie Eiken, Laboratory of Physiopharmacology, Universiteitsplein 1, B-2610 Antwerpen, Belgium

Cédéric F. Michiels   University of Antwerp – Campus Drie Eiken, Laboratory of Physiopharmacology, Universiteitsplein 1, B-2610 Antwerpen, Belgium

Tsunehiro Mizushima   Picobiology Institute, Department of Life Science, Graduate School of Life Science, University of Hyogo, 3-2-1, Kouto, Kamigori-cho, Ako-gun, Hyogo, 678-1297, Japan

Kris Nys   Translational Research in GastroIntestinal Disorders, Department of Clinical and Experimental Medicine, Faculty of Medicine, Campus Gasthuisberg, K.U. Leuven, Herestraat 49, Bus 701, B3000 Leuven, Belgium

Ozlem Oral   Sabanci University, Faculty of Engineering and Natural Sciences, Orhanli-Tuzla 34956, Istanbul, Turkey

Manuel Oropesa-Ávila   Pathophysiology Group Cell in Development and Disease, Lab 210, Andalusian Centre for Developmental Biology – CSIC UPO, Carretera de Utrera Km 1, 41013 Sevilla, Spain

Marina Villanueva Paz   Pathophysiology Group Cell in Development and Disease, Lab 210, Andalusian Centre for Developmental Biology – CSIC UPO, Carretera de Utrera Km 1, 41013 Sevilla, Spain

Carmen Pérez Calero   Pathophysiology Group Cell in Development and Disease, Lab 210, Andalusian Centre for Developmental Biology – CSIC UPO, Carretera de Utrera Km 1, 41013 Sevilla, Spain

Goran Petrovski   Department of Biochemistry and Molecular Biology, Stem Cells, Apoptosis and Genomics Research Group of the Hungarian Academy of Sciences, University of Debrecen, H-4010 Egyetem Tér 1., Debrecen, Hungary

Edward A. Ratovitski   Johns Hopkins University School of Medicine, CRB-II, Room 2M05, 1550 Orleans Street, Baltimore, Maryland 21231, USA

Ángeles Rodríguez Hernández   Pathophysiology Group Cell in Development and Disease, Lab 210, Andalusian Centre for Developmental Biology – CSIC UPO, Carretera de Utrera Km 1, 41013 Sevilla, Spain

Noemí Rubio Romero   Cell Death Research and Therapy Laboratory, Cellular & Molecular Medicine Department, Faculty of Medicine, KU Leuven (KUL), Herestraat 49, O&NI Box 802, Leuven 3000, Belgium

Emil Rudolf   Department of Medical Biology and Genetics, Charles University in Prague, Faculty of Medicine in Hradec Kralove, Simkova 870, 500 38 Hradec Kralove, Czech Republic

Dorien M. Schrijvers   University of Antwerp – Campus Drie Eiken, Laboratory of Physiopharmacology, Universiteitsplein 1, B-2610 Antwerpen, Belgium

Lokendra K. Sharma   Dr Brian Herman's Lab, University of Texas Health Science Center at San Antonio, South Texas Research Park, 8403 Floyd Curl Dr., San Antonio, Texas 78229-3904, USA

Dong-Min Shin   Infection Signaling Network Research Center, Department of Microbiology, Chungnam National University School of Medicine, 6 Munhwa-dong, Jungku, Daejeon 301-747, S. Korea

Rajesh Singh   Department of Cell Biology, School of Biological Sciences and Biotechnology, Indian Institute of Advanced Research, Gandhinagar, India

Kenji Takagi   Picobiology Institute, Department of Life Science, Graduate School of Life Science, University of Hyogo, 3-2-1, Kouto, Kamigori-cho, Ako-gun, Hyogo, 678-1297, Japan

Ying Tang   Institute of Mitochondrial Biology and Medicine, School of Life Science and Technology, Xi'an Jiaotong University, Xi'an 710049, China

S. Tariq Ahmad   Department of Biotechnology, College of Life Science and Nanotechnology, Hannam University, Dajeon 305-811, Korea

Meenakshi Tiwari   Dr Brian Herman's Lab, University of Texas Health Science Center at San Antonio, South Texas Research Park, 8403 Floyd Curl Dr., San Antonio, Texas 78229-3904, USA

Dhanendra Tomar   Department of Cell Biology, School of Biological Sciences and Biotechnology, Indian Institute of Advanced Research, Gandhinagar, India

Séverine Vermeire   Translational Research in GastroIntestinal Disorders, Department of Clinical and Experimental Medicine, Faculty of Medicine, Campus Gasthuisberg, K.U. Leuven, Herestraat 49, Bus 701, B3000 Leuven, Belgium

Keiji Wada   Department of Degenerative Neurological Diseases, National Institute of Neuroscience, National Center of Neurology and Psychiatry, 4-1-1 Ogawahigashi, Kodaira, Tokyo, 187-8502, Japan

Yuran Xie   BSEB 314, Section of Endocrinology and Diabetes, Department of Medicine, University of Oklahoma Health Sciences Center, Oklahoma City, Oklahoma 73104, USA

Zhonglin Xie   BSEB 314, Section of Endocrinology and Diabetes, Department of Medicine, University of Oklahoma Health Sciences Center, Oklahoma City, Oklahoma 73104, USA

Jae-Min Yuk   Infection Signaling Network Research Center, Department of Microbiology, Chungnam National University School of Medicine, 6 Munhwa-dong, Jungku, Daejeon 301-747, S. Korea

Ke Zen   School of Life Sciences, Nanjing University, 22 Hankou Road, Nanjing, Jiangsu 210093, China

Qipeng Zhang   School of Life Sciences, Nanjing University, 22 Hankou Road, Nanjing, Jiangsu 210093, China

List of Contributions Projected in Volumes 2–4

(incomplete)

Abbreviations and Glossary

1AP	inhibitor of apoptosis protein
3-MA	3-methyladenine, an autophagy inhibitor
3-methyladenine	an autophagic inhibitor
5-Fu	5 fluorouracil
AAP	protein that mediates selective autophagy
ACF	aberrant crypt foci
aggrephagy	degradation of ubiquitinated protein aggregates
aggresome	inclusion body where misfolded proteins are confined and degraded by autophagy
AIF	apoptosis–inducing factor
AIM	Atg8-family interacting motif
Akt	protein kinase B regulates autophagy
Alfy	autophagy-linked FYVE protein
ALIS	aggresome-like induced structures
ALR	autophagic lysosome reformation.
AMBRA-1	activating molecule in Beclin 1-regulated autophagy
AMP	adenosine monophosphate
amphisome	intermediate compartment formed by fusing an autophagosome with an endosome
AMPK	adenosine monophosphate-activated protein kinase
aPKC	atypical protein kinase C
APMA	autophagic macrophage activation
apoptosis	programmed cell death type 1
ARD1	arrest-defective protein 1
ASK	apoptosis signal regulating kinase
AT1	Atg8-interacting protein
ATF5	activating transcription factor 5
ATF6	activating transcription factor 6
Atg	autophagy-related gene or protein
Atg1	serine/threonine protein 1 kinase
Atg2	protein that functions along with Atg18
Atg3	ubiqitin conjugating enzyme analogue
Atg4	cysteine protease
Atg5	protein containing ubiquitin folds
Atg6	component of the class III PtdIns 3-kinase complex
Atg7	ubiquitin activating enzyme homologue
Atg8	ubiquitin-like protein

Atg9	transmembrane protein
Atg10	ubiquitin conjugating enzyme analogue
Atg11	fungal scaffold protein
Atg12	ubiquitin-like protein
Atg13	component of the Atg1 complex
Atg14	component of the class III PtdIns 3-kinase complex
Atg15	vacuolar protein
Atg16	component of the Atg12-Atg5-Atg16
Atg17	yeast protein
Atg18	protein that binds to PtdIns
Atg19	receptor for the Cvt pathway
Atg20	PtdIns P binding protein
Atg21	PtdIns P binding protein
Atg22	vacuolar amino acid permease
Atg23	yeast protein
Atg24	PtdIns binding protein
Atg25	coiled-coil protein
Atg26	sterol glucosyltransferase
Atg27	integral membrane protein
Atg28	coiled-coil protein
Atg29	protein in fungi
Atg30	protein required for recognizing peroxisomes
Atg31	protein in fungi
Atg32	mitochondrial outer membrane protein
Atg33	mitochondrial outer membrane protein
Atg101	Atg13-binding protein
ATM	ataxia-telangiectasia mutated protein
autolysosome protein	lysosomal associated membrane protein 2
autolysosome	formed by fusion of the autophagosome and lysosome, degrading the engulfed cell components
autophagic body	the inner membrane-bound structure of the autophagosome
autophagic flux	the rate of cargo delivery to lysosomes through autophagy
autophagosome maturations	events occurring post-autophagosome closure followed by delivery of the cargo to lysosomes
autophagosome	double-membrane vesicle that engulfs cytoplasmic contents for delivery to the lysosome
autophagy	programmed cell death type 2
AV	autophagic vacuole
axonopathy	degradation of axons in neurodegeneration
BAD	Bcl-2 associated death promoter protein
Bafilomycin	inhibitor of the vacuolar-type ATPase
Bafilomycin A1(BAF-A1)	an autophagy inhibitor
BAG	Bcl-2-associated athanogene
BAG3	Bcl2-associated athanogene 3
BAK	Bcl-2 antagonist/killer

Barkor	Beclin 1-associated autophagy-related key regulator
BATS	Barkor/Atg14(L) autophagosome targeting sequence
BAX	Bcl-2-associated X protein
Bcl-2	B cell lymphoma-2
Beclin 1	mammalian homologue of yeast Atg6, activating macroautophagy
Beclin 1	Bcl-2-interacting protein 1
BH3	Bcl-2 homology domain-3
BH3-only proteins	induce macroautopagy
BHMT	betaine homocysteine methyltransferase protein found in the mammalian autophagosome (metabolic enzyme)
BID	BH3-interacting domain death agonist
Bif-1 protein	interacts with Beclin 1, required for macroautophagy
Bim	Bcl-2 interacting mediator
BNIP	pro-apoptotic protein
BNIP3 protein	required for the HIF-1-dependent induction of macroautophagy
bortezomib	selective proteasome inhibitor
CaMKKβ protein	activates AMPK at increased cytosolic calcium concentration
CaMK	calcium/calmodulin-dependent protein kinase
CASA	chaperone-assisted selective autophagy
caspase	cysteine aspartic acid specific protease
CCI-779	rapamycin ester that induces macroautophagy
CD46 glycoprotein	mediates an immune response to invasive pathogens
chloroquine	an autophagy inhibitor which inhibits fusion between autophagosomes and lysosomes
c-Jun	mammalian transcription factor that inhibits starvation-induced macroautophagy
Clg 1	a yeast cyclin-like protein that induces macroautophagy
CMA	chaperone-mediated autophagy
COG	functions in the fusion of vesicles within the Golgi complex
COP1	coat protein complex1
CP	20S core particle
CRD	cysteine-rich domain
CSC	cancer stem cell
CTGF	connective tissue growth factor
Cvt	cytoplasm-to-vacuole targeting
DAMP	damage-associated molecular pattern molecule/ danger-associated molecular pattern molecule
DAP1	death-associated Protein 1
DAPK	death-associated protein kinase
DAPK1	death-associated protein kinase 1
DDR	DNA damage response
DEPTOR	DEP domain containing mTOR-interacting protein
DFCP1	a PtdIns (3) P-binding protein
DISC	death-inducing signaling complex

DMV	double-membrane vesicle
DOR	diabetes-and obesity-regulated gene
DRAM	damage-regulated autophagy modulator
DRAM-1	damage-regulated autophagy modulator 1 induces autophagy in a p53-dependent manner.
DRC	desmin-related cardiomyopathy
DRiP	defective ribosomal protein
DRP1	dynamin related protein 1
DUB	deubiquitinases that accumulate proteins into aggresomes
E2F1	a mammalian transcription factor
EGFR	epidermal growth factor receptor
EIF2α	eukaryotic initiation factor 2 alpha kinase
endosomes	early compartments fuse with autophagosomes to generate amphisomes
ERAA	endoplasmic reticulum-activated autophagy
ERAD	endoplasmic reticulum-associated degradation pathway
ERK	extracellular signal regulated kinase
ERK1/2	extracellular signal regulated kinase 1/2
ERT	enzyme replacement therapy
ESCRT	endosomal sorting complex required for transport
everolimus	mTOR inhibitor
FADD	Fas-associated death domain
FKBP12	FK506-binding protein 12
FoxO3	Forkhead box O transcription factor 3
FYCO1	FYVE and coiled domain containing 1
GAA	acid α-glucosidase
GABARAP	gamma-aminobutyric acid receptor-associated protein
GAS	group A streptococcus
GATE-16	Golgi-associated ATPase enhancer of 16 kDa
GFP	green fluorescent protein
glycophagy	degradation of glycogen particles
GPCR	G protein-coupled receptor
GSK-3β	glycogen synthase kinase 3 beta regulates macroautophagy
GST-BHMT	BHMT fusion protein used to assay macroautophagy in mammalian cells
HAV	heavy autophagic vacuole
HCV	hepatitis C virus
HDAC	histone deacetylase
HDAC6	histone deacetylase 6
HIF	hypoxia-inducible factor
HIF1	hypoxia-inducible factor 1
HMGB1	high mobility group box 1
HR-PCD	hypersensitive response programmed cell death
Hsc70	heat shock cognate protein
Hsp	heat shock protein

Hsp90	heat shock protein 90
HspB8	heat shock cognate protein beta-8
I13P	phosphatidylinositol
IAP	inhibitor of apoptosis protein
IKK	inhibitor of nuclear factor κB
IL3	interleukin-3
IM	isolation membrane
inflammasome	an intracellular protein complex that activates caspase-1
IRF	interferon regulatory factor
IRGM	immunity-associated GTPase family M
IRS	insulin receptor substrate
JNK/SAPK	c-Jun N-terminal kinase/stress-activated protein kinase
KRAS	an oncogene that induces autophagy in cancer cells
LAMP	lysosome-associated membrane protein
LAMP1	lysosome marker, lysosome-associated membrane protein 1
LAMP2	lysosomal-associated membrane protein 2
LAMP-2A	lysosomal-associated membrane protein 2A
LAP	LC3-associated phagocytosis
LAV	light autophagic vacole
LC3 (MAP1LC3B)	autophagosome marker microtubule-associated protein 1 light chain 3B
LC3	microtubule-associated protein light chain 3
LET	linear energy transfer
lipophagy	selective delivery of lipid droplets for lysosomal degradation
LIR	LC3 interacting region
LKB	liver kinase B
LSD	lysosomal storage disorder
lysosomotropic agent	compound that accumulates preferentially in lysosomes
macroautophagy	autophagy
macrolipophagy	regulation of lipid metabolism by autophagy
MALS	macroautophagy–lysosome system
MAPK	mitogen-activated protein kinase
MARF	mitofusion mitochondrial assembly regulatory factor
MCU	mitochondrial calcium uptake uniporter pore
MDC	monodansylcadaverine to measure autophagic flux *in vivo*
MEF	mouse embryonic fibroblast
MFN2	mitofusin 2, a mitochondrial outer membrane protein involved in fusion/fission to promote mitochondrial segregation and elimination
MHC	major histocompatibility complex
MHC-II	major histocompatibility complex class II
MiCa	mitochondrial inner membrane calcium channel
micropexophagy or macropexophagy	peroxisome degradation by autophagic machinery
MIPA	micropexophagy-specific membrane apparatus

mitofusion	mitochondrial fusion-promoting factor
mitophagy	degradation of dysfunctional mitochondria
MOM	mitochondrial outer membrane
MPS	mucopolysaccharide
MPT	mitochondrial permeability transition
mPTP	mitochondrial permeability transition pore
MSD	multiple sulfatase deficiency
MTOC	microtubule organizing center
mTOR	mammalian target of rapamycin, which inhibits autophagy and functions as a sensor for cellular energy and amino acid levels
mTORc1	mammalian target of rapamycin complex 1
MTP	mitochondrial transmembrane potential
MTS	mitochondrial targeting sequence
MVB	multivesicular body
NBR1	neighbor of BRCA1 gene 1
NDP52	nuclear dot protein 52 kDa
NEC-1	necrostatin-1
necroptosis	a form of programmed cell death by activating autophagy-dependent necrosis
Nix	a member of the Bcl-2 family required for mitophagy
NLR	NOD-like receptor
NOD	nucleotide-binding oligomerization domain
NOS	nitric oxide synthase
NOX	NADPH oxidase
Nrf2	nuclear factor 2
OCR	oxygen consumption rate
Omegasome	PI(3)P-enriched subdomain of the ER involved in autophagosome formation
OMM	outer mitochondrial membrane
OPA1	mitafusin 1 is required to promote mitochondrial fusion
Ox-LDL	oxidized low density lipoprotein is a major inducer of ROS, inflammation, and injury to endothelial cells
p62	an autophagy substrate
PAMP	pathogen-associated molecular pattern molecule
PAS	pre-autophagosomal structure
PB1 domain	Phox and Bem1 domain
PCD	programmed cell death
PDI	protein disulfide isomerase
PE	phosphatidyl ethanolamine
PERK	protein kinase-like endoplasmic reticulum kinase
PFI	proteasome functional insufficiency
Phagophore	a cup-shaped, double membraned autophagic precursor structure
PI(3)K-PKB-FOXO	a growth factor that inhibits autophagy and increases apoptosis by regulating glutamine metabolism

PI3K	phosphatidylinositol 3-kinase
PI3KC3	phosphatidylinositol-3-kinase class 3
PINK1	PTEN (phosphatase and tensin homologue deleted on chromosome 10)-induced putative kinase 1
PKA	protein kinase A
PKB	protein kinase B
PKC	protein kinase C
polyQ	polyglutamine
PQC	protein quality control
prion disease	transmissible spongiform encephalopathy
PRR	pathogen recognition receptor
PS	phosphatidyl serine
PSMB5	proteasome subunit beta type-5
PtdIns	Phosphatidylinositol
PTGS	post-transcriptional gene silencing
PUMA	p53 upregulated modulator of apoptosis
R1G	retrograde signaling pathway
Rag	GTPase that activates TORC1 in response to amino acids
RAGE	receptor for advanced glycation end product
rapamycin	a well-known autophagy inducer by suppressing mTOR
RAPTOR	regulatory-associated of mTOR
RE	recycling endosome
residual body	lysosome containing undegraded material
reticulophagy	degradation of endoplasmic reticulum
ribophagy	degradation of ribosomes
RIP	receptor-interacting protein
RISC	RNA-induced silencing complex
RLS	reactive lipid species
RNAi	RNA interference
RNS	reactive nitrogen species
ROS	reactive oxygen species
ROT	rottlerin used as a protein kinase C-delta inhibitor
RP	19 S regulatory particle
Rubicon	RUN domain and cysteine-rich domain-containing Beclin 1-interacting protein
selective autophagy	selective recruitment of substrates for autophagy
sequestosome (SQSTMI)1	P62 protein, a ubiquitin-binding scaffold protein
sequestosome 1 (p62/SQSTM1)	a multifunctional adapter protein implicated in tumorigenesis
sequestosome 1	an autophagy substrate
SESN2	sestrin-2
shRNA	small/short hairpin RNA
siRNA	small interference RNA
sirt 1	sirtuin 1 class III histone deacetylase, prevents Alzheimer's disease

SMIR	small molecule inhibitor of rapamycin
SNARE	soluble N-ethylmaleimide-sensitive factor attachment receptor
SNP	single nucleotide polymorphism
SQSTM1	sequestosome 1
Syt1	synaptotagmin1
T1DM	type 1 diabetes mellitus
TAKA	transport of Atg9 after knocking-out Atg1
TASCC	TOR-autophagy spatial coupling compartment
TCN	transe-Golgi network
TCR	T cell receptor
TECPR1	tectonin beta-propeller repeat containing 1
Tensirolimus	mTOR inhibitor
TFEB	transcript factor EB
TGFβ	transforming growth factor β that activates autophagy
TGN	trans-Golgi network
TIGR	TP53 (tumor protein 53)-induced glycolysis and apoptosis regulator
TK	tyrosine kinase
TKI	tyrosine kinase inhibitor
TLR	Toll-like receptor
TMD	transmembrane domain
TMEM166	transmembrane protein 166 that induces autophagy
TNF	tumor-necrosis factor
TNF-α	tumor necrosis factor alpha
Torin1	ATP-competitive mTOR inhibitor
TRAIL	tumor necrosis factor-regulated apoptosis-inducing ligand
TSC	tuberous sclerosis complex
TSC2	tuberous sclerosis complex 2
TSP	thrombospondin
UBA	domain: ubiquitin-associated domain
UBAN	ubiquitin-binding domain
Ubiquitin	a small protein that functions in intracellular protein breakdown and histone modification
Ubiquitination	a well-established signal for inducing autophagy of protein aggregates
Ubl	ubiquitin-like
ULK	Unc-51-like kinase complex
ULK1	putative mammalian homologue of yeast Atg1p required for macroautophagy
UPR	unfolded protein response
UPS	ubiquitin–proteasome system
UVRAG	UV-irradiation resistance-associated gene
VAchT	vesicular acetylcholine transporter
VAMP	vesicle-associated membrane protein
VCP/p97	valosin-containing protein involved in endosomal trafficking and autophagy

VEGF	Vascular endothelial growth factor
VEGFR	vascular endothelial growth factor receptor
VMP1	vacuole membrane protein 1, promotes formation of autophagosomes
VPS15	vacuolar protein sorting 15 homologue
VTAs	vascular targeting agents
VTC	vacuolar transporter chaperone
wortmannin	an autophagic inhibitor
XBP1	a component of the ER stress response that activates macroautophagy
xenophagy	degradation of invading bacteria, viruses and parasites
YFP	yellow fluorescent protein
zymophagy	lysosomal degradation of zymogen granules (digestive enzymes)

See also Klionsky, D.J., Codogno, P., Cuervo, A.M. et al. (2010). A comprehensive glossary of autophagy-related molecules and processes. Autophagy 6, 438–448.

Introduction to Autophagy: Cancer, Other Pathologies, Inflammation, Immunity, Infection and Aging, Volumes 1–4

M.A. Hayat

Abstract

Autophagy plays a direct or indirect role in health and disease. A simplified definition of autophagy is that it is an exceedingly complex process which degrades modified, superfluous (surplus) or damaged cellular macromolecules and whole organelles using hydrolytic enzymes in the lysosomes. It consists of sequential steps of induction of autophagy, formation of autophagosome precursor, formation of autophagosome, fusion between autophagosome and lysosome, degradation of cargo contents, efflux transportation of degraded products to the cytoplasm, and lysosome reformation.

This chapter discusses specific functions of autophagy, the process of autophagy, major types of autophagy, influences on autophagy, and the role of autophagy in disease, immunity and defense.

INTRODUCTION

Because the aging process is accompanied by disability and disease (for example, Alzheimer's and Parkinson's conditions) and cannot be prevented, it seems that slow aging is the only way to have a healthy longer life. In general, aging can be slowed down by not smoking or chewing tobacco, by preventing or minimizing perpetual stress (anger, competition), and by abstinence from alcoholic beverages, regular exercise, and having a healthy diet. There is no doubt that regular physical activity is associated with a reduced risk of mortality and contributes to the primary and secondary prevention of many types of diseases. Discipline is required to attain this goal.

Regarding the role of a healthy diet, a caloric restriction induces autophagy that counteracts the development of age-related diseases and aging itself. On the other hand, autophagy is inhibited by high glucose and insulin-induced P13K signaling via PKB and mTOR. Based on its fundamental roles in these and other disease processes' prevention and therapy, autophagy has emerged as a potential target for disease.

Unfortunately, inevitable death rules our lives, and a group of abnormal cells plays a part in it. Safe disposal of cellular debris is crucial to keep us alive and healthy. Our body uses autophagy and apoptosis as clearing mechanisms to eliminate malfunctioning, aged, damaged, excessive, and/or pathogen-infected cell debris that might otherwise be harmful/autoimmunogenic. However, if such a clearing process becomes uncontrollable, it can instead be deleterious. For example, deficits in protein clearance in the brain cells because of dysfunctional autophagy may lead to dementia. Autophagy can also promote cell death through excessive self-digestion and degradation of essential cellular constituents.

Cancer is associated with aging, for more than 80% of human cancers are diagnosed in people aged 55 years or older. Humans and other mammals with long lifespans unfortunately have to face the problem of getting old and the accumulation of somatic mutations over time. Most of the mutations cause diseases that eventually lead to the demise of the individual. Cancer is one of these major diseases, and is caused by a combination of somatic genetic alterations in a single cell, followed by uncontrolled cell growth and proliferation. Even a single germline deletion of or mutation in a tumor suppressor gene (e.g., *p53*) predisposes an individual to cancer. It is apparent that nature tries to ensure the longevity of the individual by providing tumor suppressor genes and other protective mechanisms. Autophagy (*Beclin 1* gene) is one of these mechanisms that plays an important role in influencing the aging process.

Autophagy research is in an explosive phase, driven by a relatively new awareness of the enormously significant role it plays in health and disease, including cancer, other pathologies, inflammation, immunity, infection, and aging. The term autophagy (*auto phagein*, from the Greek meaning self-eating) refers to a phenomenon in which cytoplasmic components are delivered to the lysosomes for bulk or selective degradation under the lysosomes' distinct intracellular and extracellular milieu. This term was first coined by de Duve over 46 years ago (Deter and de Duve, 1967), based on the observed degradation of mitochondria and other intracellular structures within lysosomes of rat liver perfused with the pancreatic hormone, glucagon.

Over the past two decades an astonishing advance has been made in the understanding of the molecular mechanisms involved in the degradation of intracellular proteins in yeast vacuoles and the lysosomal compartment in mammalian cells. Advances in genome-scale approaches and computational tools have presented opportunities to explore the broader context in which autophagy is regulated at the systems level.

A simplified definition of autophagy is that it is an exceedingly complex process which degrades modified, superfluous (surplus), or damaged cellular macromolecules and whole organelles using hydrolytic enzymes in the lysosomes. Autophagy can be defined in more detail as a regulated process of degradation and recycling of cellular constituents participating in organelle turnover, resulting in the bioenergetic management of starvation. This definition, however, still represents only some of the numerous roles played by the autophagic machinery in mammals; most of the autophagic functions are listed later in this chapter.

Autophagy plays a constitutive and basally active role in the quality control of proteins and organelles, and is associated with either cell survival or cell death. Stress-responsive autophagy can promote cell survival, whereas in certain models autophagy has been shown to be a mechanism by which cells die – a process termed autophagic or type 2 cell death. Autophagy prevents the accumulation of random molecular damage in long-lived structures, particularly mitochondria, and more generally provides a means to reallocate cellular resources from one biochemical pathway to another. Consequently, it is upregulated in conditions where a cell is responding to stress signals, such as starvation, oxidative stress, and exercise-induced adaptation. The balance between protein and lipid biosynthesis, their eventual degradation and resynthesis, is one critical components of cellular health.

Degradation and recycling of macromolecules via autophagy provides a source of building blocks (amino acids, fatty acids, sugars) that allow temporal adaptation of cells to adverse conditions. In addition to recycling, autophagy is required for the degradation of damaged or toxic material that can be generated as a result of ROS accumulation during oxidative stress. The mitochondrial electron transport chain and the peroxisomes are primary sources of ROS production in most eukaryotes.

SPECIFIC FUNCTIONS OF AUTOPHAGY (A SUMMARY)

Autophagy plays a direct or indirect role in health and disease, including control of embryonic and early postnatal development, tissue homeostasis (protein and cell organelle turnover); mitochondrial quality control; protection of cells from stresses; survival response to nutrient deprivation; cellular survival or physiological cell death during development;

involvement in cell death upon treatment with chemotherapy and radiotherapy; tissue remodeling during differentiation and development, including regulation of number of cells and cell size, endocytosed gap junctions, villous trophoblasts, cellular house-cleaning, protein, glucose, and lipid metabolism; supply of energy; anti-aging; human malignancy, tumorigenesis, tumor maintenance, inflammation, cancer (pro and anti), ovarian cancer, nasopharyngeal carcinoma, melanoma, colon cancer, and neutrophil differentiation of acute promyelocytic leukemia; lysosomal storage diseases; metabolic disorders; osteoarthritis; cardiovascular diseases; alcoholic cardiomyopathy, and steatosis in alcoholics (fatty degeneration of the heart); neurodegenerative diseases (Alzheimer's, Parkinson's, Huntington's, amyotrophic lateral sclerosis, and prion disease); muscular dystrophy; skeletal myopathy; atherosclerosis; diabetes; obesity; lipid degradation in the liver; alcoholic liver disease; pancreatitis; cellular quality control; protection of the genome; innate and adoptive immune responses to infection by microbial pathogens; defense against intracellular bacterial, parasitic, and viral infections; protection of intracellular pathogens; epileptogenesis; Pompe disease; nephropathy; reduction of liver damage during ischemia–reperfusion; regression of the corpus luteum; protection of stem cells from apoptosis during stress; and cross-talk with apoptosis.

AUTOPHAGY IN NORMAL MAMMALIAN CELLS

Although autophagy mediates cell adaptation to a range of stress conditions, including starvation, this stress is not a problem that a normal cell of a multicellular organism would face on a regular basis. The basal level of autophagy (the so-called basal or quality control autophagy) is found in most cells, and is required for the normal clearance of potentially deleterious protein aggregates that can cause cellular dysfunction. Thus, mammalian autophagy is primarily required for intracellular cleaning of misfolded proteins and damaged/old organelles. In the absence of such cleaning, neoplastic transformation is likely.

As alluded to above, starvation is uncommon in mammalian cells under normal nutritional conditions. Therefore, it is important to know the mechanism responsible for regulating autophagy under normal nutritional conditions. In mammalian cells, mTOR kinase, the target of rapamycin, mediates a major inhibitory signal that terminates autophagy under nutrient-rich conditions. Calpain 1 keeps autophagy under tight control by downregulating the levels of Atg12–Atg5 conjugate. Atg5 and Atg12–Atg5 conjugate are key signaling molecules for increasing the levels of autophagy (Xia et al., 2010). It is also known that intracellular Ca^{2+} regulates autophagy. Inhibition of Ca^{2+} influx results in the induction of autophagy. Reduction in intracellular Ca^{2+} prevents the cleavage of Atg5, which in turn increases the levels of full-length Atg5 and Atg12–Atg5 conjugate. The Atg12–Atg5 signaling molecule is regulated by calpain 1 in controlling the levels of autophagy in mammalian cells under nutrient-rich conditions. It is known that inhibition of calpains induces autophagy, and reduces the accumulation of misfolded proteins. It is further known that increased levels of LC3-II in fluspirilene-treated cells promote autophagy by increasing the levels of Atg5 and Atg12–Atg5 conjugate; fluspirilene is one of the autophagy inducers. Although autophagy is maintained at very low levels in normal mammalian cells, it can be rapidly induced within minutes upon starvation, or invasion by intracellular pathogens.

MAJOR TYPES OF AUTOPHAGIES

Based on the type of cargo delivery, there are three types of autophagy systems in mammals – macroautophagy (autophagy), microautophagy, and chaperone-mediated autophagy – each of which is discussed below. Although significant advances (some of which are included here) have been made in our understanding of different types of autophagies, many unanswered questions remain. A further understanding of the exact functions of the three types of autophagy is necessary before we can manipulate these pathways to treat human diseases.

Macroautophagy (Autophagy)

Whole regions of the cytosol are sequestered and delivered to lysosomes for degradation. Cargo sequestration occurs in the autophagosome, a double-membrane vesicle that forms through the elongation and sealing of a *de novo* generated membrane (Ohsumi and Mizushima, 2004). This limiting membrane originates from a tightly controlled series of interactions between more than 10 different proteins which resemble the conjugation steps that mediate protein ubiquitinization (Cuervo, 2009). Formation of the limiting membrane also requires the interaction between a protein and a specific lipid molecule, regulated by conjugating enzymes.

Microautophagy

Microautophagy is the direct uptake of soluble or particulate cellular constituents into lysosomes. It translocates cytoplasmic substances into the lysosomes for degradation via direct invagination, protrusion, or septation of the lysosomal limiting membrane. In other words, microautophagy involves direct invagination and fusion of the vacuolar/lysosomal membrane under nutrient limitation. The limiting/sequestering membrane is the lysosomal membrane, which invaginates to form tubules that pinch off into the lysosomal lumen.

Microautophagy of soluble components, as in macroautophagy (autophagy), is induced by nitrogen starvation and rapamycin. Microautophagy is controlled by the TOR and EGO signaling complexes, resulting in direct uptake and degradation of the vacuolar boundary membrane (Uttenweiler *et al.*, 2007). Hence, this process could compensate for the enormous influx of membrane caused by autophagy.

It seems that microautophagy is required for the maintenance of organelle size and membrane composition rather than for cell survival under nutrient restriction. Uttenweiler *et al.* (2007) have identified the vacuolar transporter chaperone, VTC complex, required for microautophagy. This complex is present on the endoplasmic reticulum and vacuoles, and at the cell periphery. Deletion of the VTC complex blocks microautophagic uptake into vacuoles.

Chaperone-Mediated Autophagy

Chaperone-mediated autophagy (CMA) has been characterized in higher eukaryotes but not in yeast. Because of the particular characteristics of this type of delivery, explained below, only soluble proteins, but not whole organelles, can be degraded through CMA (Cuervo, 2009). CMA is dependent on the constitutively expressed heat shock cognate

70 (Hsc70), shares 80% homology with the heat shock protein 70 (Hsp70), and identifies peptide sequences of cytoplasmic substrates; thus, it is more selective than autophagy in its degradation (Hoffman *et al.*, 2012). CMA serves to balance dysregulated energy, and is maximally activated by nutrient/metabolic and oxidative/nitrosative stresses. Cross-talk between CMA and autophagy is likely. CMA differs from the other two types of autophagies with respect to the mechanism for cargo selection and delivery to the lysosomal lumen for degradation. In other words, CMA is involved in the delivery of cargo, which does not require the formation of intermediate vesicles, membrane fusion, or membrane deformity of any type. Instead, the substrates are translocated from the cytosol directly into the lysosomal lumen across the membrane in a process mediated by a translocation protein complex that requires the substrate unfolding.

A chaperone protein binds first to its cytosolic target substrate, followed by a receptor on the lysosomal membrane at the site of protein unfolding. This protein is subsequently translocated into the lysosome for its degradation. In this system the substrate proteins are selectively targeted one-by-one to the lysosomes, and are then translocated across the lysosomal membrane.

Selectivity and direct lysosomal translocation have thus become trademarks of CMA. An essential requirement for a protein to become a CMA substrate is the presence of a pentapeptide motif biochemically related to KFERQ in its amino acid sequence (Dice, 1990). During CMA, proteins are directly imported into lysosomes via the LAMP-2a transporter assisted by the cytosolic and lysosomal Hsc70 chaperone that recognizes the KFERQ-like motif. Substrates of CMA carry signal peptides for sorting into lysosomes, similar to other protein transport mechanisms across membranes.

CMA is a generalized form of autophagy present in almost all cell and tissue types. All the CMA substrate proteins are soluble cytosolic proteins containing a targeting motif biochemically related to the pentapeptide KFERQ. This motif, present in ~30% of the proteins in the cytosol, is recognized by a cytosolic chaperone, the heat shock cognate protein of 73 kDa (cyt-Hsc70). The interaction with chaperone, modulated by the Hsc70 co-chaperones, targets the substrate to the lysosomal membrane, where it interacts with the lysosomal membrane protein (LAMP) type 2a (Cuervo and Dice, 1996). Substrates are required to be unfolded before translocation into the lysosomal lumen. Several cytosolic chaperones associated with the lysosomal membrane have been proposed, which assist in the unfolding (Aggarraberes and Dice, 2001). Translocation of the substrate requires the presence of a variant of Hsc70, lys-Hsc70, in the lysosomal lumen. This is followed by the rapid proteolysis of the substrate by residual lysosomal proteases (half-life of 5–10 minutes in the lysosomal lumen).

SELECTIVE AUTOPHAGIES

There are specific types of autophagy in which specific proteins or cell organelles are delivered to the autophagosome/lysosome for degradation. These autophagy types are enumerated below.

1. *Aggrephagy*: selective degradation of cellular aggregates, especially proteins (Overbye *et al.*, 2007)
2. *Axophagy*: degradation of axons (Yue, 2007)

3. *Glyophagy*: degradation of glycogen particles (Jiang *et al.*, 2011)
4. *Lipophagy*: selective degradation of lipid droplets (Singh *et al.*, 2009)
5. *Mitophagy*: selective degradation of mitochondria (Kanki, 2010; Coto-Montes *et al.*, 2012)
6. *Nucleophagy*: selective degradation of parts of the nucleus (Mijaljica *et al.*, 2010)
7. *Pexophagy*: selective degeneration of peroxisomes; dependent on PEX3 and PEX4 proteins (Klionsky, 1997)
8. *Reticulophagy*: selective degradation of rough endoplasmic reticulum to balance its expansion by unfolded proteins (Klionsky *et al.*, 2007)
9. *Ribophagy*: selective degradation of the 60S ribosomal subunit (Kraft *et al.*, 2008)
10. *Xenophagy*: defense against intracellular pathogens (Shpilka and Elazar, 2012)
11. *Zymophagy*: degradation of zymogen granules (Vaccaro, 2012).

Among these autophagy types, mitophagy plays a critical role in the well-being of cells because their autophagic delivery to lysosomes is the major degradative pathway in mitochondrial turnover.

AUTOPHAGOSOME FORMATION

Autophagy is a highly complex process consisting of sequential steps of induction of autophagy, formation of autophagosome precursor, formation of autophagosome, fusion between autophagosome and lysosome, degradation of cargo contents, efflux transportation of degraded products to the cytoplasm, and lysosome reformation.

In mammalian cells autophagosome formation begins with a nucleation step, where isolation membranes of varied origins form phagophores which then expand and fuse to form a completed double-membrane vesicle called an autophagosome (Luo and Rubinsztein, 2010). Autophagosomes are formed at random sites in the cytoplasm. They move along microtubules in a dynein-dependent fashion towards the microtubule-organizing center, where they encounter lysosomes. After fusion with lysosomes the cargo is degraded with hydrolases, followed by the reformation of lysosomes primarily by the Golgi complex.

The isolation membranes may be generated from multiple sources that include endoplasmic reticulum (ER), Golgi complex, outer mitochondrial membrane, and plasma membrane; however, the ER source is more feasible because it, along with its ribosomes, is involved in protein synthesis. The presence of many Atg proteins near the ER also suggests that ER plays an important role as a membrane source for autophagosome formation. The formation of isolation membrane is initiated by class III phosphatidylinositol 3-kinase (PI3KC)/Beclin-containing complexes. Elongation of the isolation membrane involves two ubiquitin-like conjugation systems. In one of them, Atg12 associates with Atg5 to form Atg12–Atg5–Atg16L1 molecular complexes that bind the outer membrane of the isolation membrane. In the second, LC3 is coupled with phosphatidylethanolamine to generate a lapidated LC3-II form, which is integrated in both the outer and inner membranes of the autophagosome (Fujita *et al.*, 2008). Recently, it was reported that human Atg2 homologues Atg2A and AtgB are also essential for autophagosome formation, presumably at a late stage (Velikkakath *et al.*, 2012).

Autophagosome membrane formation requires critical autophagy proteins (Atgs) along with the insertion of lapidated microtubule-associated light chain 3 (LC3) or gamma-aminobutyric acid, a receptor-associated protein (GABARAP) subfamily members. Various components in the autophagosomal compartment can be recognized by the presence of specific autophagy molecules. Atg16L1 and Atg5 are mainly present in the phagophore, while LC3 labels isolation membranes, matured autophagosomes, and autolysosomes (Gao et al., 2010). This evidence suggests that different Atg molecules participate in autophagosome biogenesis at various stages. Autophagophore substrate selectivity can be conferred by interactions between LC3 and specific cargo receptors, including sequestosome-1 (SQSTM1 p62) and a neighbor of BRCA1 (NBR1). During this process of autophagy, both lapidated LC3 (LC3-II) and the cargo receptors are degraded (Hocking et al., 2012).

In yeast, the Atg5–Atg12/Atg16 complex is essential for autophagosome formation (Romanov et al., 2012). This complex directly binds membranes. Membrane binding is mediated by Atg5, inhibited by Atg12, and activated by Atg16. All components of this complex are required for efficient promotion of Atg18 conjugation to phosphatidylethanolamine. However, this complex is able to tether (fasten) membranes independently of Atg8.

AUTOPHAGIC LYSOSOME REFORMATION

Following degradation of engulfed substrates with lysosomal hydrolytic enzymes and release of the resulting molecules (amino acids, fatty acids, monosaccharides, nucleotides), autophagic lysosome reformation (ALR) occurs. Although a great deal is known regarding the molecular mechanisms involved in the formation of autophagososomes and autolysosomes, the available information on post-degradation events, including ALR, is inadequate. The importance of such information becomes apparent considering that autophagosomes can fuse with multiple lysosomes. Thus, post-degradation of substrates might result in the depletion of free lysosomes within a cell unless free lysosomes are rapidly reformed. A cellular mechanism is required for maintaining lysosome homeostasis during and after autophagy.

Some information is available at the molecular level regarding the process of ALR. The ALR process can be divided into six steps (Chen and Yu, 2012): phospholipid conversion, cargo sorting, autophagosomal membrane budding, tubule extension, budding and fusion of vesicles, and protolysosome maturation. Initially, LAMP1-positive tubular structures extend from the autolysosomes; these appear empty, without detectable luminal contents from the autolysosomes. Lysosomal membrane proteins (LAMP1, LAMP2) only are located on these tubules; autophagosomal membrane proteins (LC3) are absent.

The role of mTOR is also relevant in the ALR. It has been found that the starvation-induced autophagy process is transient. During starvation, intracellular mTOR is inhibited before autophagy can occur, but it is reactivated after prolonged starvation, and the timing of this reactivation is correlated with the initiation of ALR and termination of autophagy (Chen and Yu, 2012). Thus, mTOR reactivation is required for ALR. ALR is blocked when mTOR is inhibited, and mTOR reactivation is linked to lysosomal degradation.

The lysosomal efflux transporter spinster is also required to trigger ALR (Rong et al., 2011); these transporters are lysosomal membrane proteins that export lysosomal degradation products. Sugar transporter activity of spinster is essential for ALR. Inhibition of spinster results in the accumulation of a large amount of undigested cytosol in enlarged autolysosomes, seen in the transmission electron microscope, as a result of over-acidification of autolysosomes (Rong *et al.*, 2011).

Clathrin is also essential for ALR. It is known that clathrin proteins play an important role in vesicular trafficking (Brodsky, 1988). Clathrin mediates budding in various membrane systems. A clathrin-PI (4,5) P2-centered pathway regulates ALR. This protein is present on autolysosomes, with exclusive enrichment on buds. Clathrin itself cannot directly anchor to membranes; instead, various adapter proteins (AP2) link clathrin to membranes. Additional studies are needed to fully understand the terminal stage of autophagy, and how this process ends in the reformation of free lysosomes.

AUTOPHAGIC PROTEINS

Cells assure the renewal of their constituent proteins through a continuous process of synthesis and degradation that also allows for rapid modulation of the levels of specific proteins to accommodate the changing extracellular environment. Intracellular protein degradation is also essential for cellular quality control to eliminate damaged or altered proteins, thus preventing the toxicity associated with their accumulation inside cells.

Autophagy essential proteins are the molecular basis of protective or destructive autophagy machinery. Some information is available regarding the signaling mechanisms governing these proteins and the opposing consequences of autophagy in mammals. Genes responsible for the synthesis of these proteins are summarized here.

Autophagy was first genetically defined in yeast, where 31 genes, referred to as autophagy-related genes (Atgs), were identified as being directly involved in the execution of autophagy (Mizushima, 2007; Xie and Klionsky, 2007). At least 16 members of this gene family have been identified in humans. The role of a large number of these genes has been deciphered. Our understanding of the molecular regulation of autophagy process originates from the characterization of these genes and proteins in yeast, many of which have counterparts in mammals. The core autophagic machinery comprises 18 Atg proteins, which represent three functional and structural units: (1) the Atg9 cycling system (Atg9, Atg1 kinase complex (Atg1 and Atg13), Atg2, Atg18, and Atg27); (2) the phosphatidylinositol 3-kinase (PI3K) complex (Atg6/VPS30), Atg14, VPS15, and VPS34; and (3) the ubiquitin-like protein system (Atg3–5, Atg7, Atg8, Atg10, Atg12, and Atg16) (Minibayeva *et al.*, 2012). In addition to these core Atg proteins, 16 other proteins are essential for certain pathways or in different species.

An alternate abbreviated system of Atg proteins follows. Autophagic proteins generally function in four major groups: the Atg1 kinase complex, the Vps34 class III phosphatidylinositol 3-kinase complex, two ubiquitin-like conjugation systems involving Atg8 and Atg12, and a membrane -trafficking complex involving Atg9 (Florey and Overholtzer, 2012). In mammalian cells, the key upstream kinase that regulates the induction of most forms of autophagy is the Atg1 homology Ulk1, which forms a complex with Atg13, Fip200, and Atg101. Among the Atg proteins, Atg9 is the only multispanning membrane protein essential for autophagosome formation.

It needs to be noted that autophagy proteins are also involved in non-autophagic functions such as cell survival, apoptosis, modulation of cellular traffic, protein secretion, cell signaling, transcription, translation, and membrane reorganization (Subramani and Malhotra, 2013). This subject is discussed in detail later in this chapter.

PROTEIN DEGRADATION SYSTEMS

There are two major protein degradation pathways in eukaryotic cells: the ubiquitin proteasome system and the autophagy–lysosome system. Both of these systems are characterized by selective degradation. The ubiquitin proteasome system (UPS) is responsible for degradation of short-lived proteins, and is involved in the regulation of various cellular signaling pathways. Autophagy is a selective regulatory mechanism for degrading large proteins with longer half-lives, aggregates, and defective cellular organelles. Ubiquitin binding proteins such as p62 and NBR1 regulate autophagy dynamics. These adaptor proteins decide the fate of protein degradation through either UPS or the autophagy–lysosome pathway. Many degenerative conditions, such as Huntington's, Parkinson's, Alzheimer's, amyotrophic lateral sclerosis, and diabetes, are due to defective clearance of mutated protein aggregates or defective organelles through autophagy.

BECLIN 1

Beclin 1 (from Bcl-2 interacting protein) is a 60-kDa coiled-coil protein that contains a Bcl-2 homology-3 domain, a central coiled-coil domain, and an evolutionary conserved domain. The function of Beclin 1 in autophagy was first suspected due to its 24.4% amino acid sequence identity with the yeast autophagy protein Atg6. Beclin 1 was found to restore autophagic activity in Atg6-disrupted yeast, becoming one of the first identified mammalian genes to positively regulate autophagy. Beclin 1 was originally discovered not as an autophagy protein but as an interaction partner for the anti-apoptotic protein Bcl-2. Subsequent studies demonstrated that Beclin 1 is a haploinsufficient tumor-suppressor gene that is either monoallelically deleted or shows reduced expression in several different cancers (Yue *et al.*, 2003).

Beclin 1 is also involved in several other biological functions, and in human conditions including heart disease, pathogen infections, development, and neurodegeneration. These functions will not be discussed in this chapter because only the role of this gene (protein) in autophagy is relevant here. The central role of Beclin 1 complexes is in controlling human VPS34-mediated vesicle trafficking pathways including autophagy. Beclin 1 and its binding partners control cellular VPS34 lipid kinase activity that is essential for autophagy and other membrane trafficking processes, targeting different steps of the autophagic process such as autophagosome biogenesis and maturation (Funderburk *et al.*, 2010). Beclin 1-depleted cells cannot induce autophagosomes for motion. In conclusion, the crucial regulator of autophagy is Beclin 1 (the mammalian homologue of yeast Atg6) which forms a multiprotein complex with other molecules such as UVRAG, AMBRA-1, Atg14L, Bif-1, Rubicon, SLAM, IP3, PINK, and Survivin; this complex activates the class III phosphatidylinositol-3-kinase (Petiot *et al.*, 2000).

NON-AUTOPHAGIC FUNCTION OF AUTOPHAGY-RELATED PROTEINS

The importance of non-autophagic biological functions of autophagy-related proteins is beginning to be realized. These proteins (e.g., ubiquitin-like proteins Atg8 and Atg12) play an important role in various aspects of cellular physiology, including protein sorting, DNA repair, gene regulation, protein retrotranslation, apoptosis, and immune response (Ding *et al.*, 2011). They also play a role in cell survival, modulation of cellular traffic, protein secretion, cell signaling, transcription, translation, and membrane reorganization (Subramani and Malhotra, 2013). Apparently, these proteins and their conjugates possess a different, broader role that exceeds autophagy.

The interactions of ubiquitin-like proteins with other autophagy-related proteins and other proteins are summarized below. For example, 6 Atg8 orthologues in humans interact with at least 67 other proteins. Non-autophagy-related proteins that interact with Atg8 and LC3 include GTPases, and affect cytoskeletal dynamics, cell cycle progression, cell polarity, gene expression, cell migration, and cell transformation (Ding *et al.*, 2011). Non-lipidated LC3 and non-lipidated Atg8 regulate viral replication and yeast vacuole fusion, respectively (Tamura *et al.*, 2010). Atg5 and Atg12–Atg5 conjugates suppress innate antiviral immune signaling. Based on these and other functions, ubiquitin-like proteins in their conjugated and unconjugated forms modulate many cellular pathways, in addition to their traditional role in autophagy (Subramani and Malhotra, 2013).

In addition to ubiquitin-like Atg proteins, other Atg-related proteins are also involved in non-autophagic functions; these are summarized below. UNC-51, the homologue of human ULK1, regulates axon guidance in many neurons. Atg16L1 positively modulates hormone secretion in PC12 cells, independently of autophagic activity (Ishibashi *et al.*, 2012). Atg161L, Atg5, Atg7, and LC3 are genetically linked to susceptibility to Crohn's disease, a chronic inflammation condition of the intestinal tract (Cadwell *et al.*, 2009). Atg5, Atg7, Atg4B, and LC3 are involved in the polarized secretion of lysosomal enzymes into an extracellular resorptive space, resulting in the normal formation of bone pits or cavities (bone resorption) (Deselm *et al.*, 2011).

The wide variety of functions of Atg-related proteins in typical non-autophagic cellular activities (some of which are enumerated here) indicates that the autophagic machinery is enormously complex and more versatile than presently acknowledged. Indeed, much more effort is needed to better understand the role of this machinery in health and disease, which eventually may allow us to delay the aging process and provide us with effective therapeutics.

MICROTUBULE-ASSOCIATED PROTEIN LIGHT CHAIN 3

Microtubule-associated protein chain 3 (LC3) is a mammalian homologue of yeast Atg8. It was the first mammalian protein discovered to be specifically associated with autophagosomal membranes. Presently, LC3 is the most widely used marker for autophagosomes. Although LC3 has a number of homologues in mammals, LC3B is most commonly used for autophagy (macroautophagy) assays. LC3 plays an indispensable role in autophagy formation, and for this reason is a suitable marker for the process.

The cytosolic fraction contains not only a precursor form (LC3-I) but also an active form (LC3-II). Immediately after synthesis of the precursor protein (pro-LC3), hAtg4B cleaves a C-terminal 22-amino acid fragment, which is the membrane-bound form. Because of its essential role in the expansion step of autophagosome formation, LC3-II is regarded as the most reliable marker protein for autophagy. After covalent linkage to phosphatidylethanolamine (PE), LC3-II localizes in both the cytosolic and intralumenal faces of autophagosomes (Karim et al., 2007). Following fusion with lysosomes, intralumenally-located LC3-II is degraded by lysosomal hydrolases, and cytosolically-oriented LC3-II is delipidated by hAtg4B, released from the membrane, and finally recycled back to LC3-I (Karim et al., 2007). Divergent roles of LC3 (or Beclin 1) in tumorigenesis have been reported. For example, LC3 expression is either decreased in brain cancer (Aoki et al., 2008) and ovary cancer (Shen et al., 2008) or increased in esophageal and gastrointestinal neoplasms (Yoshioka et al., 2008). LC3 is also associated with a poor outcome in pancreatic cancer (Fujita et al., 2008), whereas its expression is associated with a better survival in glioblastoma patients with a poor performance score (Aoki et al., 2008). It has also been reported that LC3-II protein expression is inversely correlated with melanoma thickness, ulceration, and mitotic rate (Miracco et al., 2010). These and other studies imply that the clinical impact of LC3 is associated with the tumor type, tissue context, and other factors.

MONITORING AUTOPHAGY

A number of methods are available to monitor autophagy; such monitoring can be accomplished by using electron microscopy, biochemical protocols, and detection of relevant protein modifications through SDS-PAGE and Western blotting. Autophagy can be monitored by detecting autophagosomal proteins such as LC3. LC3 is a specific marker protein of autophagic structure in mammalian cultured cells. The appearance of this protein-positive puncta is indicative of the induction of autophagy. One such method consists of monitoring autophagy by detecting LC3 conversion from LC3-I to LC3-II by immunoblot analysis because the amount of LC3-II is clearly correlated with the number of autophagosomes. Endogenous LC3 is detected as two bands following SDS-PAGE and immunoblotting: one represents cytosolic LC3-I and the other LC3-II that is conjugated with phosphatidylethanolamine, which is present on isolation membranes and autophagosomes but much less on autolysosomes (Mizushima and Yoshimori, 2007). According to Kadowaki and Karim (2009), the LC3-I to LC3-II ratio in the cytosol (cytosolic LC3 ratio), but not in the homogenate, is an easy quantitative method for monitoring the regulation of autophagy.

Another approach is use of the fluorescent protein GFP-LC3, which is a simple and specific marker. To analyze autophagy in whole animals, GFP-LC3 transgenic mice have been generated (Mizushima and Kuma, 2008). However, the GFP-LC3 method does not provide a convenient measure for assessing autophagic flux. Therefore, another alternative method, immunoelectron microscopy using antibodies against autophagosomal marker proteins, can be used.

In spite of the advantages of the LC3 method, it has some limitations. LC3 protein, for example, tends to aggregate in an autophagy-independent manner. LC3-positive dots seen in the light microscope after using the transfected GFP-LC3 method may represent protein aggregates, especially when GFP-LC3 is overexpressed or when aggregates are found within cells (Kuma *et al.*, 2007). LC3, in addition, is easily incorporated into intracellular protein aggregates – for example, in autophagy-deficient hepatocytes, neurons, or senescent fibroblasts. Also, LC3 is degraded by autophagy.

In light of the above limitations, it is important to measure the amount of LC3-II delivered to lysosomes by comparing its levels in the presence of or absence of lysosomal protease inhibitors such as E64d and pepstatin A (Mizushima and Yoshimori, 2007). These authors have pointed out pitfalls and necessary precautions regarding LC3 immunoblot analysis. A very extensive update of the assays for monitoring autophagy has been presented by Klionsky *et al.* (2012), who strongly recommend the use of multiple assays to monitor autophagy, and present 17 methods of doing so.

REACTIVE OXYGEN SPECIES (ROS)

Reactive oxygen species (ROS) are highly reactive forms of molecular oxygen, including the superoxide anion radical, hydrogen peroxide, singlet oxygen, and hydroxyl radical (Park *et al.*, 2012). ROS are generally produced during normal metabolism of oxygen inside the mitochondrial matrix that acts as the primary source of them. Basal levels of ROS serve as physiological regulators of normal cell multiplication and differentiation. If the balance of ROS increases more than the scavenging capacity of the intracellular antioxidant system, the cell undergoes a state of oxidative stress with significant impairment of cellular structures. Excessive levels of ROS, for example, can cause severe damage to DNA and proteins.

The oxidative stress especially targets mitochondria, resulting in the loss of mitochondrial membrane potential and initiating mitochondria-mediated apoptosis. Oxidative stress can also lead to the auto-oxidation of sterols, thereby affecting the cholesterol biosynthetic pathway – mainly the postlanosterol derivatives. The intracellular accumulation of oxysterols directs the cell to its autophagic fate, and may also induce it to differentiate. ROS, in fact, can play contrasting roles: they can initiate autophagic cell death and also function as a survival mechanism through induction of cytoprotective autophagy in several types of cancer cells.

MAMMALIAN TARGET OF RAPAMYCIN (mTOR)

The mammalian target of rapamycin (mTOR), also known as the mechanistic target of rapamycin or FK506-binding protein 12-rapamycin-associated protein 1 (FRAP1), is a 289-kDa protein originally discovered and cloned from *Saccharomyces cerevisiae* that shares sequence homologies with the phosphoinositide 3-kinase (PI3-kinase) family, which is the key element in response to growth factors. mTOR represents a serine threonine protein kinase that is present in all eukaryotic organisms (Wullschleger *et al.*, 2006).

Rapamycin binds to the FKBP12 protein, forming a drug–receptor complex which then interacts with and perturbs TOR. TOR is the central component of a complex signaling network that regulates cell growth and proliferation. Rapamycin does not perturb all mTOR functions because it exists in two distinct multiprotein complexes, and only one binds to FKB12-rapamycin. This complex is composed of mTOR and receptor protein; rapamycin inhibits its kinase activity. The rapamycin-insensitive complex also contains mTOR, but instead of raptor a different protein, called rictor, is involved. These complexes are involved in protein–protein interactions. The components of these complexes exist in all eukaryotes.

mTOR represents the catalytic subunit of two distinct complexes; mTORC1 and mTORC2 (Zoncu et al., 2011). mTORC1 controls cell growth by maintaining a balance between anabolic processes (e.g., macromolecular synthesis and nutrient storage) and catabolic processes (e.g., autophagy and the utilization of energy stores) (Nicoletti et al., 2011). The receptor–mTOR complex positively regulates cell growth, and its inhibition causes a significant decrease in cell size. The raptor part of the mTOR pathway modulates a large number of major processes that are listed here.

As indicated above, mTOR is multifunctional protein that plays a key role in intracellular nutrient sensing. It serves as the convergent point for many of the upstream stimuli to regulate cell growth and nutrient metabolism, cell proliferation, cell motility, cell survival, ribosome biosynthesis, protein synthesis, mRNA translation, and autophagy (Meijer and Godogno, 2004). Two mammalian proteins, S6 kinase and 4E-BP1, link raptor–mTOR to the control of mRNA translation (Sarbassov et al., 2005). mTOR is a major cellular signaling hub that integrates inputs from upstream signaling pathways, including tyrosine kinase receptors.

mTOR also governs energy homeostasis and cellular responses to stress, such as nutrient deprivation and hypoxia. Many studies have demonstrated that the Akt/mTOR-dependent pathway is involved in the process of chemical (platinum)-induced autophagy, in which mTOR is a pivotal molecule in controlling autophagy by activating mTOR (Hu et al., 2012). Another recent investigation also shows that methamphetamine causes damage to PC12 cells, but this damage can be decreased by using a supplement of taurine via inhibition of autophagy, oxidative stress, and apoptosis (Li et al., 2012).

Abundance of nutrients, including growth factors, glucose, and amino acids, activates mTOR and suppresses autophagy, while nutrient deprivation suppresses mTOR, resulting in autophagy activation. In other words, triggering of autophagy relies on the inhibition of mammalian mTOR, an event that promotes the activation of several autophagy proteins (Atgs) involved in the initial phase of membrane isolation. Among many signaling pathways controlling mTOR activation, phosphoinositide 3-kinase (PI3K) is the key element in response to growth factors. In mammalian cells, the complex containing ULK1 (the Atg1 homologue) and Atg13 is directly controlled by mTOR, and is a critical part of the autophagy machinery in response to nutritional status (Jung et al., 2009). Among the numerous factors involved in the regulation of autophagy and growth, mTOR is a key component that coordinately regulates the balance between growth and autophagy in response to nutritional status, growth factor, and stress signals. mTORC1 and Atg1–ULK complexes constitute the central axis of the pathways that coordinately regulate growth and autophagy in response to cellular physiological and nutritional conditions. The negative regulation of mTORC1 by Atg1–ULK stresses further the intimate cross-talk between autophagy and cell growth pathways (Jung *et al.*, 2010).

ROLE OF AUTOPHAGY IN TUMORIGENESIS AND CANCER

Malignant neoplasms constitute the second most common cause of death in the United States, and malignant brain tumors contribute 2.4% of cancer-related deaths. An estimated 20,340 new cases of primary central nervous system tumors were diagnosed in 2012 in the United States alone, and resulted in approximately 13,110 deaths. Despite considerable advances in multimodal treatment of tumors in the past five decades, there has been only a minimal improvement in the median survival time of brain-malignancy patients. Causative factors for the poor survival rate include the highly invasive nature of brain malignant tumors, making them intractable to complete surgical resection, and resistance to standard chemotherapy and radiotherapy. This difficulty in remedying cancer underscores the need to pursue prosurvival signaling mechanisms that contribute to the resistance of cancer development; such alternative therapies include the use of autophagy.

Autophagy defects are linked to many diseases, including cancer, and its role in tumorigenesis, being tissue- and genetic context-dependent, is exceedingly complex. Metabolically stressed tumor cells rely on autophagy for survival and reprogramming of their metabolism to accommodate rapid cell growth and proliferation (Lozy and Karantza, 2012). To accomplish this goal, specific catabolic reactions (e.g., aerobic glycolysis and glutaminolysis) are upregulated to provide needed energy and rebuild new complex macromolecules such as proteins, nucleic acids, and lipids.

Autophagy has complex and paradoxical roles in antitumorigenesis, tumor progression, and cancer therapeutics. Initially, two principal lines of evidence connected autophagy and cancer: it was found that (1) the *BECL1* gene is monoallelically deleted in several types of cancers, and (2) autophagy can function to promote tumor cell survival, but can also contribute to cell death. In other words, autophagy can be both tumorigenic and tumor suppressive. Its exact role in each case is dependent on the context and stimuli. Autophagy can be upregulated or suppressed by cancer therapeutics, and upregulation of autophagy in cancer therapies can be either prosurvival or prodeath for tumor cells.

It is known that autophagy maintains cellular integrity and genome stability. Loss of autophagy genes perturbs this homeostasis, thereby potentially priming the cell for tumor development. The following autophagy genes are frequently mutated in human cancers (Liu and Ryan, 2012): *BECN1*, *UVRAG*, *SH3GLB1* (Bif-1), *Atg2B*, *Atg5*, *Atg9B*, *Atg12*, and *RAB7A*. Mutations in *Atg2B*, *Atg5*, *Atg9B*, and *Atg12* have been reported in gastric and colorectal cancers (Kang *et al.*, 2009). The expression of Bif-1 is downregulated in gastric and prostate cancers (Takahashi *et al.*, 2010). Mutations of *UVRAG* have been found in colon cancer (Knaevelsrud *et al.*, 2010).

Autophagy is associated with both cancer progression and tumor suppression. The molecular mechanisms underlying these two phenomena have been elucidated. It is known that cancer cells generally tend to have reduced autophagy compared with their normal counterparts and premalignant lesions. Therefore, for autophagy to induce cancer progression, it will have to be activated. This is accomplished, for example, by the KRAS oncogene, which is known to induce autophagy. It has been shown that autophagy is activated constitutively in oncogenic KRAS-driven tumors, and that this cellular event is required for the development of pancreatic tumors (Yang *et al.*, 2011).

The discovery that the autophagic-related gene *Beclin 1* suppresses tumor growth stimulated significant interest from cancer biologists in this previously unexplored therapeutic process. This interest has resulted in both intensive and extensive research efforts to understand the role of autophagy in cancer initiation, progression, and suppression. Pharmacological or genetic inactivation of autophagy impairs KRAS-mediated tumorigenesis. It has been shown that transmembrane protein VMP1 (vacuole membrane protein 1), a key mediator of autophagy, is a transcriptional target of KRAS signaling in cancer cells (Lo Ré *et al.*, 2012). It regulates early steps of the autophagic pathway. In fact, KRAS requires VMP1 not only to induce but also to maintain autophagy levels in cancer. PI3K–AKT1 is the signaling pathway mediating the expression and promoter activity of VMP1 upstream of the GLI3–p300 complex.

The *Beclin 1* gene is deleted in ~40% of prostate cancers, ~50% of breast cancers, and ~75% of ovarian cancers (Liang *et al.*, 1999). In addition, reduced expression of Beclin 1 has been found in other types of cancers, including human colon cancer, brain tumors, hepatocellular carcinoma, and cervical cancer. It can be concluded that a defective autophagic process is clearly linked to cancer development.

However, it should be noted that the role of autophagy in cancer development is exceedingly complex. In tumorigenesis, autophagy is a double-edged sword acting as either a tumor suppressor or a supporter of cancer cell survival, depending on the stimulus and cell type. Thus, autophagy can function as an anticancer or procancer mechanism. In the latter case, autophagy enables tumor cells to survive stressors in the tumor microenvironment. Indeed, some types of cancer cells induce autophagy as a means of adapting to the unfavorable tumor microenvironment, which is characterized by hypoxia, limited nutrients, and metabolic stress. Autophagy, in addition, may block the toxicity of certain anticancer drugs.

Autophagy is associated with resistance to chemotherapeutics such as 5-fluorouracil and cisplatin. It is recognized that tumors and the immune systems are intertwined in a competition where tilting the critical balance between tumor-specific immunity and tolerance can finally determine the fate of the host (Townsend *et al.*, 2012). It is also recognized that defensive and suppressive immunological responses to cancer are exquisitely sensitive to metabolic features of rapidly growing tumors.

On the other hand, autophagy may increase the effectiveness of anticancer radiotherapy. It is known that some malignancies become relatively resistant to repeated radiotherapy, and may eventually recover self-proliferative capacity. This problem can be diminished by inducting autophagy through Beclin 1 overexpression in conjunction with radiotherapy. It is known that autophagy enhances the radiosensitization of cancer cells rather than protecting them from radiation injury and cell death. It is also known that autophagy inhibits the growth of angiogenesis in cancer cells. It should also be noted that autophagic cell death occurs in many cancer types in response to various anticancer drugs. In other words, autophagy can serve as a pathway for cellular death. Based on the two opposing roles of autophagy, it is poised at the intersection of life and death. It is apparent that we need to understand and modulate the autophagy pathway to maximize the full potential of cancer therapies.

Depending on the cell type and context, macroautophagy (autophagy from here on) has different roles; in fully transformed cancer cells it functions as a tumor suppressor, as defective autophagy is associated with malignant transformation and carcinogens. In contrast, in normal cells and in some cancer cells it functions as a protective mechanism against cellular stress, and yet the induction of autophagy is associated with cell death in some types of cancers.

Cancer cells often display a reduced autophagic capacity compared to their normal counterparts. Cancer cells express lower levels of autophagy-related proteins LC3-II and Beclin 1 than those in normal cells. Heterozygous disruption of Beclin 1 promotes tumorigenesis, while overexpression of this protein inhibits tumorigenesis, supporting the contention that defective autophagy or its inhibition plays a role in malignant transformation.

As mentioned earlier, autophagy is frequently upregulated in cancer cells following standard treatments (chemotherapy, radiotherapy), showing prosurvival or prodeath for cancer cells (reviewed by Liu and Ryan, 2012). Treatment with rapamycin, rapamycin analogues, and imatinib shows a prodeath effect, while treatment with radiation, tamoxifen, camptothecan, and proteasome inhibitors results in the survival of cancer cells. The effect of autophagy seems to be different in distinct tumor types, at various stages of tumor development, and even within different regions of the same tumor. It is concluded that, generally, either overactivation or underactivation of autophagy contributes to tumorigenesis, and that autophagy limits tumor initiation, but promotes establishment and progression.

ROLE OF AUTOPHAGY IN IMMUNITY

The eradication of invading pathogens is essential in multicellular organisms, including humans. During the past two decades there has been rapid progress in the understanding of the innate immune recognition of microbial components and its critical role in host defense against infection. The innate immune system is responsible for the initial task of recognizing and destroying potentially dangerous pathogens. Innate immune cells display broad antimicrobial functions that are activated rapidly upon encountering microorganisms (Franchi *et al.*, 2009).

Autophagy can function as a cell's defense against intracellular pathogens. It is involved in almost every key step, from the recognition of a pathogen to its destruction and the development of a specific adaptive immune response to it. Autophagy, in addition, controls cell homeostasis and modulates the activation of many immune cells, including macrophages, dendritic cells, and lymphocytes, where it performs specific functions such as pathogen killing or antigen processing and presentation (Valdor and Macian, 2012).

Autophagy pathways are linked to one or more aspects of immunity. Studies have shown that autophagy is regulated by these pathways that are critical for the function and differentiation of cells of the immune system, including Toll-like receptors (TLRs). TLRs were the first class of immune receptors identified as regulators in cells of the innate immune system, and play a crucial role in many aspects of the immune response. They are broadly expressed in immune cells, particularly in antigen-presenting cells, and recognize pathogen-associated molecular patterns such as lipopolysaccharides, viral double-stranded RNA, and unmethylated CPG islands (Harashima *et al.*, 2012). Initiation of TLR signaling induces release of inflammatory cytokines, maturation of dendritic cells, and activation of adaptive immunity. Cancer cells also express functional TLRs. TLR4 signaling, for example, promotes escape of human lung cancer cells from the immune system by inducing immune suppressive cytokines and promoting resistance to apoptosis (He *et al.*, 2007). In contrast, TRL3 signaling induces antitumor effects. Akt activation can render cancer cells resistant to antitumor cellular immunity (Hähnel *et al.*, 2008). The implication is that Akt inactivation increases the susceptibility of cancer cells to immune surveillance.

TLRs also have been shown to induce autophagy in several cell types, including neutrophils (Xu *et al.*, 2007). Activation of the TLR downstream signaling proteins MyD88 and Trif appears to be involved in the induction of autophagy. These proteins are recruited together with Beclin 1 to TLR4, which promotes the dissociation of the Beclin 1–Bc12 complex and induces autophagosome formation (Shi and Kehri, 2008). MyD88 and Trif target Beclin 1 to trigger autophagy in macrophages. TLRs have also been shown to promote a process involving the autophagy machinery termed LC3-associated phagocytosis (Valdor and Macian, 2012). The uptake of cargo containing TLR ligands by macrophages leads to the recruitment of LC3 on the phagosome surface, promoting degradation of the pathogens by enhancing phagosome–lysosome fusion in the absence of autophagosome formation (Sanjuan *et al.*, 2009).

In fact, the study of TLRs showed that pathogen recognition by the innate immune system is specific, relying on germline-encoded pattern-recognition receptors that have evolved to detect components of foreign pathogens (Akira *et al.*, 2006). TLRs recognize conserved structures in pathogens, which leads to the understanding of how the body senses pathogen invasion, triggers innate immune responses, and primes antigen-specific adaptive immunity (Kawai and Akira, 2010). The adaptive immune system relies on a diverse and specific repertoire of clonally selected lymphocytes. Additional studies are needed to better understand the mechanisms that regulate autophagy in immune cells and the role this process plays in the establishment of immune responses against foreign pathogens.

ROLE OF AUTOPHAGY IN VIRAL DEFENSE AND REPLICATION

Viruses and other pathogens induce dramatic changes in the intracellular environment. Infected cells activate certain defense pathways to combat these pathogens. Conversely, pathogens interfere with defense processes and utilize cellular supplies for pathogen propagation. Autophagy, for example, plays an antiviral role against the mammalian vesicular stomatitis virus, and the phosphatidylinositol 3-kinase–Akt signaling pathway is involved in this defense process (Shelly *et al.*, 2009). Many virus types, including herpes simplex virus 1 and Sindbus virus, have been observed inside autophagic compartments for degradation (Orvedahl *et al.*, 2007).

Autophagy is an essential component of *Drosophila* immunity against the vesicular stomatitis virus (Shelly *et al.*, 2009). Recently, an interesting role of the RNAse L system and autophagy in the suppression or replication of the encephalomyocarditis virus or vesicular stomatitis virus was reported (Chakrabarti *et al.*, 2012). At a low multiplicity of infection, induction of autophagy by RNAse L suppresses virus replication; however, in subsequent rounds of infection, autophagy promotes viral replication. RNAse is a virus-activated host

RNAse pathway that disposes of or processes viral and cellular single-stranded RNAs. However, it has not been established whether autophagy itself is sufficient to control viral replication in all cases; the participation of other cell death phenomena in this defense process cannot be disregarded. On the other hand, autophagy is, for example, actively involved in influenza A virus replication (Zhou *et al.*, 2009). Mouse hepatitis virus and polio virus sabotage the components of the mammalian autophagy system, which normally is important in innate immune defense against intracellular pathogens. In other words, autophagic machinery (which normally would function to eliminate a virus) may promote viral assembly (Jackson *et al.*, 2005). However, Zhao *et al.* (2007) indicate that mouse hepatitis virus replication does not require the autophagy gene Atg5.

The survival of HIV depends on its ability to exploit the host cell machinery for replication and dissemination, to circumvent the cell's defense mechanisms or to use them for its replication. Autophagy plays a dual role in HIV-1 infection and disease progression. Direct effects of HIV on autophagy include the subversion of autophagy in HIV-infected cells and the induction of hyper-autophagy in bystander CD4+ T cells. HIV proteins modulate autophagy to maximize virus production (Killian, 2012). On the other hand, HIV-1 protein also disrupts autophagy in uninfected cells and thus contributes to CD4+ T cell death and viral pathogenesis.

It has also been reported that HIV-1 downregulates autophagy regulatory factors, reducing both basal autophagy and the number of autophagosomes per cell (Blanchet *et al.*, 2010). The HIV negative elongation factor (Nef) protein protects HIV from degradation by inhibiting autophagosome maturation (Kyei *et al.*, 2009). It has been shown that the foot and mouth disease virus induces autophagosomes during cell entry to facilitate infection, but does not provide membranes for replication (Berrym *et al.*, 2012).

Another example of a virus that uses a component of autophagy to replicate itself is the hepatitis C virus (HCV) (Sir *et al.*, 2012). HCV perturbs the autophagic pathway to induce the accumulation of autophagosomes in cells (via the class III PI3K-independent pathway) and uses autophagosomal membranes for its RNA replication. Other positive-strand RNA viruses (poliovirus, dengue virus, rhinoviruses, and nidoviruses) also use the membrane of autophagic vacuoles for their RNA replication (Sir and Ou, 2010). Suppression of LC3 and Atg7 reduces the HCV RNA replication level; these two proteins are critical for autophagosome formation. There is still controversy regarding the contrasting roles of autophagy in pathogen invasion; the mechanisms governing activation of autophagy in response to virus infection require further elucidation.

ROLE OF AUTOPHAGY IN INTRACELLULAR BACTERIAL INFECTION

Post-translation modifications of cell proteins (e.g., ubiquitination) regulate the intracellular traffic of pathogens. Ubiquitin is a small protein that is widely expressed in all eukaryotic cells, and ubiquitination involves the addition of ubiquitin to the lysine residues of target proteins, resulting in endocytosis and sorting events (Railborg and Stenmark, 2009). Several strategies have been developed by pathogenic bacteria to interfere with the host's ubiquitination and thus to achieve successful infection. Some types of bacteria act directly on the ubiquitination pathway by mimicking host cell proteins, while others (e.g., *Escherichia coli*, *Shigella flexneri*) act indirectly by expressing or interfering with the host ubiquitinating pathway. The other defense by the cell against bacterial infection is through autophagy; this is described below.

Autophagy serves as a double-edged sword; on the one hand it eliminates some pathogens and bacterial toxins, while on the other hand some pathogens can evade or exploit autophagy for survival and replication in a host. Recently, it has become clear that the interaction between autophagy and intracellular pathogens is highly complex. The components of the autophagy machinery also play roles in infection in a process different from the canonical autophagy pathway (formation of a double-membrane autophagosome and the involvement of more than 35 autophagy-related proteins, including the LC3 mammalian autophagy marker). There is an alternative autophagy pathway that is relevant to infection. For example, a subset of autophagy components can lead to LC3 conjugation onto phagosomes (Cemma and Brumell, 2012). In other words, the process of LC3-associated phagocytosis (LAP) results in the degradation of the cargo by promoting phagosome fusion with lysosomes. It is likely that both the LAP process and the canonical system operate simultaneously or selectively as host defenses against infection. Examples of bacteria the growth of which is suppressed by autophagy include *Escherichia coli* (Cooney *et al.*, 2010), *Salmonella typhimurium* (Perrin *et al.*, 2004), *Streptococcus pyogenes* (Virgin and Levine, 2009), and *Mycobacterium tuberculosis* (Randow, 2011); examples of bacteria that exploit autophagy for replication include *Staphylococcus aureus*, *Legionella pheumophila*, and *Yersinia pseudotuberculosis*; examples of bacteria that can evade targeting by autophagy/LAP include *Listeria monocytogenes* (Randow, 2011), *Shigella flexneri* (Virgin and Levine, 2009), and *Burkholderia pseudomallei*.

ROLE OF AUTOPHAGY IN HEART DISEASE

Heart failure is one of the leading causes of morbidity and mortality in industrialized countries. Myocardial stress due to injury, valvular heart disease, or prolonged hypertension induces pathological hypertrophy, which contributes to the development of heart failure and sudden cardiac death (Ucar *et al.*, 2012).

It has been reported that autophagy is an adaptive mechanism to protect the heart from hemodynamic stress. In fact, autophagy plays a crucial role in the maintenance of cardiac geometry and contractile function (Nemchenko *et al.*, 2011). Cardiac-specific loss of autophagy causes cardiomyopathy. Impaired autophagy has been found in a number of heart diseases, including ischemia/reperfusion injury. Excessive and uncontrolled autophagy leads to loss of functional proteins, depletion of essential organic molecules, oxidative stress, loss of ATP, the collapse of cellular catabolic machinery, and, ultimately, the death of cells in the heart. Autophagic elimination of damaged organelles, especially mitochondria, is crucial for proper heart function, whereas exaggerated autophagic activity may foster heart failure. Therefore, a delicate balance of autophagy maintains cardiac homeostasis, whereas an imbalance leads to the progression of heart failure.

A consensus on whether autophagy is cardioprotective or leads to hypertrophy and heart failure is lacking. In any case, autophagy is an important process in the heart. Various studies indicate that autophagy has a dual role in the heart, where it can protect against or contribute to cell death depending on the stimulus. It occurs at low basal levels under normal conditions, and is important for the turnover of organelles. Autophagy is upregulated in the heart in response to stress such as ischemia/reperfusion. Studies of ischemia/reperfusion injury indicate that ROS and mitochondria are critical targets of injury, as opening of the mitochondrial permeability transition pore culminates in cell death. However, Sciarretta *et al.* (2011) indicate that autophagy is beneficial during ischemia but harmful during reperfusion.

It has been shown that mitophagy mediated by Parkin is essential for cardioprotection (Huang *et al.*, 2011). The sequestration of damaged mitochondria depends on Parkin, which averts the propagation of ROS-induced ROS release and cell death. The implication is that mitochondrial depolarization and removal through mitophagy is cardioprotective. The sequestration of damaged cell materials into autophagosomes is essential for cardioprotection. An increased number of autophagosomes is a prominent feature in many cardiovascular diseases, such as cardiac hypertrophy and heart failure (Zhu *et al.*, 2007). Recently, Gottlieb and Mentzer (2012) have ably reconciled contradictory findings and concluded that the preponderance of evidence leans towards a beneficial role of autophagy in the heart under most conditions.

Recently, it was reported that autophagy plays a role in the onset and progression of alcoholic cardiopathy (Guo and Ren, 2012). Adenosine monophosphate-activated protein kinase (AMPK) plays a role in autophagic regulation and subsequent changes in cardiac function following an alcoholic challenge. It is known that AMPK promotes autophagy via inhibition of mTORC1 by phosphorylating the mTORC1-associated protein Raptor and tuberous sclerosis complex 2.

MicroRNAs (miRNAs) also play a role in cardiomyopathy and heart failure. These endogenous small molecules regulate their target gene expression by post-transcriptional regulation of messenger RNA. Recently, it was demonstrated that hypertrophic conditions induced the expression of the miR-212/132 family in cardiomyocytes, and both of these molecules regulated cardiac hypertrophy and cardiomyocyte autophagy (Ucar *et al.*, 2012). Cardiac hypertrophy and heart failure in mice can be rescued by using a pharmacological inhibitor of miR-132.

Inflammation is also implicated in the pathogenesis of heart failure. Some information is available regarding the mechanism responsible for initiating and integrating inflammatory responses within the heart. Mitochondrial DNA plays an important role in inducing and maintaining inflammation in the heart. Mitochondrial DNA that escapes from autophagy cell autonomously leads to Toll-like receptor (TLR) 9-mediated inflammatory responses in cardiomyocytes, and is capable of inducing myocarditis and dilated cardiomyopathy (Oka *et al.*, 2012). Pressure overload induces the impairment of mitochondrial cristae morphology and functions in the heart. It is known that mitochondria damaged by external hemodynamic stress are degraded by the autophagy/lysosome system in cardiomyocytes (Nakai *et al.*, 2007). It is also known that increased levels of circulating proinflammatory cytokines are associated with disease progression and adverse outcomes in patients with chronic heart failure.

ROLE OF AUTOPHAGY IN NEURODEGENERATIVE DISEASES

Before discussing the role of autophagy in neurodegenerative diseases, a brief description of their characteristics is presented. Alzheimer's disease (AD), Parkinson's disease (PD), and

Huntington's disease (HD) are the major neurodegenerative conditions causing dementia and movement disorders in the aging population. When AD and PD disorders overlap, the condition is called Lewy body disease. All three diseases are characterized by the presence of abnormal protein aggregate and neuronal death, although the etiology of AD is distinct from that of PD and HD.

It is known that epigenetic dysregulation and transcriptional dysregulation are pathological mechanisms underlying neurological diseases. It is also known that histone deacetylase (HDAC) inhibitor 4b preferentially targets HDAC1 and HDAC3, ameliorating, for example, HD (Jia et al., 2012). HDACs are enzymes that remove acetyl groups from lysine amino acid on a histone. Several studies have identified HDAC inhibitors (4b) as candidate drugs for the treatment of neurodegenerative diseases, including HD.

Familial AD mutations increase the amyloidogenicity of the amyloid beta peptide, placing disruption of amyloid precursor protein (APP) metabolism and amyloid beta production at the center of AD pathogenesis (Pickford et al., 2008). An increase in the production of both APP and amyloid beta, and a decrease in the degradation of APP, contribute to AD.

PD is a progressive neurodegenerative disorder caused by the interaction of genetic and environmental factors. It is characterized by the loss of dopaminergic neurons. The available evidence indicates that mitochondrial dysfunction, environmental toxins, oxidative stress, and abnormal accumulation of cytoplasmic proteinaceous materials can contribute to disease pathogenesis. These proteins tend to aggregate within Lewy bodies. The loss of dopaminergic neurons in the substantia nigra may be partly due to the accumulation of aggregated or misfolded proteins or mitochondrial dysfunction. Prevention of such accumulation or degeneration of dysfunctional mitochondria might prevent the occurrence of apoptosis. Mutations in the DJ-1 oncogene are also implicated in the pathogenesis of this disease. This oncogene is neuroprotective by activating the ERK1/2 pathway and suppressing mTOR in the dopaminergic neurons, leading to enhanced autophagy.

One of the major constituents of Lewy bodies is a protein called alpha-synuclein. This protein is likely to be a toxic mediator of pathology in PD because wild-type alpha-synuclein gene duplications, which increase its expression levels, cause rare cases of autosomal dominant PD (Winslow and Rubinsztein, 2011). Overexpression of alpha-synuclein increases mutant huntingtin aggregation. Mutant huntingtin is an autophagy substrate, and its level increases when autophagy is compromised. Even physiological levels of this protein negatively regulate autophagy.

HD is characterized by the accumulation of mutant huntingtin (the protein product of the IT15 gene) in intraneuronal inclusions, primarily in the brain but also peripherally. The increase is caused by the appearance of cytoplasmic (neutrophil) and nuclear aggregates of mutant huntingtin, and selective cell death in the striatum and cortex (DiFiglia et al., 1997). HD is recognized as a toxic gain-of-function disease, where the expansion of the polyQ stretch within huntingtin confers new deleterious functions on the protein. Loss of normal huntingtin function is thought to be responsible for HD.

Amyotrophic lateral sclerosis (ALS) is the fourth common neurodegenerative disease. It is characterized by progressive loss of upper and motor neurons. The following genes and proteins have been reported to be involved in familial ALS: superoxide dismutase 1, als2, TAR DNA binding protein 43 kDa, fused in sarcoma, and optineurin (Da Cruz and Cleveland, 2011). Accumulation of ubiquitinated inclusions containing these gene products is a common feature in most familial ALS models, and is also a pathologic hallmark of sporadic ALS. Failure to eliminate detrimental proteins is linked to pathogenesis of both familial and sporadic types of ALS. Dysfunction of 26S proteasome in motor neurons is sufficient to induce cytopathological phenotypes of ALS (Tashiro *et al.*, 2012). This evidence indicates that dysfunction of the ubiquitin–proteasome system primarily contributes to the pathogenesis of sporadic ALS. In other words, proteasomes, but not autophagy, fundamentally govern the development of ALS, in which TDP-43 and FUS proteinopathy plays a crucial role (Tashiro *et al.*, 2012). The role of autophagy in AD, PD, and HD is further elaborated below.

Loss of autophagy-related genes results in neurodegeneration and abnormal protein accumulation. Autophagy is important to avoid, or at least delay, the development of age-related diseases such as neurodegeneration and cancer. In fact, autophagy is an essential pathway in postmitotic cells such as neurons; cells that are particularly susceptible to the accumulation of defective proteins and organelles. Neuron-specific disruption of autophagy results in neurodegenerative diseases, including AD, PD, HD, ALS, and prion diseases. Tissue-specific genetic manipulation of autophagy of the brain causes neuronal accumulation of misfolded proteins and an accelerated development of neurodegeneration.

One of the prominent features of AD is the accumulation of autophagic vacuoles in neurons, suggesting dysfunction in this degradation pathway. Autophagy is normally efficient in the brain, as reflected by the low number of brain autophagic vacuoles at any given moment (Nixon and Yang, 2011). In contrast, brains of AD patients exhibit prominent accumulation of such vacuoles in association with dystrophic neuritis and deformed synaptic membranes (Yu *et al.*, 2005).

The majority of PD is idiopathic, with no clear etiology. The available evidence indicates that mitochondria dysfunction, environmental toxins, oxidative stress, and abnormal protein accumulation can contribute to disease pathogenesis. The loss of dopaminergic neurons in the substantia nigra may be partly due to the accumulation of aggregated or misfolded proteins, or mitochondrial dysfunction. Prevention of such accumulations or degradation of dysfunctional mitochondria might prevent the occurrence of apoptosis. Mutations in the DJ-1 oncogene are also implicated in the pathogenesis of this disease. DJ-1 is neuroprotected by activating the ERL1/2 pathway and suppressing mTOR in the dopaminergic neurons, leading to enhanced autophagy. Upregulation of autophagy has the potential to be a therapeutic strategy for disorders. This genetic method for autophagy upregulation is mTOR-independent. The development of genetic-based therapeutic strategies aimed at stimulating the autophagic clearance of aggregated proteins can be used both in the treatment of neurodegenerative diseases and in lifespan extension (Zhang *et al.*, 2010). Several studies have identified histone deacetylase (HDAC) inhibitors (4b) as candidate drugs for the treatment of neurological diseases, including HD.

CROSS-TALK BETWEEN AUTOPHAGY AND APOPTOSIS

The cross-talk between autophagy and apoptosis is exceedingly complex, and various aspects of this phenomenon are still being understood. A brief introduction to the apoptosis pathway is in order. The significant functions of apoptosis (type 1 programmed cell death) are embodied in its maintenance of organism homeostasis and metabolic balance, and organ development. Morphological changes and death in apoptotic cells are caused by caspases, which cleave 400 proteins. The earliest recognized morphological changes in apoptosis involve condensation of cytoplasm and chromatin, DNA fragmentation, and cell shrinkage. The plasma membrane convolutes or blebs in a florid manner, producing fragments of a cell (apoptotic bodies). The fragments are membrane bound, and contain nuclear parts. The apoptotic bodies are rapidly taken up by nearby cells and degraded within their lysosomes.

There are two established signaling pathways that result in apoptosis. In the extrinsic pathway, apoptosis is mediated by death receptors on the cell surface, which belong to the TNF receptor superfamily and are characterized by extracellular cysteine-rich domains and extracellular death domains. In other words, the extrinsic pathway is induced by cell death receptor pathways such as TRAIL or FAS ligand. The cell surface receptors form a multiprotein complex called the death-inducing signaling complex (DISC).

The intrinsic pathway, on the other hand, is mediated by mitochondria in response to apoptotic stimuli, such as DNA damage, irradiation and some other anticancer agents (Zhan et al., 2012), serum deprivation, cytochrome c, SMAC/DIABLO (a direct inhibitor of apoptosis-binding protein), AIF (apoptosis-inducing factor that promotes chromatin condensation), and EndoG (endonuclease G facilitates chromatin condensation). Cytochrome c binds to and activates Apaf-1 (apoptotic protease activating factor-1) protein in the cytoplasm. This induces the formation of an apoptosome that subsequently recruits the initiator procaspase-9, yielding activated caspase-9, and finally mediates the activation of caspase-3 and caspase-7 (Tan et al., 2009). It is apparent that diverse stimuli cause release of mitochondrial proteins to activate the intrinsic apoptosis pathway leading to MOMP and the release of cytochrome c and other apoptogenic proteins; MOMP is regulated by the Bcl family of proteins. In summary, in both pathways activated caspases cleave and activate other downstream cellular substrates as explained above.

Under stress conditions, prosurvival and prodeath processes are simultaneously activated and the final outcome depends on the complex cross-talk between autophagy and apoptosis. Generally, autophagy functions as an early induced cytoprotective response, favoring stress adaptation by removing damaged subcellular constituents. It is also known that apoptotic stimuli induce a rapid decrease in the level of the autophagic factor activating molecule in Beclin 1-regulated autophagy (Ambra 1) (Pagliarini et al., 2012). Such Ambra 1 decrease can be prevented by the simultaneous inhibition of caspases and calpains. Caspases cleave Amba 1 at the D482 site, while calpains are involved in complete Ambra 1 degradation. Ambra 1 levels are critical for the rate of apoptosis induction.

Autophagy can trigger caspase-independent cell death by itself, or by inducing caspase-dependent apoptosis. Autophagy can protect cells by preventing them from undergoing apoptosis. Autophagy also protects cells from various other apoptotic stimuli. Although the exact mechanism underlying this protection is not known, the role of damaged mitochondrial sequestration has been suggested; this prevents released cytochrome c from being able to form a functional apoptosome in the cytoplasm (Thorburn, 2008). There is a close connection between the autophagic machinery and the apoptosis machinery. Is it possible that there is simultaneous activation of these two types of death processes? In fact, autophagy is interconnected with apoptosis, as the two pathways share key molecular regulators (Eisenberg-Lener et al., 2009). For example, it has been reported that autophagy regulates neutrophil apoptosis in an inflammatory context-dependent manner, and mediates the early pro-apoptotic effect of TNF-α in neutrophils. Neutrophils are a major subset of circulating leukocytes, and play a central role in defense against bacterial and fungal infections.

The concept of the presence of cross-talk between autophagy and apoptosis is reinforced by the indication that common cellular stresses activate various signaling pathways which regulate both of these two cell death programs. ROS induce apoptosis and regulate Atg4, which is essential for autophagy induction. In addition, Atg5 promotes both apoptosis and autophagy induction. In addition to Atg5, several other signal transduction pathways (Bcl2 regulator) can elicit both of those cell death mechanisms. The transcription factor p53 is another such molecule.

Several additional recent studies have revealed additional information regarding the molecular mechanisms underlying the cross-talk between autophagy and apoptosis. An interesting study of the effect of ganoderic acid (a natural triterpenoid) on melanoma cells was recently carried out by Hossain et al. (2012). This study indicated that ganoderic acid induced orchestrated autophagic and apoptotic cell death as well as enhanced immunological responses via increased HLA class II presentation in melanoma cells. In other words, this treatment initiated a cross-talk between autophagy and apoptosis as evidenced by increased levels of Beclin 1 and LC3 proteins.

Another study investigated the effect of taurine on methamphetamine (METH)-induced apoptosis and autophagy in PC12 cells, and the underlying mechanism (Li et al., 2012). METH, a commonly abused psychostimulant, induces neuronal damage by causing ROS formation, apoptosis, and autophagy. Taurine, in contrast, decreases METH-induced damage by inhibiting autophagy, apoptosis, and oxidative stress through an mTOR-dependent pathway. It is known that mTOR is the major negative regulator of autophagy.

The cross-talk between autophagy and apoptosis is indicated by the involvement of Beclin 1 in both of these programmed cell death types. Autophagy and apoptosis are two dynamic and opposing (in most cases) processes that must be balanced to regulate cell death and survival. Available evidence clearly indicates that cross-talk between autophagy and apoptosis does exist, and that in its presence the former precedes the latter. Also, autophagy may delay the occurrence of apoptosis. Many studies indicate that cancer cells treated with an anticancer drug induce both autophagy and apoptosis. In addition, normal cells exposed to cancer-causing agents tend to invoke defense by inducing both autophagy and apoptosis. Moreover, cancer cells exposed to anticancer agents induce autophagy, but in the absence of autophagy these cells develop apoptosis. This concept is confirmed by a recent study by Li et al. (2012), which indicated that oridonin (an anticancer agent) upregulates p21 (an antitumor gene) expression and induces autophagy and apoptosis in human prostate cancer cells, and that autophagy precedes apoptosis, thus protecting such treated cells from apoptosis by delaying the onset of the latter. To substantiate the above conclusions, several other recently published reports are described below.

Co-regulation of both autophagy and apoptosis using bis-benzimidazole derivatives has been reported (Wang et al., 2012). These compounds are potent antitumor agents. The implication is that autophagy and apoptosis act in synergy to exert tumor cell death. In another study, it was shown that low-density lipoprotein receptor-related protein-1 (LRP1) mediates autophagy and apoptosis caused by Helicobacter pylori in the gastric epithelial cell line AZ-521 (Yahiro et al., 2012). This study also proposes that the cell surface receptor, LRP1, mediates vacuolating cytotoxin-induced autophagy and apoptosis; this toxin induces mitochondrial damage leading to apoptosis. In these cells, the toxin triggers formation of autophagosomes, followed by autolysosome formation. Recently it was reported that death-associated protein kinase (DAPK) induces autophagy in colon cancer cells in response to treatment with histone deacetylase inhibitor (HDACi), while in autophagy-deficient cells DAPK plays an essential role in committing cells to HDACi-induced apoptosis (Gandesiri *et al.*, 2012).

Further evidence supporting the cross-talk between autophagy and apoptosis was recently reported by Visagie and Joubert (2011). They demonstrated the induction of these two programmed cell death mechanisms in the adenocarcinoma cell line MCF-7, which was exposed to 2-methoxyestradiol-bis-sulfamate (2-MeDE2bis MATE), a 2-methoxyestradiol derivative (an anticancer agent). The presence of apoptosis was indicated in this morphological study by growth inhibition, presence of a mitotic block, membrane blebbing, nuclear fragmentation, and chromatin condensation, which are hallmarks of this type of cell death. Simultaneously, this drug induced autophagy, shown by increased lysosomal staining.

Organic compounds have also been used to determine the cross-talk between autophagy and apoptosis. A few examples follow. Pterostilbene (a naturally occurring plant product) activates autophagy and apoptosis in lung cancer cells by inhibiting epidermal growth factor receptor and its downstream pathways (Chen *et al.*, 2012). Gui *et al.* (2012) used glyphosate (a herbicide linked to Parkinson's disease) to induce autophagy and apoptosis in PC12 cells, and found that the *Beclin 1* gene was involved in cross-talk between the mechanisms governing the two programmed cell death types. Two plant products, dandelion root extract and quinacrine, mediate autophagy and apoptosis in human pancreatic cancer cells and colon cancer cells, respectively (Mohapatra *et al.*, 2012; Ovadje *et al.*, 2012). Hirsutanol A compound from the fungus *Chondrostereum* inhibits cell proliferation, elevates the ROS level, and induces autophagy and apoptosis in breast cancer MCF-7 cells (Yang *et al.*, 2012).

A switch from apoptosis to autophagy is not uncommon during chemoresistance by cancer cells. It is known that defective apoptosis is an important mechanism underlying chemoresistance by cancer cells. Such resistance is associated with profound changes in cell death responses, and a likely switch from apoptosis to autophagy. This switch involves balancing the deletion of multiple apoptotic factors by upregulation of the autophagic pathway and collateral sensitivity to the therapeutic agent. Ajabnoor *et al.* (2012) have reported that reduction of apoptosis occurring in the MCF-7 breast cancer cells upon acquisition of paclitaxel resistance is balanced by upregulation of autophagy as the principal mechanism of cytotoxicity and cell death; this sensitivity is associated with mTOR inhibition. Upregulation of the autophagic pathway gives rise to rapamycin resistance. Also, loss of expression of caspase-7 and caspase-9 is observed in these cells.

It is known that the cell survival mechanism is driven by Beclin 1-dependent autophagy, while cell death is controlled by caspase-mediated apoptosis. Both of these processes share regulators such as Bcl2, and influence each other through feedback loops. The question is whether autophagy and apoptosis coexist at the same time at the same stress level. To elucidate the role of regulatory components involved in both autophagy and apoptosis, and better understand the cross-talk between these two programmed cell death mechanisms, Kapuy *et al.* (2013) have explored the systems level properties of a network comprising cross-talk between autophagy and apoptosis, using a mathematical model. They indicate that a combination of Bcl2-dependent regulation and feedback loops between Beclin 1 and caspases strongly enforces a sequential activation of cellular responses depending upon the intensity and duration of stress levels (transient nutrient starvation and growth factor withdrawal). This study also shows that amplifying loops for caspase activation involving Beclin 1-dependent inhibition of caspases and cleavage of Beclin 1 by caspases not only make the system bistable but also help to switch off autophagy at high stress levels. In other words, autophagy is activated at lower stress levels, whereas caspase activation is restricted to higher levels of stress. Apparently, autophagy precedes apoptosis at lower stress levels, while at a very high stress level apoptosis is activated instantaneously and autophagy is inactivated. According to this observation, autophagy and apoptosis do not coexist at the same time at the same stress level.

In summary, it is clear that a close relationship exists between autophagy and apoptosis, and that autophagy and apoptosis are not mutually exclusive pathways. They can act in synergy, or can counteract or even balance each other. Both share many of the same molecular regulators (Bcl2). However, stress (e.g., nutrient deficiency, growth factor withdrawal) levels tend to affect autophagy and apoptosis differently from each other, resulting in mutual balancing. Thus, in a clinical setting it is difficult to predict the outcome of inhibition or activation of one form of programmed cell death (autophagy) without considering that of the other (apoptosis) (Eisenberg-Lerner *et al.*, 2009). Because autophagy is involved not only in cell death but also (and mostly) in cell survival, and apoptosis leads only to cell death, an understanding of the critical balance between these two types of cellular processes is required to design anticancer therapeutics. The dual role of autophagy depends on the context and the stimuli. It has even been proposed that not only autophagy and apoptosis but also programmed necrosis may jointly decide the fate of cells of malignant neoplasms (Ouyang *et al.*, 2012).

References

Agarraberes, F.A., Dice, J.F., 2001. A molecular chaperon complex at the lysosomal membrane is required for protein translocation. J. Cell Biol. 114, 2491–2499.

Ajabnoor, G.M.A., Crook, T., Coley, H.M., 2012. Paclitaxel resistance is associated with switch from apoptotic to autophagic cell death in MCF-7 breast cancer cells. Cell Death Dis. 3, 1–9.

Akira, S., Uematsu, S., Takeuchi, O., 2006. Pathogen recognition and innate immunity. Cell 124, 783–801.

Aoki, H., Kondo, Y., Aldape, K., et al., 2008. Monitoring autophagy in glioblastoma with antibody against isoform B of human microtubule-associated protein 1 light chain 3. Autophagy 4, 467–475.

Berrym, S., Brooks, E., Burman, A., et al., 2012. Foot-and-mouth disease virus induces autophagosomes during cell entry via a Class III phosphatidylinositol 3-kinase-independent pathway. J. Virol. 86, 12940–12953.

Blanchet, F.P., Morris, A., Nikolic, D.S., et al., 2010. Human immunodeficiency virus-1 inhibition of immuno-amphisomes in dendritic cells impairs early innate and adaptive immune responses. Immunity 32, 654–669.

Brodsky, F.M., 1988. Living with clathrin: its role in intracellular membrane traffic. Science 242, 1396–1402.

Cadwell, K., Patel, K.K., Komatsu, M., et al., 2009. A common role for Atg16L1, Atg5, and Atg7 in small intestinal Paneth cells and Crohn disease. Autophagy 5, 250–252.

Cemma, M., Brumell, J.H., 2012. Interactions of pathogenic bacteria with autophagy systems. Cur. Biol. 22, 540–545.

Chakrabarti, A., Gosh, P.K., Banerjee, S., et al., 2012. RNase L triggers autophagy in response to viral infections. J. Virol. 86, 11311–11321.

Chen, G., Hu, X., Zhang, W., et al., 2012. Mammalian target of rapamycin regulates isoliquiritigenin-induced autophagic and apoptotic cell death in adenoid cystic carcinoma cells. Apoptosis 17, 90–101.

Chen, Y., Yu, L., 2012. Autophagic lysosome reformation. Exp. Cell Res. 319, 142–146.

Cooney, R.J., Baker, O., Brain, B., et al., 2010. NOD2 stimulation induces autophagy in dendritic cells influences bacterial handling and antigen presentation. Nat. Med. 16 (1), 90–97.

Coto-Montes, A., Boga, J.A., Rosales-Corral, S., et al., 2012. Role of melatonin in the regulation of autophagy and mitophagy; a review. Mol. Cell. Endocrin. 361, 12–23.

Cuervo, A.M., 2009. Chaperone-mediated autophagy: selectivity pays off. Trends Endocrinol. Metab. 21, 142–150.

Cuervo, A.M., Dice, J.F., 1996. A receptor for the selective uptake and degradation of proteins by lysosomes. Science 273, 501–503.

Da Cruz, S., Cleveland, D., 2011. Understanding the role of TDP-43 and FUS/TLS in ALS and beyond. Curr. Opin. Neurobiol. 21, 904–919.

DeSelm, C.J., Miller, B.C., Zou, W., et al., 2011. Autophagy proteins regulate the secretory component of osteoclastic bone resorption. Dev. Cell 21, 966–974.

Deter, R.L., de Duve, C., 1967. Influence of glucagon, and inducer autophagy, on some physical properties of rat liver lysosomes. J. Cell Biol. 33, 437–499.

Dice, J., 1990. Peptide sequences that target cytosolic proteins for lysosomal proteolysis. Trends Biochem. Sci 15, 305–309.

DiFiglia, M., Sapp, E., Chase, K.O., et al., 1997. Aggregation of Huntingtin in neuronal intranuclear inclusions and dystrophic neurites in brain. Science 277, 1990–1993.

Ding, F., Yin, Z., Wang, H.R., 2011. Ubiquitination in Rho signaling. Curr. Top. Med. Chem. 11, 2879–2887.

Eisemberg-Lerner, A., Bialik, S., Simon, H.-U., et al., 2009. Life and death partners: apoptosis, autophagy, and the cross-talk between them. Cell Death Differ. 16, 966–975.

Florey, O., Overholtzer, M., 2012. Autophagy proteins in macroendocytic engulfment. Trends Cell Biol. 22, 376–380.

Franchi, L., Eigenbrod, T., Munoz-Planillo, R., et al., 2009. The inflasome: a caspase-1 activation platform regulating immune responses and disease pathogenesis. Nat. Immunol. 10, 241–255.

Fujita, N., Itoh, T., Omori, H., et al., 2008. The Atg16L complex specifies the site of LC3 lipidation for membrane biogenesis in autophagy. Mol. Biol. Cell 19, 2092–2100.

Funderburk, S.F., Wang, Q.J., Yue, Z., 2010. The Beclin 1-VPS34 complex at the crossroads of autophagy and beyond. Trends Cell Biol. 20, 355–362.

Gandesiri, M., Chakilam, S., Ivanovska, J., et al., 2012. Dapk plays an important role in panobinostat-induced autophagy and commits cells to apoptosis under autophagy deficient conditions. Apoptosis 17, 1300–1315.

Gao, W., Kang, J.H., Liao, Y., et al., 2010. Biochemical isolation and characterization of tubulovesicular LC3-positive autophagosomal compartment. J. Biol. Chem. 285, 1371–1383.

Gottlieb, R.A., Mentzer, Jr, R.M., 2012. Autophagy: an affair of the heart. doi: 10.1007/s10741-012-9367-2.3.

Gui, Y.-X., Fan, X.-N., Wang, H.-m., et al., 2012. Glyphosate induced cell death through apoptotic mechanisms. Neurot. Terat. 34, 344–349.

Guo, R., Ren, J., 2012. Deficiency in AMK attenuates ethanol-induced cardiac contractile dysfunction through inhibition of autophagosome formation. Cardiovas. Res. 94, 480–491.

Hähnel, P.S., Thaler, S., Antunes, E., et al., 2008. Targeting AKT signaling sensitizes cancer to cellular immunotherapy. Cancer. Res. 68 (10), 3899–3906.

Harashima, N., Inao, T., Imamura, R., et al., 2012. Roles of PI3K/Akt pathway and autophagy in TLR3 signaling-induced apoptosis and growth arrest of human prostate cancer. Cancer Immunol. Immunother. 61, 667–676.

He, W., Liu, Q., Wang, L., et al., 2007. TLR4 signaling promotes immune escape of human lung cancer cells by inducing immunosuppressive cytokines and apoptosis resistance. Mol. Immunol. 44, 258.

Hocking, L.J., Whitehouse, A., Helfrich, M.H., 2012. Autophagy: a new player in skeletal maintenance? J. Bone Min. Res. 27, 1439–1447.

Hoffman, W.H., Shacka, J.J., Andjelkovic, A.V., 2012. Autophagy in the brains of young patients with poorly controlled TIDM and fatal diabetic ketoacidosis. Exp. Mol. Path. 93, 273–280.

Hossain, A., Radwan, F.F.Y., Doonan, B.P., et al., 2012. A possible crosstalk between autophagy and apoptosis in generating an immune response in melanoma. Apoptosis 17, 1066–1078.

Hu, S.-Y., Tai, C.C., Li, Y.H., et al., 2012. Progranulin compensates for blocked IGF-1 signaling to promote myotube hypertrophy in C2C12 myoblast via the PI3K/Akt/mTOR pathway. FEBS Lett. 586 (19), 3485–3492.

Huang, C., Andres, A.M., Ratliff, E.P., et al., 2011. Preconditioning involves selective mitophagy mediated by Parkin and p26/SQSTM1. PLos ONE 6, 20975.

Ishibashi, K., Uemura, T., Waguri, S., et al., 2012. Atg16L1, an essential factor for canonical autophagy, participates in hormone secretion from PC12 cells independently of autophagic activity. Mol. Cell Biol. 23, 3193–3202.

Jackson, W.T., Giddings Jr., T.H., Taylor, M.P., et al., 2005. Subversion of cellular autophagosomal machinery by RNA viruses. Plos Biol. 3, 861–871.

Jia, H., Kast, R.J., Steffan, J.S., et al., 2012. Selective histone deacetylase (HDAC) inhibition imparts beneficial effects in Huntington's disease mice: implications for the ubiquitin-proteasomal and autophagy systems. Human. Mol. Genet. 21, 5280–5293.

Jiang, S., Wells, C.D., Roach, P.J., 2011. Starch-binding domain-containing protein 1 (Stbd1) and glycogen metabolism: Identification of the Atg8 family interacting motif (AIM) in Stbd1 required for interaction with GABARAPL1. Biol. Chem. Res. Commun. 413, 420–425.

Jung, C.H., Jun, C.B., Ro, S.H., et al., 2009. ULK–Atg13–FIP200 complexes mediate mTOR signaling to the autophagy machinery. Mol. Biol. Cell 20, 1992–2003.

Jung, C.H., Ro, S.H., Cao, J., et al., 2010. mTOR regulation of autophagy. FEBS Lett. 585, 1287–1295.

Kadowaki, M., Karim, M.R., 2009. Cytosolic LC3 ratio as a quantitative index of macroautophagy. Methods Enzymol. 452, 199–213.

Kang, M.R., Kim, M.S., Oh, J.E., et al., 2009. ATG2B, ATG5, ATG9B, and ATG12 in gastric and colorectal cancers with microsatellite instability. J. Pathol. 217, 702–706.

Kanki, T., 2010. Nix, a receptor protein for mitophagy in mammals. Autophagy 63, 433–435.

Kapuy, O., Vinod, P.K., Mandl, J., et al., 2013. A cellular stress-directed bistable switch controls then crosstalk between autophagy and apoptosis. Mol. BioSyst. 9, 296–306.

Karim, R., Kanazawa, T., Daigaku., Y., et al., 2007. Cytosolic LC3 ratio as a sensitive index of macroautophagy in isolated rat hepatocytes and H4-11-E cells. Autophagy 3, 553–560.

Kawai, T., Akira, S., 2010. The role of pattern-recognition receptors in innate immunity: update on Toll-like receptors. Nat. Immunol. 11, 373–384.

Killian, M.S., 2012. Dual role of autophagy in HIV-1 replication and pathogenesis. Aids Res. Therap. 9, 1–13.

Klionsky, D.J., 2012. A human autophagy interaction network. Autophagy 8 (4), 439–441.

Klionsky, D.J., 1997. Protein transport from the cytoplasm into the vacuole. J. Membr. Biol. 157, 105–115.

Klionsky, D.J., Cuervo, A.M., Seglen, P.O., 2007. Methods for monitoring autophagy from yeast to human. Autophagy 3 (3), 181–206.

Klionsky, D.J., Abdalla, F.C., Abeliovich, H., et al., 2012. Guidelines for the use and interpretation of assays for monitoring autophagy. Autophagy 8 (4), 445–544.

Knaevelsrud, H., Ahlquist, T., Merok, M.A., et al., 2010. UVRAG mutations associated with microsatellite unstable colon cancer do not affect autophagy. Autophagy 6, 863–870.

Kraft, C., Deplazes, A., Sohrman, M., et al., 2008. Mature ribosomes are selectively degraded upon starvation by an autophagy pathway requiring the Ubp3p/Bre5p ubiquitin protease. Nat. Cell Biol. 10, 602–610.

Kuma, A., Matsui, M., Mizushima, N., 2007. LC3, and autophagosome marker, can be incorporated into protein aggregates independent of autophagy. Autophagy 3, 323–328.

Kyei, G.B., Dinkins, C., Davis, A.S., et al., 2009. Autophagy pathway intersects with HIV-1 biosynthesis and regulates viral yields in macrophages. J. Cell Biol. 186, 255–268.

Li, Y., Hu, Z., Chen, B., et al., 2012. Taurine attenuates methamphetamine-induced autophagy and apoptosis in PC12 cells through mTOR signaling pathway. Toxicol. Lett. 215, 1–7.

Liang, X.H., Jackson, S., Seaman, M., et al., 1999. Induction of autophagy and inhibition of tumorigenesis by Beclin 1. Nature 402, 672–676.

Liu, E.Y., Ryan, K.M., 2012. Autophagy and cancer: issues we need to digest. J. Cell Sci. 125, 2349–2358.

Lo Ré, A.E., Fernández-Barrena, M.G., Almada, L.L., et al., 2012. Novel AKT1-GL13-VWP1 pathway mediates KRAS oncogene-induced autophagy in cancer cells. J. Biol. Chem. 287, 25325–25334.

Lozy, F., Karantza, V., 2012. Autophagy and cancer cell metabolism. Rev. Cell Dev. Biol. 23, 395–401.

Luo, S., Rubinsztein, D.C., 2010. Apoptosis blocks Beclin 1-dependent autophagosome synthesis: an effect rescued by Bcl-xL. Cell Death Differ. 17 (268), 277.

Meijer, A.J., Godogno, P., 2004. Regulation and role of autophagy in mammalian cells. Int. J. Biochem. Cell Biol. 36, 2445–2462.

Mijaljica, D., Prescott, M., Devenish, R.J., 2010. The intricacy of nuclear membrane dynamics during nucleophagy. Nucleus 1, 213–223.

Minibayeva, F., Dmitrieva, S., Ponomareva, A., et al., 2012. Oxidative stress-induced autophagy in plants: the role of mitochondria. Plant Physiol. Biochem. 59, 11–19.

Miracco, C., Meng, G.C., Franchi, A., et al., 2010. Beclin 1 and LC3 autophagic gene expression in cutaneous melanocytic lesins. Hum. Pathol. 41, 503–512.

Mizushima, N., 2007. Autophagy: process and function. Genes Dev. 21, 2861–2973.

Mizushima, N., Kuma, A., 2008. Autophagosomes in GFP-LC3 transgenic mice. Methods Mol. Biol. 445, 119–124.

Mizushima, N., Yoshimori, T., 2007. How to interprete LC3 immunoblotting? Autophagy 3, 542–545.

Mohapatra, P., Preet, R., Das, D., et al., 2012. Quinacrine-mediated autophagy and apoptosis in colon cancer cells is through a p53-and p21-dependent mechanism. Oncol. Res. 20, 81–91.

Nakai, A., Yamaguchi, O., Takeda, T., et al., 2007. The role of autophagy in cardiomyocytes in the basal state and in response to hemodynamic stress. Nat. Med. 13, 619–624.

Nemchenko, A., Chiong, M., Turer, A., et al., 2011. Autophagy as a therapeutic target in cardiovascular disease. J. Mol. Cell. Cardiol. 300, H2123–H2134.

Nicoletti, F., Fagone, P., Meroni, P., et al., 2011. mTOR as a multifunctional therapeutic target in HIV infection. Drug Discov. Today 16, 715–721.

Nixon, R.A., Yang, D.S., 2011. Autophagy failure in Alzheimer's disease – locating the primary defect. Neurobiol. Dis. 43, 38–45.

Ohsumi, Y., Mizushima, N., 2004. Two ubiquitin-like conjugation systems essential for autophagy. Semin. Cell Develop. Biol. 15, 231–236.

Oka, T., Hikoso, S., Yamaguchi, O., et al., 2012. Mitochondrial DNA that escapes from autophagy causes inflammation and heart failure. Nature 485, 251–256.

Orvedahl, A., Alexander, D., Talloczy, Z., et al., 2007. HSV-1 1CP34.5 confers neurovirulence by targeting the Beclin 1 autophagy protein. Cell Host Microbe 1, 23–35.

Ouyang, L., Shi, Z., Zhao, S., et al., 2012. Programmed cell death pathways in cancer: a review of apoptosis, autophagy, and programmed necrosis. Cell Prolif. 45, 487–498.

Ovadje, P., Chochkeh, M., Akbari-Asl, P., et al., 2012. Selective induction of apoptosis and autophagy through treatment with dandelion root extract in human pancreatic cancer cells. Pancreas 41, 1039–1047.

Overbye, A., Fengsrud, M., Seglen, P.O., 2007. Proteomic analysis of membrane-associated proteins from rat liver autophagosome. Autophagy 3, 300–322.

Pagliarini, V., Wirawan, E., Romagnoli, A., et al., 2012. Proteolysis of Ambra1 during apoptosis has a role in the inhibition of the autophagic pro-survival response. Cell Death Differ. 19, 1495–1504.

Park, S.-H., Kim, J.-H., Chi, G.Y., et al., 2012. Induction of apoptosis and autophagy by sodium selenite in A549 human lung carcinoma cells through generation of reactive oxygen species. Toxicol. Lett. 212, 252–261.

Perrin, A.J., Jiang, X., Birmingham, C.L., et al., 2004. Recognition of Bacteria in the cytosol of Mammalian cells by the ubiquitin system. Curr. Biol. 14, 806–811.

Petiot, A., Ogier-Denis, E., Blommaart, E.F., et al., 2000. Distinct classes of phosphatidylinositol 3'-kinases are involved in signaling pathways that control macroautophagy in HT-29 cells. J. Biol. Chem. 275, 992–998.

Pickford, F., Masliah, E., Britschgi, M., 2008. The autophagy-related protein beclin 1 shows reduced expression in early Alzheimer disease and regulates amyloid β accumulation in mice. J. Clin. Invest. 118, 2190–2199.

Railborg, C., Stenmark, H., 2009. The ESCRT machinery in endosomal sorting of ubiquitylated membrane proteins. Nature 458, 445–452.

Randow, F., 2011. How cells deploy ubiquitin and autophagy to defend their cytosol from bacterial invasion. Autophagy 7 (3), 304–309.

Romanov, J., Walczak, M., Lbiricu, I., et al., 2012. Mechanism and functions of membrane binding by the Atg5–Atg12/Atg16 complex during autophagsome formation. EMBO J. 31, 4304–4317.

Rong, Y., McPhee, C.K., Deng, S., et al., 2011. Spinster is required for autophagic lysosome reformation and mTOR reactivation following starvation. Proc. Natl Acad. Sci. U.S.A. 108, 7826–7831.

Sanjuan, M.A., Milasta, S., Green, D.R., 2009. Toll-like receptor signaling in the lysosomal pathways. Immunol. Rev. 227, 203–220.

Sarbassov, D.D., Ali, S.M., Sabatini, D.M., 2005. Growing roles for the mTor pathway. Curr. Opin. Biol. 17, 596–603.

Sciarretta, S., Hariharan, N., Monden, Y., et al., 2011. Is autophagy in response to ischemia and reperfusion protective or detrimental for the heart? Pediatr. Cardiol. 32, 275–281.

Shelly, S., Lukinova, N., Bambina, S., et al., 2009. Autophagy is an essential component of *Drosophila* immunity against vesicular stomatitis virus. Immunity 30, 588–598.

Shen, Y., Li, D.D., Wang, L.L., et al., 2008. Decreased expression of autophagy-related proteins in malignant epithelial ovarian cancer. Autophagy 16, 1067–1068.

Shi, C.S., Kehri, J.H., 2008. MyD88 and Trif target Beclin 1 to trigger autophagy in macrophages. J. Biol. Chem. 283, 33175–33182.

Shpilka, T., Elazar, Z., 2012. Essential role for the mammalian ATG8 isoform LC3C in xenophagy. Mol. Cell. 48 (3), 325–326.

Singh, R., Kaushik, S., Wang, Y., et al., 2009. Autophagy regulates lipid metabolism. Nature 458, 1131–1135.

Sir, D., Ou, J.H., 2010. Autophagy in viral replication and pathogenesis. Mol. Cells 29, 1–7.

Sir, D., Kuo, C.-F., Tian, Y., et al., 2012. Replication of hepatitis C virus RNA on autophagosomal membranes. J. Biol. Chem. 287, 18036–18043.

Subramani, S., Malhotra, V., 2013. Non-autophagic roles of autophagic-related proteins. EMBO Rep. 14, 143–151.

Takahashi, Y., Coppola, D., Matsushita, N., et al., 2010. Bif-1 interacts with Beclin 1 through UVRAG and regulates autophagy and tumorigenesis. Nat. Cell Biol. 9, 1142–1151.

Tamura, N., Oku, M., Sakai, Y., 2010. Atg8 regulates vacuolar membrane dynamics in a lipidation-independent manner in *Pichia pastoris*. J. Cell Sci. 123, 4107–4116.

Tan, M.L., Ooi, J.P., Ismail, N., et al., 2009. Programmed cell death pathways and current antitumor targets. Pharmaceut. Res. 26, 1547–1560.

Tashiro, Y., Urushitani, M., Inoue, H., et al., 2012. Motor neuron-specific disruption of proteasome, but not autophagy replicates amyotrophic lateral sclerosis. J. Biol. Chem. 287, 42984–42994.

Thorburn, A., 2008. Apoptosis and autophagy: regulatory connections between two supposedly different processes. Apoptosis 13 (1), 1–9.

Townsend, K.N., Hughson, L.R., Schlie, K., et al., 2012. Autophagy inhibition in cancer therapy: metabolic considerations for antitumor immunity. Immunol. Rev. 249, 176–194.

Ucar, A., Gupta, S.K., Fiedler, J., et al. 2012. The miRNA-212/132 family regulates both cardiac hypertrophy and cardiomyocyte autophagy. doi: 10.1038/ncomms2090.

Uttenweiler, A., Schwarz, H., Neumann, H., et al., 2007. The vacuolar transporter chaperone (VTC) complex is required for microautophagy. Mol. Biol. Cell 18, 166–175.

Vaccaro, M.I., 2012. Zymophagy: selective autophagy of secretory granules. Int. J. Cell. Biol. April doi: 10.1155/2012/396705.

Valdor, R., Macian, F., 2012. Autophagy and the regulation of the immune response. Pharmacol. Res. 66, 475–483.

Velikkakath, A.K.G., Nishimora, T., Oita, E., et al., 2012. Mammalian Atg2 proteins are essential for autophagosome formation and important for regulation of size and distribution of lipid droplets. Mol. Biol. Cell 23, 896–909.

Virgin, H.W., Levine, B., 2009. Autophagy genes in immunity. Nat. Immunol. 10, 461–470.

Visagie, M.H., Joubert, A.M., 2011. 2-Methoxyestradiol-bis-sulfamate induces apoptosis and autophagy in a tumorigenic breast epithelial cell line. Mol. Cell Biochem. 357, 343–352.

Wang, X.-J., Chu, N.-Y., Wang, Q.-H., 2012. Newly synthesized bis-benzimidazole derivatives exerting anti-tumor activity through induction of apoptosis and autophagy. Biorg. Meg. Chem. Lett. 22, 6297–6300.

Winslow, A.R., Rubinsztein, D.C., 2011. The Parkinson disease protein α-synuclein inhibits autophagy. Autophagy 7, 429–431.

Wullschleger, S., Loewith, R., Hall, M.N., 2006. TOR signaling in growth and metabolism. Cell 124, 471–484.

Xia, H.G., Zhang, L., Chen, G., et al., 2010. Control of basal autophagy by calpain1 mediated cleavage of ATG5. Autophagy 6 (1), 61–66.

Xie, Z., Klionsky, D.J., 2007. Autophagosome formation: core machinery and adaptations. Nat. Cell Biol. 9, 1102–1109.

Xu, Y., Jagannath, C., Liu, X.D., et al., 2007. Toll-like receptor 4 is a sensor for autophagy associated with innate immunity. Immunity 27, 135–144.

Yahiro, K., Satoh, M., Nakano, M., et al., 2012. Low-density lipoprotein receptor-related protein-1 (LRP1) mediates autophagy and apoptosis caused by *Helicobacter pylori* VacA. J. Biol. Chem. 287, 31104–31115.

Yang, F., Chen, W.D., Deng, R., et al., 2012. Hirsutanol A induces apoptosis and autophagy via reactive oxygen species accumulation in breast cancer MCF-7 cells. J. Pharmacol. Sci. 119, 214–220.

Yang, S., Wang, X., Contino, G., et al., 2011. Pancreatic cancers require autophagy for tumor growth. Genes Dev. 25, 717–729.

Yoshioka, A., Miyata, H., Doki, Y., et al., 2008. LC3: and autophagosome marker, is highly expressed in gastrointestinal cancer. Int. J. Oncol. 33, 461–475. 468.

Yu, W.H., Cuervo, A.M., Kumar, A., et al., 2005. Macroautophagy – a novel Beta-amyloid peptide-generating pathway activated in Alzheimer's disease. J. Cell Biol. 171, 87–98.

Yue, Z., 2007. Regulation of neuronal autophagy in axon. Autophagy 3 (2), 139–141.

Yue, Z., Jin, S., Yang, C., et al., 2003. Beclin 1, an autophagy gene essential for early embryonic development, is a haploinsufficient tumor suppressor. Proc. Natl. Acad. Sci., U.S.A. 100, 15077–15082.

Zhan, Y., Gong, K., Chen, C., et al., 2012. P38 MAP kinase functions as a switch in MS-275-induced reactive oxygen species-dependent autophagy and apoptosis in human colon cancer cells. Free Rad. Biol. Med. 53, 532–543.

Zhang, S., Clabough, E.B.D., Sarkar, S., et al., 2010. Deletion of the Huntingtin polyglutamine stretch enhances neuronal autophagy and longevity in mice. PLos Genet. 6, 1–15.

Zhao, Z., Trackray, L.B., Miller, B.C., et al., 2007. Coronavirus replication does not require the autophagy gene Atg5. Autophagy 3 (6), 581–585.

Zhou, Z., Jiang, X., Liu, D., et al., 2009. Autophagy is involved in influenza A virus replication. Autophagy 5, 321–328.

Zhu, H., Tannous, P., Johnstone, J.L., et al., 2007. Cardiac autophagy is a maladaptive response to hemodynamic stress. J. Clin. Invest. 117, 1782–1793.

Zoncu, R., Efevan, A., Sabatini, D.M., 2011. mTOR: from growth signal integration to cancer, diabetes and ageing. Nat. Rev. Mol. Cell Biol. 12, 21–35.

PART I

GENERAL DISEASES

Mechanisms of Regulation of p62 in Autophagy and Implications for Health and Diseases

Kenji Takagi and Tsunehiro Mizushima

Abstract

Autophagy refers to bulk degradation processes responsible for the turnover of long-lived proteins, disposal of damaged organelles, and clearance of aggregate prone proteins. Aberrant autophagy causes the formation of cytoplasmic inclusion bodies, leading to liver injury and neurodegeneration. However, details of abnormalities related to impaired autophagy are largely unknown. The efficiency of the autophagy pathway relies on cargo receptors to identify the ubiquitinated targets destined for the degradation pathway. For instance, p62 promotes the formation of protein aggregates and their association with the autophagosome. Recent studies showed that murine p62 contains a highly conserved LC3 recognition sequence (LRS). Structural analysis of the LC3–LRS complex revealed an interaction between Trp^{340} and Leu^{343} of p62 and two hydrophobic pockets (hp1 and hp2) on the ubiquitin fold of LC3. The LRS motif of NBR1, autophagy

© 2014 Elsevier Inc. All rights reserved.

receptor, presents differences to this classical LRS motif with a tyrosine residue and an isoleucine residue substituting Trp and Leu, respectively. NMR studies of NBR1–LRS complexed with GABARAPL, another Atg8 homologue, indicated that the presence of tryptophan residue in the LRS motif increases the binding affinity, but other substitutions have little effect on the binding affinity due to enthalpy–entropy compensation. The aforementioned results indicate that each autophagic receptor has a unique interaction form. Most recently, it has been demonstrated that the selectivity of the autophagy receptor NDP52 for LC3C is crucial for innate immunity. Other than those listed above, many autophagy receptors and Atg8 homologue binding proteins are reported.

In vivo experiments showed that cells expressing p62 mutants lacking LC3 binding ability accumulate ubiquitin-positive inclusion bodies, instead of autophagosomes, as in hepatitis and neurodegenerative diseases. These data demonstrate that cellular levels of p62 are tightly regulated by autophagy through direct interaction with LC3, and that selective turnover of p62 via autophagy prevents inclusion body formation.

INTRODUCTION

Macroautophagy (hereafter referred to as autophagy) is an evolutionary conserved pathway for the intracellular bulk degradation of cytoplasmic substrates. In this process, cytoplasmic portions containing macromolecules and/or organelles are engulfed by a double-membrane vesicle called an autophagosome. The autophagosome then fuses with lysosomes, which degrade their contents using various hydrolytic enzymes (Levine and Kroemer, 2008; Mizushima, 2007).

Over 30 autophagy (atg) genes have been identified in yeasts, most of which are essential for autophagy and have orthologues in higher eukaryotes (Levine and Klionsky, 2004). Among them, the ubiquitin-like proteins Atg12 and Atg8 are a part of the highly conserved machinery involved in the formation of the phagophore, a crescent-shaped double membrane that expands and fuses to form the autophagosome (Johansen and Lamark, 2011). The Atg5–Atg12–Atg16 complex and E1 enzyme (Atg7) assist in the anchoring of Atg8 to the phagophore through the interaction between the C-terminal of Atg8 and the amino group of phosphatidylethanolamine (PE) in the membrane. This conjugation drives the expansion of the phagophore and hemifusion of the lipid membranes to complete the autophagosome (Ohsumi, 2001; Xie and Klionsky, 2007). In mammals, this process is supported by several Atg8 homologues: LC3 (LC3A, LC3B, and LC3C), GABARAP (GABARAP, GABARAPL-1, and GABARAPL-2), and GATE-16 (He *et al.*, 2003; Xin *et al.*, 2001).

Autophagy serves two physiological purposes: adaptive autophagy and constitutive (basal) autophagy. Growing lines of evidence point to the importance of the latter, which operates constitutively at low rates even under a nutrient-rich environment and plays a vital role in the maintenance of cellular homeostasis (Hara *et al.*, 2006; Komatsu *et al.*, 2005, 2006, 2007a). Turnover of long-lived proteins, disposal of excess or damaged organelles, and clearance of aggregate-prone proteins are regulated by constitutive autophagy (Elmore *et al.*, 2001; Iwata *et al.*, 2006). Studies using mouse genetics have highlighted that autophagy-deficient mice exhibit remarkable Ub- and p62-positive proteinaceous inclusions followed by hepatocytic and neuronal cell death, irrespective of nutrient stresses (Hara *et al.*, 2006; Komatsu *et al.*, 2005, 2006).

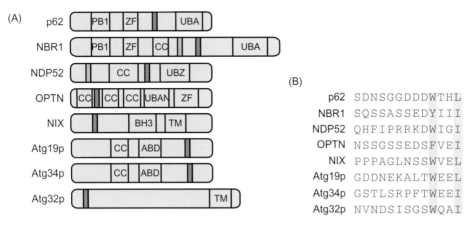

FIGURE 2.1   (A) A schematic map of the known characterized autophagy receptors. Phox and Bem1 (PB1), zinc finger (ZF), ubiquitin-associated (UBA), coiled-coil (CC), ubiquitin-binding zinc finger (UBZ), ubiquitin-binding in ABIN and NEMO (UBAN), Bcl-2 homology 3 (BH3), Ams1-binding (ABD), and transmembrane (TM) domains are represented. (B) Sequence alignments of functional LRS motif in autophagy receptors. Essential residues (Trp and Leu in p62) in the LRS motif are highlighted in yellow.

The autophagic adaptors, p62 and possibly NBR1 (neighbor of the *BRCA1* gene), act as cargo receptors for the degradation of ubiquitinated substrates (Kirkin *et al.*, 2009). For instance, proteins selected by chaperones for autophagy are ubiquitinated, and then aggregated by p62, which recruits a phagophore through direct interaction with LC3. The cellular contents in p62 and NBR1 are continuously regulated by autophagic clearance (Bjorkoy *et al.*, 2005; Kirkin *et al.*, 2009; Pankiv *et al.*, 2007). In models of autophagy deficiency, p62 accumulates and drives the formation of ubiquitin-positive inclusion body formation in the cytoplasm of hepatocytes and neurons, which leads to hepatitis and neurodegeneration (Komatsu *et al.*, 2007b). However, the molecular relationship between the autophagic removal of p62 and inclusion body formation remains undetermined. This chapter reviews the interactions between p62 and LC3, the mechanism of p62 degradation, and the role of p62 in the formation of ubiquitin-positive inclusion. It also explores other autophagy receptors, such as NBR1, as possible substitutions for p62 in autophagy.

LC3 RECOGNITION BY p62

Interacting Region between LC3 and p62

The autophagosomal marker protein LC3 is localized on the inner and outer membranes of phagophores and autophagosomes (Itakura and Mizushima, 2012). The inner membrane fraction is degraded after fusion of the autophagosome with lysosomes. Proteomic analysis revealed that LC3 interacts directly with p62, a multifunctional protein composed of three domains: the N-terminal Phox and Bem1 (PB1) domain, the zinc finger domain (zinc), and the C-terminal ubiquitin-associated (UBA) domain (Figure 2.1A). The PB1 domain exhibits self-oligomerization, and the UBA domain binds to the ubiquitinated proteins selected for autophagy to promote aggregation (Lamark *et al.*, 2009). Several reports suggest that p62 is sequestered in the autophagosome by direct interaction with LC3 (Komatsu *et al.*, 2007b; Pankiv *et al.*, 2007). Mutagenesis studies in mice identified the interacting linker on p62 as 11 amino acids (334–344) between the zinc finger and UBA domains (Ichimura *et al.*, 2008). This region, named the LRS (LC3 recognition sequence), is essential and sufficient for p62–LC3 interaction. The LRS linker contains two highly conserved motifs involved in the interaction: acidic cluster (337–339; DDD or DEE) and hydrophobic residues (340 and 343; WXXL or WXXV). Though structurally diverse, all known autophagy receptors (Atg19, Atg32, Atg34, p62, NBR1, NDP52, OPTN, Nix, and Atg32) share a common small peptide motif, which binds to the Atg8 docking site (Figure 2.1B) mediating direct receptor–Atg8 interaction (Noda *et al.*, 2010). Therefore, the direct p62–LC3 interaction is well established as an essential part of autophagy.

Furthermore, several adaptor proteins facilitating cargo-receptor–Atg8 assembly on incipient autophagic membrane are also implicated; Atg11 in yeasts, and Alfy in mammals. Atg11 binds Atg19, Atg32, and Atg34, whereas Alfy binds p62 via the C-terminal BEACH domain (Simonsen *et al.*, 2004). However, their specific functions are not well characterized. Further investigations are required.

Overall Structure of the LC3–p62–LRS Complex

The LC3–p62 complex, determined by X-ray crystallography, consists of full length LC3 (residues 1–125) bound to the LRS of p62 (residues 334–344) (PDB 2ZJD) (Figure 2.2A) (Ichimura *et al.*, 2008). The structure of LRS-bound LC3 is essentially identical to the structures of apo-LC3 (PDB 1UGM) with an RMSD of 1.15. The crystal structure shows that the LRS arm of p62 is inserted into a narrow channel of the LC3 groove (Figure 2.2B). The dominant interaction is the indole ring of Trp^{340} inserted into a site surrounded by a conserved group of hydrophilic and hydrophobic residues: Asp^{19}, Ile^{23}, Pro^{32}, Lys^{51}, Leu^{53}, and Phe^{108}. The second major interaction is Leu^{343} making van der Waals contacts with Ile^{35}, Phe^{52}, Val^{54}, Leu^{63}, and Ile^{66} and the aliphatic portion of Arg^{70}. The third interaction site is between the N-terminal portion of LRS and the basic cluster (Arg^{10}, Arg^{11}, and Lys^{49}) at the surface of LC3. In the contact area, several charged and hydrophilic residues provided by both p62 and LC3 could potentially form salt bridges and hydrogen bonds between the two molecules (Figure 2.2C).

Mutational studies designed based on this information indicate that the hydrophobic (Trp^{340} and Leu^{343}) and acidic (Asp^{337}–Asp^{339}) clusters of p62 are important for LC3 binding. Complementary mutations of LC3 residues at R10A, R11A, K51A, F52A, L53A, I66A, and R70A, and N-terminal helix deletion, all significantly compromised binding affinity in pull-down assays. These data are in agreement with the above crystal structure analysis.

Characterization of Atg8 Homologue–LRS Domain

Members of the Atg8 family of proteins, including LC3, contain a ubiquitin-fold domain at the C-terminus. The structure of the receptor docking bay includes an exposed β-strand (β1) within the ubiquitin-fold, and two adjacent hydrophobic pockets (hp1 and hp2) (Behrends and Fulda, 2012). These pockets are involved in the interaction between p62 and LC3. The residues Trp340 and Leu343 of LRS in p62 insert deeply into these pockets to form an intermolecular β-sheet with LC3.

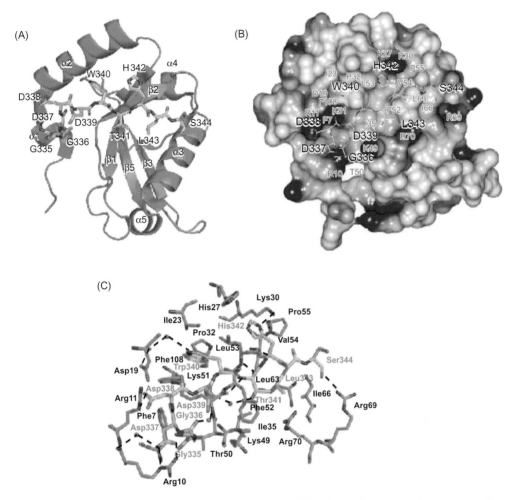

FIGURE 2.2   (A) Overall structure of the LC3–p62 complex (PDB code 2ZJD). The secondary structure elements for LC3 are labeled. (B) Electrostatic surface representation of the p62-binding site of LC3 with LRS. (C) Close-up view of the LC3–LRS interface showing amino acids of LC3 (green), LRS (yellow), and water molecules (red).

The autophagy receptor NBR1 also contains LC3- and ubiquitin-binding domains, with some modifications. The LRS of NBR1 presents as a tyrosine residue and an isoleucine residue, substituting for the tryptophan residue and leucine residue, respectively. The crystal structure of the GABARAPL-1–NBR1–LRS complex was recently determined by solution NMR (Figure 2.3A,B) (Rozenknop *et al.*, 2011). The overall configuration and binding mode appears to be almost identical to the LC3–p62 complex. The replacement of a tryptophan with a tyrosine residue in the LRS motif increased binding affinity. However, substitution of this residue by other aromatic amino acids, or increasing the number of negatively charged residues at the N-terminus of the LRS motif, has little effect on binding affinity due to enthalpy–entropy compensation. These manipulations indicate that the presence of a

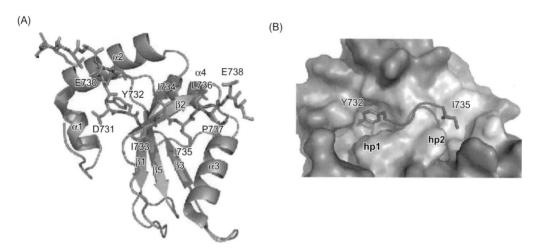

FIGURE 2.3   (A) Structure of the GABARAPL1–NBR1–LRS (pdb code:2ZJD) complex. (B) LRS binding site of GABARAPL1.

tryptophan residue in the LRS motif increases the binding affinity, but different LRSs can interact with autophagy modifiers with unique binding properties.

The binding mechanism between the LRS peptide and another Atg8 homologue, GATE-16, has been also elucidated by computer modeling (Ichimura *et al.*, 2008). The complex model of GATE-16 and p62-LRS was created using the structure of bovine GATE-16 and the MOE program (version 2005.06; Chemical Computing Group, Montreal, Canada). In this model, although GATE-16 contributes to the major interaction sites Trp^{340} and Leu^{343}, the basic surface on the α1 helix of LC3 interacting with the acidic cluster Asp^{337}–Asp^{339} is different from that of the corresponding GATE-16 region. However, MBP pull-down assays showed equivalent interactions of p62 with LC3, GABARAP, and GATE-16, suggesting that these Atg8 homologues have similar affinities for p62 *in vitro*.

Very recently, the structure of the NDP52–LC3C complex has also been determined (see also Figure 4C of von Muhlinen *et al.*, 2012). Although NDP52 binds selectively to the LC3C isoform, the selectivity of this interaction is conferred by a non-canonical LRS motif, which comprises the tripeptide Leu–Val–Val.

ROLE OF p62 AS AN AUTOPHAGY RECEPTOR

Autophagic Degradation of p62

A cell reporter system was developed to monitor the degradation of p62 by autophagy using green fluorescent protein (GFP)-p62 (Ichimura *et al.*, 2008). When mutants of p62 reducing the LC3–p62 interaction (W340A, L343A, D338A/D339A, and D337A/D338A/D339A) were expressed into $p62^{-/-}$ mouse embryonic fibroblasts (MEFs), the degradation rates of GFP-p62 were significantly slower compared with wild-type p62. Nevertheless, these degradation rates were still higher than GFP-p62 in Atg7/p62 double knockout MEFs, implying a partial defect in the degradation of these mutants. Interestingly, an *in vitro* binding assay revealed no significant difference in LC3-binding ability among the p62 mutants, except for the triple D337A/D338A/D339A mutation, which dramatically reduced LC3 interaction. However, these degradation rates were comparable *in vivo*, suggesting an equal contribution of the hydrophobic (Trp^{340} and Leu^{343}) and acidic (Asp^{337}–Asp^{339}) clusters to the p62–LC3 interaction. Taken together, these studies strongly suggest that the loss of interaction between LC3 and p62 is sufficient to impair p62 degradation.

It has been postulated that p62 deficiency results in the accumulation of ubiquitinated proteins through the loss of autophagy. However, the level of ubiquitinated protein in p62-knockout tissues was significantly lower than in autophagy-deficient tissues (Komatsu *et al.*, 2007b; Ramesh Babu *et al.*, 2008; Wooten *et al.*, 2008). A possible explanation for this discrepancy could be the presence of another autophagic adaptor, namely NBR1. First, NBR1 and p62 share short peptides binding LC3 and ubiquitinated proteins. Second, NBR1 is thought to be sequestered in the autophagosome via LC3 interaction and/or p62 interaction, and accumulates markedly in autophagy-deficient animals. Furthermore, the autophagic clearance of NBR1 also depends on the LRS region of NBR1. While p62 and NBR1 interact, p62-independent mechanisms of autophagic degradation have been identified for NBR1 (Kirkin *et al.*, 2009). Unfortunately, an LRS deletion mutant of NRB1 is currently unable to explore the contribution of this pathway to ubiquitinated protein autophagy.

Requirement of the PB1 Domain for p62 Degradation

The PB1 domains are scaffold modules with a beta-grasp topology that allows proteins like p62 to self-oligomerize, as the front end of one PB1 domain binds the back end of another PB1 domain. The K7A/D69A mutant of p62, which has a compromised PB1 surface interaction, cannot self-oligomerize, and is associated with a significant delay in p62 degradation compared with wild-type p62. However, the degradation rate of p62K7A/D69A was still higher than in *Atg7/p62* double knockout MEFs, indicating that p62 monomers are degraded, at least in part, by autophagy. Actually, p62 mutations disrupting LC3 binding accelerated delay of p62 degradation. These data suggest that, in addition to LC3 interaction, self-oligomerization is required for the effective degradation of p62 by autophagy (Ichimura *et al.*, 2008).

The NBR1 adaptor also has a PB1 domain, but self-oligomerizes using a CC1 domain. The impact of the CC1 domain on the efficiency of NBR1 degradation has not yet been reported. Nonetheless, it is possible that p62 and NBR1 cooperate in the recognition and clearance of ubiquitinated cargo. First, they have been shown to bind together via their PB1 domains. Second, they may interact indirectly by recognizing Ub chains via their UBA domains, and by binding proteins of the Atg8 family on autophagosomes. The latter is supported by immunoprecipitation experiments showing reduced association between NBR1 with LC3 in *p62−/−* MEFs and in the liver of *p62−/−* mice (Kirkin *et al.*, 2009).

Arabidopsis thaliana is commonly used as a model organism for studying NBR1 homologue expression in the absence of p62 homologues. The NBR1 homologue expressed by this plant, AtNBR1, is more similar to mammalian NBR1 than p62 in amino acid sequence and domain architecture. However, AtNBR1 self-polymerizes via the PB1 domain, like p62. Accordingly, AtNBR1 presents hybrid properties between mammalian NBR1 and p62, which makes it an interesting model to investigate the roles of the PB1 and CC1 domains. Further investigation is required to uncover autophagosome maturation in this plant (Svenning *et al.*, 2011).

Ubiquitin- and p62-Positive Inclusion Formation

Immunofluorescence studies confirmed the intracellular co-localization of p62 and LC3. In models of authophagy deficiency, the impairment of p62 turnover led to the accumulation of p62-positive inclusions in the cytoplasm, and loss of co-localization of the two proteins (see also Figure 4D of Ichimura *et al.*, 2008). In addition, the expression of GFP-p62 mutants with low binding affinity for LC3 was associated with the formation of p62-positive inclusions, which were negative for LC3, and these p62-positive inclusions were filled with ubiquitinated proteins.

In *p62* knockout MEFs expressing GFP-p62, only a few ubiquitin-positive areas could be detected in autophagosomes, suggesting that the ubiquitin-positive aggregates were trapped in the autophagosomes before they could become large aggregates/inclusions. On the other hand, autophagosome formation and degradation of long-lived proteins in *p62* knockout cells are apparently comparable with those in wild-type cells. These results suggest that impairment of p62–LC3 interaction alone is sufficient to promote the formation of ubiquitin- and p62-positive inclusions – i.e., the loss of the interaction triggers inclusion body formation. Based on oligomerization activity at the PB1 domain, and the ubiquitin-binding ability of the UBA domain, it is postulated that p62 plays an important role in the formation of cytoplasmic inclusions containing polyubiquitinated proteins. Indeed, when GFP-p62K7AD69A lacking self-oligomerization activity was expressed into *Atg7/p62* double knockout MEFs, inclusion formation was completely prevented, compared with those expressing wild-type p62. These data support an essential role for the PB1 domain in the formation of p62-positive cytoplasmic inclusions concentrating polyubiquitinated proteins (Ichimura *et al.*, 2008).

A recent study showed that p62 localizes on ER-associated autophagosome formation sites using a self-oligomerization-dependent mechanism, and independently of the presence of LC3 in the membrane. These results support the concept that p62 recruits the phagophore to the site of a ubiquitinated aggregate, which then triggers the events leading to LC3 binding to the membrane (Itakura and Mizushima, 2012).

Presently, it is unclear whether NBR1 can substitute for any of the functions mediated by p62, or can generate ubiquitinated-positive inclusion bodies.

DISCUSSION

In this chapter, we have focused on the binding mechanism of LC3–p62 toward p62 degradation, and the formation of ubiquitin-positive inclusions by p62, and considered other autophagy receptors as possible substitutions for p62 in the autophagy mechanism. The recent elucidation of the crystal structure of p62–LRS–LC3 and related complexes sheds important light on the mechanism of autophagy.

Structure comparison of LC3 homologues revealed high similarity, as LRS structurally aligned on the two hydrophobic pockets and their ubiquitin-fold domains. While the amino acid sequence of the N-terminal of LC3 is not shared by other Atg8 homologues, they present similar affinities for p62. Furthermore, LC3, GABARAP, and GATE-16 have similar biochemical characteristics, and all localize to autophagosomes. However, Atg8 homologues exhibit different responses to nutrient restrictions. On the other hand, autophagy receptors share a common, short linear peptide motif, which binds to Atg8 docking sites. While the binding affinity of each autophagy receptor has not been compared by functional assays, the newly discovered structures of GABARAPL-1 and NBR1 suggest that a single tryptophan residue in the LRS regulates binding affinity. This indicates that different LRS motifs can interact with autophagy modifiers with unique binding properties.

Among the autophagy receptor proteins, NDP52 was reported to bind selectively to LC3C. Structural analysis revealed that the selectivity of NDP52 for LC3 is conferred by a non-canonical LRS motif, which contains no aromatic residue. This case suggests that the specificity of the interactions between autophagy receptors and the autophagy machinery are functionally important to execute selective autophagy.

There is now substantial evidence that interactions between p62 and LC3 are critical for the efficient degradation of ubiquitinated proteins. Nonetheless, the level of ubiquitinated proteins in p62-knockout tissues was considerably lower than in autophagy-deficient tissues, supporting the contribution of other receptor(s), such as NBR1, in autophagy. Self-oligomerization through the PB1 domain also emerges as an important promoter of p62 degradation through autophagy. Since NBR1 self-oligomerizes using its CC1 domain, NBR1 and p62 may work together to support autophagic processes, and prevent the formation of cytoplasmic ubiquitin-positive inclusions associated with serious disorders such as hepatitis and neurogenerative diseases.

References

Behrends, C., Fulda, S., 2012. Receptor proteins in selective autophagy. Int. J. Cell. Biol. 2012, Art. ID 673290.

Bjorkoy, G., Lamark, T., Brech, A., et al., 2005. p62/SQSTM1 forms protein aggregates degraded by autophagy and has a protective effect on huntingtin-induced cell death. J. Cell. Biol. 171, 603–614.

Elmore, S.P., Qian, T., Grissom, S.F., et al., 2001. The mitochondrial permeability transition initiates autophagy in rat hepatocytes. FASEB J 15, 2286–2287.

Hara, T., Nakamura, K., Matsui, M., et al., 2006. Suppression of basal autophagy in neural cells causes neurodegenerative disease in mice. Nature 441, 885–889.

He, H., Dang, Y., Dai, F., et al., 2003. Post-translational modifications of three members of the human MAP1LC3 family and detection of a novel type of modification for MAP1LC3B. J. Biol. Chem. 278, 29278–29287.

Ichimura, Y., Kumanomidou, T., Sou, Y.S., et al., 2008. Structural basis for sorting mechanism of p62 in selective autophagy. J. Biol. Chem. 283, 22847–22857.

Itakura, E., Mizushima, N., 2012. p62 Targeting to the autophagosome formation site requires self-oligomerization but not LC3 binding. J. Cell. Biol. 192, 17–27.

Iwata, J., Ezaki, J., Komatsu, M., et al., 2006. Excess peroxisomes are degraded by autophagic machinery in mammals. J. Biol. Chem. 281, 4035–4041.

Johansen, T., Lamark, T., 2011. Selective autophagy mediated by autophagic adapter proteins. Autophagy 7, 279–296.

Kirkin, V., Lamark, T., Sou, Y.S., et al., 2009. A role for NBR1 in autophagosomal degradation of ubiquitinated substrates. Mol. Cell. 33, 505–516.

Komatsu, M., Waguri, S., Ueno, T., et al., 2005. Impairment of starvation-induced and constitutive autophagy in Atg7-deficient mice. J. Cell. Biol. 169, 425–434.

Komatsu, M., Waguri, S., Chiba, T., et al., 2006. Loss of autophagy in the central nervous system causes neurodegeneration in mice. Nature 441, 880–884.

Komatsu, M., Ueno, T., Waguri, S., et al., 2007a. Constitutive autophagy: vital role in clearance of unfavorable proteins in neurons. Cell. Death Differ. 14, 887–894.

Komatsu, M., Waguri, S., Koike, M., et al., 2007b. Homeostatic levels of p62 control cytoplasmic inclusion body formation in autophagy-deficient mice. Cell 131, 1149–1163.

Lamark, T., Kirkin, V., Dikic, I., et al., 2009. NBR1 and p62 as cargo receptors for selective autophagy of ubiquitinated targets. Cell Cycle 8, 1986–1990.

Levine, B., Klionsky, D.J., 2004. Development by self-digestion: molecular mechanisms and biological functions of autophagy. Dev. Cell 6, 463–477.

Levine, B., Kroemer, G., 2008. Autophagy in the pathogenesis of disease. Cell 132, 27–42.

Mizushima, N., 2007. Autophagy: process and function. Genes Dev. 21, 2861–2873.

Noda, N.N., Ohsumi, Y., Inagaki, F., 2010. Atg8-family interacting motif crucial for selective autophagy. FEBS Lett. 584, 1379–1385.

Ohsumi, Y., 2001. Molecular dissection of autophagy: two ubiquitin-like systems. Nat. Rev. Mol. Cell. Biol. 2, 211–216.

Pankiv, S., Clausen, T.H., Lamark, T., et al., 2007. p62/SQSTM1 binds directly to Atg8/LC3 to facilitate degradation of ubiquitinated protein aggregates by autophagy. J. Biol. Chem. 282, 24131–24145.

Ramesh Babu, J., Lamar Seibenhener, M., Peng, J., et al., 2008. Genetic inactivation of p62 leads to accumulation of hyperphosphorylated tau and neurodegeneration. J. Neurochem. 106, 107–120.

Rozenknop, A., Rogov, V.V., Rogova, N.Y., et al., 2011. Characterization of the interaction of GABARAPL-1 with the LIR motif of NBR1. J. Mol. Biol. 410, 477–487.

Simonsen, A., Birkeland, H.C., Gillooly, D.J., et al., 2004. Alfy, a novel FYVE-domain-containing protein associated with protein granules and autophagic membranes. J. Cell. Sci. 117, 4239–4251.

Svenning, S., Lamark, T., Krause, K., et al., 2011. Plant NBR1 is a selective autophagy substrate and a functional hybrid of the mammalian autophagic adapters NBR1 and p62/SQSTM1. Autophagy 7, 993–1010.

von Muhlinen, N., Akutsu, M., Ravenhill, B.J., et al., 2012. LC3C, bound selectively by a noncanonical LIR motif in NDP52, is required for antibacterial autophagy. Mol. Cell. 48, 329–342.

Wooten, M.W., Geetha, T., Babu, J.R., et al., 2008. Essential role of sequestosome 1/p62 in regulating accumulation of Lys63-ubiquitinated proteins. J. Biol. Chem. 283, 6783–6789.

Xie, Z., Klionsky, D.J., 2007. Autophagosome formation: core machinery and adaptations. Nat. Cell. Biol. 9, 1102–1109.

Xin, Y., Yu, L., Chen, Z., et al., 2001. Cloning, expression patterns, and chromosome localization of three human and two mouse homologs of GABA(A) receptor-associated protein. Genomics 74, 408–413.

Molecular Mechanisms Underlying the Role of Autophagy in Neurodegenerative Diseases

S. Tariq Ahmad and Jin-A. Lee

Abstract

Autophagy is a highly regulated process that promotes vital cellular homeostasis by allowing bulk non-specific degradation of the cytoplasmic contents, mainly damaged and/or surplus organelles and proteins. Autophagy is ubiquitous in eukaryotes, highly conserved from yeast to mammals, and occurs in all mammalian tissues. Historically, autophagy was characterized as the coping response to limited energy resources (starvation), to generate additional biomolecular raw materials. However, research in the past

© 2014 Elsevier Inc. All rights reserved.

two decades has demonstrated the indispensible roles of autophagy in eukaryotic physiology and pathology with respect to wide-ranging processes such as development, differentiation, aging, immunity, cancer biology, and neurodegenerative disorders. In this chapter, we will provide an overview of the types of autophagy and mechanisms of the autophagy pathway followed by a discussion of the current understanding of the role of autophagy in neuronal physiology, pathology of neurodegenerative disorders, and potential therapeutic approaches.

AUTOPHAGY OVERVIEW AND TYPES

Autophagy is a highly regulated, conserved, ubiquitous eukaryotic delivery system for moving the cytoplasmic cargo to lysosomes (vacuoles in yeast) for degradation. The cargo can be surplus biomolecules for recycling during nutrient/growth factor-deprived conditions, undesirable constituents like protein aggregates and faulty organelles, and, a more recent addition to the list, pathogens (Levine *et al.*, 2011). On the basis of cargo identification, sequestration, and delivery to the lysosomes, autophagy can be broadly classified as microautophagy, chaperone-mediated (CMA), or macroautophagy (Mizushima and Komatsu, 2011; Rubinsztein *et al.*, 2012; Wirawan *et al.*, 2012). Microautophagy can be considered the simplest form of autophagy, which essentially is the non-selective sequestration and delivery of the cytoplasmic content by invagination of the lysosomal membrane into its lumen. Chaperone-mediated autophagy involves a selective interaction between proteins with exposed an KFERQ-like motif and chaperones (Hsc70 complex, etc.), followed by direct infusion of the cargo–chaperone complex into the lysosomal lumen mediated by the LAMP-2A (*Lysosomal-Associated Membrane Protein-2A*) complex on the lysosomal membrane. Macroautophagy (referred to as autophagy in this chapter) is the most studied, versatile (in terms of cargo), and complex (in terms of the mechanism and components involved) form of autophagy. Autophagy is mostly non-specific in terms of cargo, which includes ubiquitinated protein aggregates and organelles. However, some selectivity in cargo recognition is emerging and thus subtypes are being defined (e.g., mitophagy for mitochondria, pexophagy for peroxisomes, nucleophagy for nucleus, reticulophagy for endoplasmic reticulum, and xenophagy for pathogens) (Wirawan *et al.*, 2012). The cargo is sequestered by encapsulation in a specialized double-membrane organelle, known as an autophagosome, through a highly concerted and regulated interplay of numerous proteins, followed by translocation of the autophagosome onto the microtubule network and fusion with the lysosomes. The mechanism of autophagy, as currently understood, is described below. Components and the modulators of the components involved in every aspect of autophagosome biology, from trigger for biosynthesis to fusion with lysosomes, are currently being studied extensively to gain an understanding of the process and of potential targets for therapeutic intervention in autophagy-associated pathology.

For a precise and detailed mechanistic understanding regarding every step of any biological process, it is important to establish a set of guidelines through rigorous review of the paradigms and biomarkers acceptable in conducting studies. Such consensus minimizes confusion in the scientific community, and allows for rapid enhancement in the understanding of the fundamental concepts. Over the past decade there has been an exponential increase in autophagy-related studies, which has necessitated a consortium to establish guidelines and biomarkers to properly observe, document, and interpret the autophagy process (Klionsky *et al.*, 2012).

PATHWAY AND MECHANISM FOR AUTOPHAGY

The core process for autophagy is the formation of a 300- to 900-nm diameter double-membrane organelle, the autophagosome. Autophagosome biogenesis can be divided into the following stages: (1) trigger/initiation; (2) nucleation – assembly of an isolation membrane (phagophore); (3) elongation/extension of the phagophore; and (4) maturation of the phagophore by membrane closure (phagosome) followed by fusion with the lysosome (Figure 3.1). The process has essentially emerged over the past couple of decades; the major breakthrough came with the identification of autophagy-related (Atg) genes in yeast (Yang and Klionsky, 2009, 2010). The stages for autophagosome biology are described below, with an emphasis of mammalian autophagy.

Initiation

The core machinery involved at this stage includes the mTORC (*mammalian Target of Rapamycin Complex*, which consists of mTOR, DEPTOR (*DEP-domain containing mTOR interacting protein*), RAPTOR (*Regulatory Associated Protein of mTOR*), PRAS40, and GβL) and ULK (*Uncoordinated (unc-51) Like Kinase*, which consists of ULK1/2, Atg13, FIP200 (*Focal Adhesion Kinase (FAK) family Interacting Protein of 200kDa*), and Atg101) complex. The master regulator for the initiation of autophagy is mTORC. However, mTOR-independent autophagy has also been described (Wirawan *et al.*, 2012). Under nutrient-rich conditions, autophagosome biosynthesis is downregulated by maintaining mTORC in an active phosphorylated state by PI3KC1 kinase (*Class I phosphatidyl-3-inositol kinase*). Active mTORC through mTOR kinase activity in turn phosphorylates ULK1 and Atg13 of the ULK complex, resulting in the suppression of phagophore initiation. The inhibitory interaction of mTORC with the ULK complex is dependent on the presence of an autophagy stimulus. Autophagy can be triggered by a variety of stimuli, which can be physiological (e.g., starvation), pharmacological (e.g., rapamycin, etoposide), or pathological (e.g., protein aggregates, pathogens). Upon appropriate stimulation, such as starvation, mTOR is inhibited and dissociates from the ULK complex, resulting in activation of the latter (Figure 3.1). Active ULK1 phosphorylates other members of the ULK complex, namely FIP200 and Atg13. Other substrates of ULK1 include myosin II motor protein (regulates trafficking of mAtg9 – a transmembrane protein considered to promote lipid assembly for the growing phagophore) and AMBRA1 (*Activating Molecule in Beclin 1-Regulated Autophagy* – a constituent of the PI3KC3 (*Class III Phosphatidyl-3-Inositol Kinase*) complex) – core proteins involved in autophagophore nucleation (Mizushima and Komatsu, 2011; Rubinsztein *et al.*, 2012; Yang and Klionsky, 2010; Wirawan *et al.*, 2012).

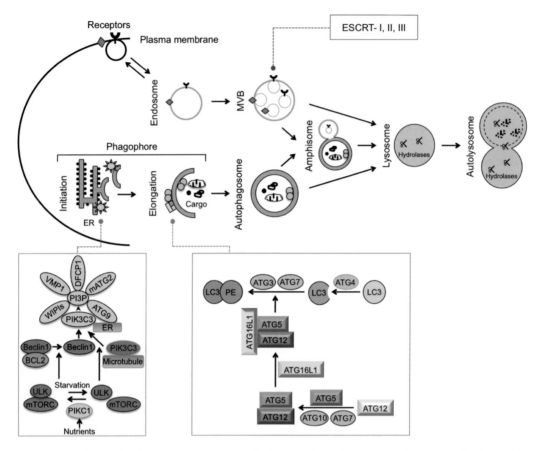

FIGURE 3.1   **The molecular mechanism of the autophagy pathway.** The process of autophagy begins with the initiation of phagophore formation, which entails budding of a limiting membrane from the endoplasmic reticulum (ER) and/or other intracellular membranes. Initiation of the phagophore is tightly regulated by the interplay of protein complexes and pathways sensitive to autophagy stimuli, such as starvation, organelle damage, misfolded proteins, etc. Under normal nutrient-rich conditions, PI3KC1 kinase activates mTOR in the mTORC complex, which interacts with the ULK complex thereby limiting its activity. During starvation and other triggers for autophagy, mTOR is inhibited, thereby activating the ULK complex, which in turn activates the PI3KC3 complex and translocates it from the microtubules to the ER. Starvation also releases Beclin 1 from the anti-autophagic interaction with the anti-apoptotic protein BCL2. Beclin 1, together with other components of the PI3KC3 complex, Atg14 and UVRAG, promotes PI3KC3 kinase activity. Activated PI3KC3 kinase generates PI3P, which in turn recruits WIPI1–4, VMP1, DFCP1, mAtg2, and transmembrane mAtg9 to nucleate the phagophore in the proximity of the cargo. Elongation of the phagophore to extend the limiting membrane around the cargo is regulated by the Atg5–Atg12–Atg16L1 and LC3–PE conjugation systems. To this end, Atg7 and Atg10, E1- and E2-ligase, respectively, modify Atg12. Modified Atg12 binds Atg5 followed by Atg16L1 binding to form the Atg5–Atg12–Atg16L1 complex. The LC3–PE complex formation is initiated by the cleavage of LC3 by Atg4 followed by coordinated interaction with the Atg7, Atg3 (an E2 ligase), and Atg5–Atg12–Atg16L1 complex to generate LC3–PE on the inner and outer phagophore membranes. The conjugation systems also contribute to the curvature and closure of the phagophore membrane to form an autophagosome. Subsequently, Atg4 unconjugates LC3–PE from the outer membrane only. The continued presence of LC3–PE on the inner membrane until fusion with the lysosome makes it a useful marker to study the autophagy flux. The autophagosome outer membrane can then directly fuse with the single-membrane lysosome to expose its contents to the digestive hydrolases in the lysosomal lumen, resulting in

Nucleation

The core machinery involved in nucleation includes the Beclin 1/PI3KC3 complex (Beclin 1 (*Bcl2 interacting protein 1*), PI3KC3, AMBRA1, p150, UVRAG (*UV Radiation Resistance Associated Gene*), and Atg14). Nucleation can be defined as the PI3KC3-mediated synthesis of phosphatidyl-inositol-3-phosphate (PI3P), which in turn enables recruitment of other Atg proteins at the phagophore assembly site. These proteins include DFCP1 (*Double FYVE-Containing Protein 1*), WIPI 1-4 (*WD repeat domain Phosphoinositide Interacting*), mAtg2, VMP1 (*Vacuole Membrane Protein 1*), and Atg9. During nutrient-rich conditions, the PI3KC3 complex resides on the microtubules due to the AMBRA1–microtubule associated–dynein interaction. Upon induction of autophagy, activated ULK1 phosphorylates AMBRA1 thereby translocating the PI3KC3 complex from microtubules to the endoplasmic reticulum (ER), which serves as an important source of the membrane for the nascent phagophore (Figure 3.1). Phagophores can bud out of the ER membrane and remain continuous with the ER lumen, leading to the term "omegasomes" for their shape, which is similar to the Greek letter omega. The mitochondrial outer membrane, Golgi apparatus, and plasma membrane can also contribute membrane to the growing phagophore.

Beclin 1, through interactions with its multiple modifiers, regulates PI3KC3 kinase activity and autophagy induction. The most studied and well-characterized interaction of Beclin 1 is with the anti-apoptotic proteins BCL2 (*B-cell Lymphoma*) and BCL-X$_L$ through direct binding via its BCL2 homology domain-3 (BH3) (Levine *et al.*, 2011). This interaction negatively regulates autophagy. During starvation JNK-mediated phosphorylation separates BCL2 and Beclin 1, resulting in the activation of autophagy (Figure 3.1). Interaction of Beclin 1 with Atg14 and UVRAG promotes PI3KC3 kinase activity. Interaction of Beclin 1 with Bif1 via UVRAG, besides promoting PI3KC3 kinase activity, may also contribute to the membrane curvature of the autophagosome (Mizushima and Komatsu, 2011; Rubinsztein *et al.*, 2012; Yang and Klionsky, 2010; Wirawan *et al.*, 2012).

Elongation

The core machinery for elongation and closure of phagophores to form autophagosome includes two ubiquitin-like conjugation systems, Atg12–Atg5–Atg16L1 (Atg12, Atg7, Atg10, Atg5, and Atg16L1) and LC3–PE (*microtubule associated Light Chain 3-Phosphatidyl Ethanolamine*, consisting of LC3, Atg4, Atg7, and Atg3) complex. Both these complexes are crucial for efficient expansion of the phagophore, with additional roles of the Atg12–Atg5–Atg16L1 complex in supporting phagophore membrane curvature and as an E3 ligase allowing conjugation of the LC3–PE complex to the phagophore membrane. The LC3–PE system

the degradation of the cargo and thereby completing the autophagy process. Alternatively, it has been suggested that the autophagosome, prior to fusion with the lysosome, can fuse with a multivesicular body (MVB), a critical component of the endosome–lysosome pathway. The endosome–lysosome pathway, responsible for the turnover of the plasma membrane receptors, begins with invagination of the plasma membrane bearing receptors into the cytoplasm (endosome). The endosome then undergoes another round of membrane invagination to form MVBs. The MVB biogenesis is a highly coordinated process mainly regulated by the endosomal sorting complex required for transport-I, -II, and -III (ESCRT). The MVBs either can directly fuse with a lysosome, thereby releasing their cargo for degradation, or may fuse with an autophagosome to form an amphisome.

also plays an important role in phagophore closure, and its interaction with p62/SQSTM1 (*Sequestosome 1*), NBR1 (*Neighbor of BRCA1 gene*), and NDP52 (*Nuclear Dot Protein 52*) imparts some specificity in cargo recognition. Due to its presence on the inner and outer membranes of the phagophore and inner membrane of the mature autophagosome, LC3–PE (LC3-II) is also considered a *bona fide* marker for the autophagy-related structures to measure autophagy flux (Klionsky *et al.*, 2012). However, some studies have indicated the presence of Atg5-, Atg7-, and LC3-independent autophagy (Nishida *et al.*, 2009). To this end, mouse embryonic fibroblasts (MEFs) from *Atg5* and *Atg7* knockout mice formed functional autophagosomes, originating from the Golgi and endosomal membranes, in an LC3-independent process (Nishida *et al.*, 2009).

Atg12–Atg5–Atg16L1 complex formation begins with the sequential activation of Atg12 by Atg7 (an E1 ligase) and Atg10 (an E2 ligase), respectively, followed by covalent linking to Atg5. The Atg12–Atg5 complex is then linked to Atg16L1 to form a trimer (Figure 3.1). These trimers homodimerize to form large multimeric complexes, which interact with other PI3P-recruited proteins at the expanding phagophore membrane.

LC3–PE complex formation begins with the proteolytic cleavage of LC3 by Atg4, a cysteine protease. Cleaved LC3 (LC3-I) is then conjugated to PE by the concerted activity of Atg7, Atg3 (an E2 ligase), and the Atg12–Atg5–Atg16L1 complex to form LC3-PE (LC3-II) (Figure 3.1). During autophagosome maturation Atg4 deconjugates LC3–PE from the outer membrane, which plays an important role in sealing off the phagophore ends. However, LC3–PE linkage with the inner membrane is maintained until autophagosome degradation in the lysosomal lumen (Mizushima and Komatsu, 2011; Rubinsztein *et al.*, 2012; Yang and Klionsky, 2010; Wirawan *et al.*, 2012).

Maturation/Fusion with Lysosomes

The autophagy process culminates with the fusion of the autophagosome double-membrane vesicle with the single-membrane lysosome to form an autolysosome. The outer membrane of the autophagosome fuses with the lysosome membrane, thereby exposing the inner membrane and its contents in the lumen to the degradative hydrolases of the lysosome (Figure 3.1). Although it is unclear how autophagosomes fuse with the lysosomes, several proteins are known for their involvement in this process. These include LAMP2, the Rubicon–UVRAG complex, SNAREs (*soluble N-ethylmalemide sensitive factor attachment protein receptor*), Rab (*Ras (rat sarcoma) like in rat brain*), and LC3. Besides the possibility of direct fusion between autophagosomes and lysosomes, studies have linked autophagosomes with the endosomal–lysosomal pathway, thereby suggesting an interesting alternate mechanism for the fusion process. These studies suggest that autophagosomes fuse with endosomes or MVBs (*MultiVesicular Bodies*) to form an amphisome, which fuses with the lysosome (Figure 3.1) (Lee and Gao, 2012; Lee *et al.*, 2007).

The endosome–lysosome system is responsible for sequestering membrane proteins (especially receptors) in vesicles (endosomes), followed by their trafficking either to the lysosome for degradation through MVB formation or back to the plasma membrane through recycling endosomes (Figure 3.1). Plasma membrane proteins on the endosomes destined for lysosomes are ubiquitinated, which triggers another round of invagination of the endosomal membrane into the endosomal lumen to form MVBs (i.e., vesicles within vesicles). Multivesicular body formation constitutes a critical and highly regulated step in the endosome–lysosome pathway, and occurs through a concerted activity of conserved heteromeric protein complexes known as the endosomal protein complex required for transport-I, -II, and -III (ESCRTs) (Figure 3.1). Numerous studies in a variety of model organisms have shown that defects in the ESCRT components are associated with the accumulation of autophagosomes in the cytoplasm, thereby indicating faulty fusion of the autophagosomes with lysosomes (Lee and Gao, 2012). This notion of the convergence of autophagy and endosome–lysosome pathways at the pre-autophagosome–lysosome fusion stage has added an extremely significant aspect to the regulation of autophagy, which could potentially be targeted to regulate autophagy in therapeutic strategies.

PHYSIOLOGICAL ROLES OF AUTOPHAGY

Autophagy is essential to maintain homeostasis, especially during nutrient-deficient conditions, by degrading cytoplasmic components to replenish biomolecules for building the components in demand, such as proteins involved in alternate energy metabolism pathways. However, over the past two decades autophagy has gained additional prominence for its crucial involvement in non-starvation related pathways (sometimes referred to as basal autophagy); i.e., constitutive autophagy at relatively low levels during normal nutrient availability. Understandably, disruption of basal autophagy can lead and/or contribute to pathology. The pathophysiological roles of autophagy include protein and organelle quality control, development and differentiation, aging, cell death, tumor biology, and immunity (Levine *et al.*, 2011; Rubinsztein *et al.*, 2012). In this chapter we will focus on the pathophysiological roles of autophagy in neurons.

AUTOPHAGY AND NEURONAL PHYSIOLOGY

Both major roles of autophagy (i.e., maintenance of nutrient and biomolecular homeostasis, and removal of unwanted components) are especially crucial for neurons because of their postmitotic status. Neurons therefore require efficient organelle and protein turnover. Consequently, a lack of autophagy in neurons can cause a biomolecular traffic jam, especially at the synapse. Studies using transgenic mouse expressing GFP-LC3 showed differential regulation of autophagy in neurons; the brain does not upregulate autophagy upon starvation (Mizushima and Levine, 2010). However, some recent studies have indicated the presence of a specialized autophagy (lipophagy) in the brain under nutrient-deficient conditions (Mizushima and Komatsu, 2011). Nevertheless, the lack of the widespread starvation-induced response in the brain is likely due to an uninterrupted supply of nutrients to the brain from other tissues even during nutrient emergencies because of a premium placed on the brain's ability to receive constant energy. Additionally, rapamycin and lithium chloride treatment, used to induce mTOR-dependent and -independent autophagy, respectively, do not increase LC3 levels in cultured primary neurons, thereby indicating differential regulation of autophagy between neurons and other cell types (Mitra *et al.*, 2009).

Quality Control

At any given moment in the life of a cell there is tremendous anabolic and catabolic activity in the transcriptome and proteome to maintain a healthy pool of biomolecules. Concurrently, cells expend a lot of energy and other resources for quality control of their biomolecules, especially DNA and proteins, with the defective ones either repaired (mostly for DNA) or degraded in the case of proteins. Ubiquitination mediated by molecular chaperones and ubiquitin ligases, followed by degradation by the proteasome assembly, is well characterized and considered to be the mechanism of choice for recognizing, degrading, and recycling misfolded proteins. Autophagy is emerging as another mechanism for the degradation of misfolded proteins especially when misfolded proteins form aggregates, thereby surpassing the substrate size limit of the proteasome. Studies limiting autophagy in cell culture and Atg-knockout mice models have shown an accumulation of misfolded ubiquitinated protein aggregates. The study using neuron specific $Atg^{-/-}$ or $Atg7^{-/-}$ deficient mice showed abnormal protein accumulation and eventual neurodegeneration in the central nervous system, indicating that autophagy is constitutively active and essential for neuronal survival (Hara et al., 2006; Komatsu et al., 2006; Mizushima and Levine, 2010).

Additionally, as mentioned previously, autophagy plays a prominent role in clearing defective organelles. Elimination of defective mitochondria (mitophagy) has been shown to depend on ubiquitination by Parkin, an E3 ubiquitin ligase. This ubiquitin tag is also suggested to impart specificity and selectivity in target recognition for autophagic removal. Recently, p62 has been suggested to contribute to the recognition of ubiquitinated substrates by autophagosomes. Also, p62 can bind both ubiquitin and LC3 on the autophagosome membrane, thereby possibly serving as a linker between cargo and autophagosome (Mizushima and Komatsu, 2011).

Development and Differentiation

Recent studies have indicated a crucial role of autophagy-related genes in the development and maturation of axons, dendrites, and synapses. Studies using mice with a specific loss of $Atg7$ in the Purkinje neurons in the cerebellum show accumulation of aberrant membrane-bound organelles and membrane structures in dystrophic axonal terminals in a cell-autonomous manner. Additionally, in Drosophila larvae autophagy facilitates synaptic development at the neuromuscular junctions (NMJs) (Shen and Ganetzky, 2010). These authors have shown that limiting basal autophagy by Atg mutants shrinks NMJ synapse and reduces bouton number, and overexpression of Atg1 results in NMJ overgrowth and surplus boutons. Autophagy downregulates the Hiw level, an E3 ligase acting as a negative regulator of NMJ synapses.

These studies highlight a specialized role of autophagy in membrane homeostasis within the axon terminal, and raise a lot of interesting questions that need to be addressed in order to uncover the exact roles of autophagy in this terminal. What are the additional substrates for autophagy in the axon terminal? How does autophagy regulate membrane homeostasis in the axon terminal? Are there any differences in the autophagy pathway between the cell body, dendrites, and axons within a neuron? From the current understanding, it appears that neuronal autophagy in the axon terminal may play an important role in the homeostasis of synaptic vesicles or membrane-bound structures abundant in the axon. In particular, synaptic vesicles are interesting candidate organelles regulated by the autophagy pathway because they are highly regulated in the axon terminal by synaptic activity. Autophagy in the axon terminal may also be involved in growth cone remodeling during axonal development, or in the regenerative process after injury. Future work to explore the role of neuronal autophagy in the axon terminal will enable us to further define neuronal autophagy, as well as disease progression associated with dysfunctional autophagy.

Besides development, studies have indicated a role of autophagy in neuronal differentiation. Genetic (AMBRA1 haploinsufficiency) and pharmacological (wortmanin, 3-methyladenine) inhibition of autophagy impaired neurogenesis in the mice olfactory bulb cell culture. Treatment with 3-methyladenine also demonstrated impaired neurogenesis in chicken otic epitilial cells (Aburto *et al.*, 2012). Autophagy impairment limits neuroblastoma differentiation into neurons and glioma stem/progenitor cells (Zhao *et al.*, 2010). Although a detailed mechanism is not known, these studies indicate an intriguing role of autophagy in neuronal differentiation and neurogenesis.

AUTOPHAGY AND NEURODEGENERATIVE DISEASES

Autophagy is generally considered a prosurvival process because of its historically defined roles in starvation and other neutralizing stressful conditions such as oxidative damage and organelle damage. A massive accumulation of autophagic vacuoles including autophagosomes or autolysosomes has been observed in the affected brain region in several neurodegenerative disorders. However, the role of autophagy in each neurodegenerative disease has not been well defined. Accumulated autophagosomes in the degenerating neurons could be due to an increase or decrease in the autophagic flux (as measured by actual degradation of cytosolic contents) (Figure 3.2). Sustained overactivation of autophagy, impairment of the balance between autophagosome formation and lysosomal fusion, and impairment of lysosomal components are considered to contribute to the degeneration of the nervous system, which is more vulnerable to protein misregulation due to the postmitotic status of neurons. Furthermore, insufficient autophagic degradation due to excessive autophagic demand because of abnormal protein aggregation (a hallmark of most neurodegenerative disorders) could cause autophagic stress associated with neurodegeneration (Figure 3.2). Finding out how autophagic stress occurs in each neurodegenerative disease would be the first important step toward understanding the molecular pathogenesis and association between neurodegenerative diseases and autophagy, and investigating new therapeutic strategies to treat neurodegenerative diseases. This section briefly summarizes the current understanding of how the autophagy pathway is associated with the pathogenic mechanism of the most common neurodegenerative diseases.

Alzheimer's Disease

Alzheimer's disease (AD) is the most common neurodegenerative disease. The symptoms of AD include loss of spatial memory, confusion, irritability, and trouble with language. Its pathogenesis is characterized by the accumulation of extracellular plaques containing aggregated amyloid-β (Aβ) peptide and intracellular tangles containing hyperphosphorylated Tau protein. Under normal conditions, Aβ is produced by cleavage of the amyloid precursor

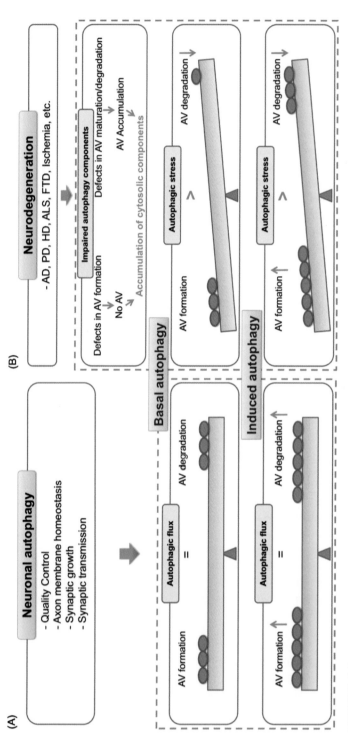

FIGURE 3.2 **Autophagic regulation in physiology and pathophysiology in neurons.** Autophagic flux reflects the balance between autophagosome formation and degradation. (A) Basal autophagy is activated in neurons to control the quality of cytosolic components, or regulate axon membrane morphology, synaptic growth, or synaptic transmission. Once autophagy is induced by various signals, autophagosome formation as well as autophagic degradation is enhanced to balance autophagic flux. (B) Any disruption of autophagic processes, such as autophagosome formation, maturation, and degradation, causes impairment of autophagy. Either deletion of early components of autophagosomes formation or defects in the molecular machinery for maturation or degradation of autophagy induces accumulation of cytosolic components, leading to neurodegeneration due to loss of autophagy. Furthermore, less efficient autophagic degradation during basal or activated autophagy causes the accumulation of autophagic vacuoles (AVs) associated with many neurodegenerative diseases.

protein by beta- and gamma-secretase, and localized in the endosomal/autophagosomal–lysosomal pathway. However, under a diseased state Aβ clearance is likely impeded due to the autophagic stress caused by impaired maturation or transport of the autophagosomes (reduced fusion or altered endocytic pathway) (Boland *et al.*, 2008). Indeed, autophagic vacuoles have been found to accumulate in the dystrophic neurites and in the cell body of AD-affected neurons (Nixon, 2005). Mutations in Presenilin-1, a constituent of the gamma-secretase complex, are a major risk factor for hereditary AD. Recently it has been reported that the failure of Presenilin-1 dependent trafficking of v-ATPase (*vacuolar-type H+-ATPase*, required for lysosomal acidification) from ER to lysosome could impair autophagosome–lysosome fusion, resulting in the accumulation of autophagosomes, which could contribute to the pathogenesis of AD (Lee *et al.*, 2010). Furthermore, Beclin 1 expression is decreased in the AD brain. Beclin 1 deficiency is associated with an increase in Aβ production, accumulation, and neurodegeneration leading to AD (Pickford *et al.*, 2008).

Mechanisms correlating altered autophagy and AD are not known in detail, and are likely to be complex and multifactorial. Nevertheless, induction and activation of autophagy using pro-autophagy proteins and chemicals such as Beclin 1 and rapamycin, respectively, could promote Aβ clearance and reduce AD pathology. Success in such strategies will raise the possibility of autophagy inducers as a therapeutic target of AD (Caccamo *et al.*, 2010). Moreover, since the impaired clearance of the autophagic vacuoles has been observed in AD animal models and patients, targeting the autophagosome–lysosome fusion stage of the autophagy pathway could yield promising results for therapeutic intervention.

Parkinson's Disease

Parkinson's disease (PD) is characterized by progressive degeneration of the dopaminergic neurons in the substantia nigra. The symptoms of PD include tremors, rigidity, and impaired balance and coordination. Mutations in α-synuclein (A53T and A30P), LRRK2 (*Leucine Rich Repeat 2*), PINK1 (*PTEN-induced putative kinase 1*), and Parkin are associated with familial cases of PD. The major component of the Lewy bodies, one of the pathological hallmarks of PD, is α-synuclein. α-Synuclein is normally degraded by CMA and macroautophagy (Cuervo *et al.*, 2004; Vogiatzi *et al.*, 2008). Interestingly, recent studies have demonstrated that mutant α-synuclein, likely due to the propensity to form aggregates, is degraded via the compensatory activation of macroautophagy instead of CMA (Cuervo *et al.*, 2004). Therefore, autophagic modulation for the restoration of the CMA function may be an effective therapeutic strategy in PD. Beclin 1 is also suggested to be involved in the degradation of α-synuclein. Accordingly, ectopic overexpression of Beclin 1 in the α-synuclein transgenic mouse model rescued the morphological defects and reduced α-synuclein accumulation (Spencer *et al.*, 2009).

A growing body of evidence shows that the dysfunctional turnover of the mitochondria might be a major cause of pathogenesis in PD. It has been shown that Parkin and PINK1, whose mutations cause an autosomal recessive form of PD, play important roles in mitophagy. Interestingly, the selective targeting of Parkin into damaged mitochondria during mitophagy is dependent on wild-type PINK1 but not mutant PINK1, suggesting a regulatory role of Parkin and PINK1 in mitophagy (Dagda *et al.*, 2009). Thus, the efficient turnover of dysfunctional mitochondria by modulation of the autophagy pathway could also be considered to be one of the therapeutic targets in PD.

Huntington's Disease

Huntington's disease (HD) is one of the most common polyglutamine (PolyQ) diseases inherited by autosomal dominant mutant expansion (more than 35 repeats) in the CAG tri-nucleotide repeats in the Huntingtin (*Htt*) gene. This disease causes neuronal loss in the striatum and cortex leading to a progressive disruption of the voluntary motor coordination. It has been generally accepted that intranuclear or cytosolic aggregates generated by an expanded polyglutamine tract in the N-terminus of *Htt* are associated with neuronal toxicity. These insoluble aggregates or toxic oligomers of mutant *Htt* are degraded by autophagy (Ravikumar *et al.*, 2004). Recent studies have shown that the stimulation and activation of autophagy reduces toxicity in various *in vivo* and *in vitro* models of HD (Lansbury and Lashuel, 2006). Additionally, modifiers of the mTOR-dependent or -independent pathway could lead to neuro-protection in the cellular and animal HD model by reducing polyglutamine aggregation (Ravikumar *et al.*, 2004). Histone deacetylases (HDACs) and microtubules have been demonstrated to facilitate the effective clearance of polyglutamine aggregates by the autophagy pathway (Pandey *et al.*, 2007). The finding that reduction of Beclin 1 or polymorphism in Atg7 (V471A) is associated with the pathogenesis of HD further supports that stimulation of autophagy promotes the degradation of aggregates (Metzger *et al.*, 2010; Shibata *et al.*, 2006). Moreover, facilitation of CMA by the selective targeting of mutant *Htt* using a fusion molecule consisting of polyglutamine binding peptide 1 (QBP1) and Hsc70-binding motifs *in vitro* and *in vivo* enhanced the degradation of aggregates and reduced disease phenotypes in a HD animal model (Bauer *et al.*, 2010). Therefore, induction of macroautophagy or CMA could be an attractive strategy for HD therapy.

Amyotrophic Lateral Sclerosis

Amyotrophic Lateral Sclerosis (ALS) is characterized by the degeneration of motor neurons leading to respiratory failure and fatality. Autophagosomes are abundant in the postmortem spinal cord of sporadic and familial ALS patients (Hetz *et al.*, 2009). Recent studies have shown that autophagy was elevated for the compensatory degradation of increased misfolded proteins or dysfunctional organelles in motor neurons (Okamoto *et al.*, 2010). However, in contrast, there are other studies that showed defective autophagy in motor neurons (Caccamo *et al.*, 2010). Although the involvement of autophagy in ALS has been extensively reported, its functional significance in neuronal survival remains speculative. However, autophagic clearance of mutant SOD1 (*superoxide dismutase1*) using heat shock protein HspB8 is beneficial for motor neuron loss in an ALS animal model (Crippa *et al.*, 2010). According to a recent report, ALS2/alsin, whose mutations are associated with recessive ALS2, could be a therapeutic target of ALS due to its function in the regulation of the autophagy–endolysosomal protein degradation pathway (Hadano *et al.*, 2010). Furthermore, autophagy induction and its subsequent activation using rapamycin or lithium might be an important therapeutic target for ALS.

Frontotemporal Dementia

Frontotemporal dementia (FTD), characterized by progressive degeneration of the frontal and temporal lobes, is the second most common dementia in those under 65 years of age. The symptoms of FTD include defects in personality, alteration of social behavior, and aggressiveness. It has been reported that a mutation in CHMP2B, an ESCRT-III subunit, causes the accumulation of ubiquitinated protein aggregates and autophagosomes due to the impairment of autophagosomes maturation and fusion with lysosomes, eventually leading to neurodegeneration (Lee *et al.*, 2007). The reduction of autophagic stress by inhibiting autophagosome biogenesis delayed neuronal cell loss, indicating that excessive autophagosomes can contribute to disease pathogenesis associated with CHMP2B.

Another gene linked to FTD is p97/VCP (*Valosin Containing Protein*), a type II AAA ATPase (ATPase associated with diverse cellular activity), which regulates vesicle fusion, the proteasomal pathway, and autophagy (Seelaar *et al.*, 2011). Several studies have implicated the autophagy pathway in VCP-associated FTD. Either overexpression of VCP mutants (R155H, A232E) or dominant negative VCP caused accumulation of the immature form of autophagosomes in an *in vitro* or *in vivo* animal model, suggesting that VCP regulates the maturation of autophagosomes (Tresse *et al.*, 2010). Although reduction of autophagic stress by inhibiting autophagy temporally delays neurodegeneration, a selective method of facilitating the delivery of autophagic components into lysosomes to assist autophagic clearance under the pathological condition should be further investigated.

Cerebral Ischemia (Injury)

Cerebral ischemia is a severe neurodegenerative condition that, depending on the area affected, could impede a variety of physiological functions, including cognitive and motor functions. Although the existence of autophagy in cerebral ischemia is well documented, the exact functions and influence of autophagy in cerebral ischemia remain elusive. Whether the activation of autophagy is beneficial or detrimental in cerebral ischemia injury largely depends on the balance between autophagy induction and autophagic degradation of the cellular substrates. A recent study showed that the HDAC inhibitor with the BH3-mimetic GX15-070 abolished the neuroprotection of ischemic preconditioning, implying a neuroprotective effect of autophagy (Wei *et al.*, 2010). Also, trauma or pharmacological injury has been linked to the autophagy pathway (Balduini *et al.*, 2012). Another report showed that inhibition of the excessive induction of autophagy in injury models seems to protect or delay neurodegeneration, indicating a possible role of autophagy in promoting neuronal cell death. However, further studies should be done in a time- and a context-dependent manner to understand the contribution of autophagy in injuries and chronic neurodegenerative diseases.

CONCLUSIONS AND FUTURE PERSPECTIVE

There has been a tremendous increase in our understanding of the autophagy pathway, its regulation, and its role in physiology and diseases. Autophagy can be primarily protective against neuronal cell death under physiological or pathological conditions. Thus, dysfunction of basal autophagy can lead to neurodegeneration, indicating its physiological role in cell survival and homeostasis. Under certain stressful conditions, autophagy may be highly active for cellular reconstruction. However, autophagy can be also strongly induced and activated to remove toxic components in several neurodegenerative diseases. Under these disease conditions, autophagy with a balanced autophagic flux could improve neuronal cell viability. In contrast, insufficient autophagy can cause autophagic stress leading to neurodegeneration. Therefore, understanding of the molecular mechanism of neuronal autophagy as well as identification of the specific role of autophagy in many neurodegenerative diseases in a context-dependent manner is needed to complement therapeutic approaches based on modulation of the autophagy pathway. The autophagy pathway is a very plausible and attractive target for therapeutic strategies to limit and eliminate the incidence and progression of neurodegenerative disorders. Thus, further studies to explore better approaches to modulate autophagy are necessary beside simple induction or inhibition of autophagy. The targets to identify drug candidates for autophagy manipulation include selective trafficking of toxic substrates into lysosomes, enhancement of autophagosome–lysosome fusion, or facilitating the delivery of autophagic vacuoles to lysosomes. Moreover, the strategies whereby the autophagy pathway can be accurately balanced and maintained within the physiological level in neurodegenerative diseases also need to be investigated. Future studies will provide a broad spectrum of potential drug targets in various neurodegenerative diseases, as well as a better understanding of the molecular mechanism of autophagy.

Acknowledgments

We thank Dr D. J. Jang and colleagues for their comments on the manuscript. This work was supported by grants from the National Center for Research Resources, INBRE 5P20RR016463-12 (to Colby College – STA) and National Institute of General Medical Sciences 8 P20 GM103423-12 from the National Institutes of Health (to Colby College – STA); a Science Division Grant, Colby College (to STA); and the Basic Science Research Program through the NRF 2010-0010824 & 2011-0022813 (to JAL).

References

Aburto, M.R., Sanchez-Calderon, H., Hurle, J.M., et al., 2012. Early otic development depends on autophagy for apoptotic cell clearance and neural differentiation. Cell Death. Dis. 3, e394.

Balduini, W., Carloni, S., Buonocore, G., 2012. Autophagy in hypoxia-ischemia induced brain injury. J. Matern. Fetal Neonatal Med. 25 (Suppl. 1), 30–34.

Bauer, P.O., Goswami, A., Wong, H.K., et al., 2010. Harnessing chaperone-mediated autophagy for the selective degradation of mutant huntingtin protein. Nat. Biotechnol. 28, 256–263.

Boland, B., Kumar, A., Lee, S., et al., 2008. Autophagy induction and autophagosome clearance in neurons: relationship to autophagic pathology in Alzheimer's disease. J. Neurosci. 28, 6926–6937.

Caccamo, A., Majumder, S., Richardson, A., et al., 2010. Molecular interplay between mammalian target of rapamycin (mTOR), amyloid-beta, and Tau: effects on cognitive impairments. J. Biol. Chem. 285, 13107–13120.

Crippa, V., Sau, D., Rusmini, P., et al., 2010. The small heat shock protein B8 (HspB8) promotes autophagic removal of misfolded proteins involved in amyotrophic lateral sclerosis (ALS). Hum. Mol. Genet. 19, 3440–3456.

Cuervo, A.M., Stefanis, L., Fredenburg, R., et al., 2004. Impaired degradation of mutant alpha-synuclein by chaperone-mediated autophagy. Science 305, 1292–1295.

Dagda, R.K., Cherra III, S.J., Kulich, S.M., et al., 2009. Loss of PINK1 function promotes mitophagy through effects on oxidative stress and mitochondrial fission. J. Biol. Chem. 284, 13843–13855.

Hadano, S., Yoshii, Y., Otomo, A., et al., 2010. Genetic background and gender effects on gross phenotypes in congenic lines of ALS2/alsin-deficient mice. Neurosci. Res. 68, 131–136.

Hara, T., Nakamura, K., Matsui, M., et al., 2006. Suppression of basal autophagy in neural cells causes neurodegenerative disease in mice. Nature 441, 885–889.

Hetz, C., Thielen, P., Matus, S., et al., 2009. XBP-1 deficiency in the nervous system protects against amyotrophic lateral sclerosis by increasing autophagy. Genes. Dev. 23, 2294–2306.

Klionsky, D.J., Abdalla, F.C., Abeliovich, H., et al., 2012. Guidelines for the use and interpretation of assays for monitoring autophagy. Autophagy 8, 445–544.

Komatsu, M., Waguri, S., Chiba, T., et al., 2006. Loss of autophagy in the central nervous system causes neurodegeneration in mice. Nature 441, 880–884.

Lansbury, P.T., Lashuel, H.A., 2006. A century-old debate on protein aggregation and neurodegeneration enters the clinic. Nature 443, 774–779.

Lee, J.A., Gao, F.B., 2012. Neuronal Functions of ESCRTs. Exp. Neurobiol. 21, 9–15.

Lee, J.A., Beigneux, A., Ahmad, S.T., et al., 2007. ESCRT-III dysfunction causes autophagosome accumulation and neurodegeneration. Curr. Biol. 17, 1561–1567.

Lee, J.H., Yu, W.H., Kumar, A., et al., 2010. Lysosomal proteolysis and autophagy require presenilin 1 and are disrupted by Alzheimer-related PS1 mutations. Cell 141, 1146–1158.

Levine, B., Mizushima, N., Virgin, H.W., 2011. Autophagy in immunity and inflammation. Nature 469, 323–335.

Metzger, S., Saukko, M., Van Che, H., et al., 2010. Age at onset in Huntington's disease is modified by the autophagy pathway: implication of the V471A polymorphism in Atg7. Hum. Genet. 128, 453–459.

Mitra, S., Tsvetkov, A.S., Finkbeiner, S., 2009. Protein turnover and inclusion body formation. Autophagy 5, 1037–1038.

Mizushima, N., Komatsu, M., 2011. Autophagy: renovation of cells and tissues. Cell 147, 728–741.

Mizushima, N., Levine, B., 2010. Autophagy in mammalian development and differentiation. Nat. Cell Biol. 12, 823–830.

Nishida, Y., Arakawa, S., Fujitani, K., et al., 2009. Discovery of Atg5/Atg7-independent alternative macroautophagy. Nature 461, 654–658.

Nixon, R.A., 2005. Endosome function and dysfunction in Alzheimer's disease and other neurodegenerative diseases. Neurobiol. Aging 26, 373–382.

Okamoto, K., Fujita, Y., Mizuno, Y., 2010. Pathology of protein synthesis and degradation systems in ALS. Neuropathology 30, 189–193.

Pandey, U.B., Nie, Z., Batlevi, Y., et al., 2007. HDAC6 rescues neurodegeneration and provides an essential link between autophagy and the UPS. Nature 447, 859–863.

Pickford, F., Masliah, E., Britschgi, M., et al., 2008. The autophagy-related protein beclin 1 shows reduced expression in early Alzheimer disease and regulates amyloid beta accumulation in mice. J. Clin. Invest. 118, 2190–2199.

Ravikumar, B., Vacher, C., Berger, Z., et al., 2004. Inhibition of mTOR induces autophagy and reduces toxicity of polyglutamine expansions in fly and mouse models of Huntington disease. Nat. Genet. 36, 585–595.

Rubinsztein, D.C., Codogno, P., Levine, B., 2012. Autophagy modulation as a potential therapeutic target for diverse diseases. Nat. Rev. Drug Discov. 11, 709–730. (p. 4, 7, 8, 9, 11).

Seelaar, H., Rohrer, J.D., Pijnenburg, Y.A., et al., 2011. Clinical, genetic and pathological heterogeneity of frontotemporal dementia: a review. J. Neurol. Neurosurg. Psychiatr. 82, 476–486.

Shen, W., Ganetzky, B., 2010. Nibbling away at synaptic development. Autophagy 6, 168–169.

Shibata, M., Lu, T., Furuya, T., et al., 2006. Regulation of intracellular accumulation of mutant Huntingtin by Beclin 1. J. Biol. Chem. 281, 14474–14485.

Spencer, B., Potkar, R., Trejo, M., et al., 2009. Beclin 1 gene transfer activates autophagy and ameliorates the neurodegenerative pathology in alpha-synuclein models of Parkinson's and Lewy body diseases. J. Neurosci. 29, 13578–13588.

Tresse, E., Salomons, F.A., Vesa, J., et al., 2010. VCP/p97 is essential for maturation of ubiquitin-containing autophagosomes and this function is impaired by mutations that cause IBMPFD. Autophagy 6, 217–227.

Vogiatzi, T., Xilouri, M., Vekrellis, K., et al., 2008. Wild type alpha-synuclein is degraded by chaperone-mediated autophagy and macroautophagy in neuronal cells. J. Biol. Chem. 283, 23542–23556.

Wei, Y., Kadia, T., Tong, W., et al., 2010. The combination of a histone deacetylase inhibitor with the BH3-mimetic GX15-070 has synergistic antileukemia activity by activating both apoptosis and autophagy. Autophagy 6, 976–978.

Wirawan, E., Vanden Berghe, T., Lippens, S., et al., 2012. Autophagy: for better or for worse. Cell Res. 22, 43–61.

Yang, Z., Klionsky, D.J., 2009. An overview of the molecular mechanism of autophagy. Curr. Top. Microbiol. Immunol. 335, 1–32.

Yang, Z., Klionsky, D.J., 2010. Mammalian autophagy: core molecular machinery and signaling regulation. Curr. Opin. Cell. Biol. 22, 124–131.

Zhao, Y., Huang, Q., Yang, J., et al., 2010. Autophagy impairment inhibits differentiation of glioma stem/progenitor cells. Brain Res. 1313, 250–258.

Roles of Multiple Types of Autophagy in Neurodegenerative Diseases

Tomohiro Kabuta, Yuuki Fujiwara, and Keiji Wada

Abstract

To date, three forms of autophagy – macroautophagy, microautophagy, and chaperone-mediated autophagy (CMA) – have been identified. Recently, we discovered a novel type of autophagy, "RNautophagy," in which RNA is taken up directly into lysosomes for degradation. Gain of toxic functions of accumulated misfolded proteins or abnormal RNAs in CNS participate to a considerable degree in the pathogenesis of various neurodegenerative diseases. Thus, degradation and clearance of the toxic species by autophagy systems may be important for the maintenance of neurons and prevention of neurodegenerative diseases. We showed that amyotrophic lateral sclerosis (ALS)-linked mutant SOD1 is degraded not only by the proteasome but also by macroautophagy, and that macroautophagy reduces mutant SOD1-mediated toxicity. We found that Parkinson's disease-associated mutant UCH-L1 interacts with LAMP-2A and Hsc70, which are the components of CMA machinery, and inhibits CMA. Because RNAs containing aberrant repeats are thought to cause some of ALS or spinocerebellar ataxia (SCA), RNautophagy may also play significant roles in the pathology of neurodegenerative diseases.

© 2014 Elsevier Inc. All rights reserved.

DEGRADATION OF ALS-LINKED MUTANT SOD1 BY MACROAUTOPHAGY

Amyotrophic lateral sclerosis (ALS) is a progressive neurodegenerative disease caused by selective loss of the upper and lower motor neurons. The prevalence of individuals with ALS is 4–8:100,000 (Traynor *et al.*, 1999). Most cases of ALS are sporadic, but approximately 10% of ALS cases run in families. Dominant missense mutations in the gene that encodes the Cu/Zn superoxide dismutase (SOD1) are responsible for 20% of familial ALS cases. Transgenic mice overexpressing mutant SOD1 exhibit an ALS-like phenotype comparable to ALS, whereas SOD1-deficient mice do not (Gurney *et al.*, 1994; Reaume *et al.*, 1996). From these observations, it is generally thought that SOD1 mutants cause motor neuron degeneration by toxic gain of functions. Thus, studies of the degradation process of mutant SOD1 could provide important insights into understanding the mechanisms that underlie the pathology of familial ALS, and into developing novel therapies for familial ALS by removing toxic species of mutant SOD1.

Cytoplasmic proteins are mainly degraded by two pathways: autophagy, and the ubiquitin–26S proteasome pathway. It has been reported that mutant SOD1 proteins are turned over more rapidly than wild-type (WT) SOD1, and a proteasome inhibitor increases the level of mutant SOD1 proteins (Hoffman *et al.*, 1996; Johnston *et al.*, 2000). Two distinct ubiquitin ligases, Dorfin and NEDL1, have been reported to ubiquitinate mutant but not WT SOD1 (Miyazaki *et al.*, 2004; Niwa *et al.*, 2002). These observations indicate that mutant SOD1 is at least partly degraded by the ubiquitin–26S proteasome pathway. The 20S proteasome, a component of the 26S proteasome, is known to be able to degrade proteins without a requirement for ubiquitination. A recent study has reported that mutant SOD1 is degraded by the 20S proteasome (Di Noto *et al.*, 2005).

Autophagy is an intracellular process in which intracellular components are degraded inside lysosomes, and where the macromolecular constituents are recycled. To date, three forms of autophagy – macroautophagy, microautophagy, and chaperone-mediated autophagy (CMA) – have been identified (Mizushima and Komatsu, 2011). Macroautophagy is the most well studied form of autophagy. Macroautophagy begins with a sequestration step, in which cytoplasmic macromolecules are engulfed by a membrane sac called the isolation membrane. This membrane results in a double-membrane structure known as an autophagosome, which fuses with the lysosome. The inner membrane of the autophagosome and its contents are degraded by lysosomal hydrolases.

Although macroautophagy can be induced by starvation, this pathway takes place constitutively in mammals. Indeed, macroautophagy plays an important role in the maintenance of neurons in mice (Hara *et al.*, 2006; Komatsu *et al.*, 2006). Therefore, we hypothesized that mutant SOD1 is degraded not only by the proteasome but also by macroautophagy.

To confirm whether mutant SOD1 is degraded by the proteasome pathway, we assessed the effect of epxomicin, a selective proteasome inhibitor, on SOD1 protein clearance (Kabuta *et al.*, 2006). We examined protein clearance of human SOD1 in Neuro2a cells transfected with mutant SOD1 in the presence of the translation inhibitor cycloheximide. The degradation of mutant SOD1 was suppressed by epoxomicin treatment, indicating that mutant SOD1 is degraded at least partly by the proteasome.

We then investigated whether mutant SOD1 is degraded by macroautophagy, using 3-methyladenine (3-MA), an inhibitor of macroautophagy. Treatment of Neuro2a cells overexpressing G93A mutant SOD1 with 3-MA promoted the accumulation of mutant SOD1 proteins. In the presence of cycloheximide, the degradation of mutant SOD1 was suppressed by treatment with 3-MA, indicating that the accumulation of SOD1 proteins by 3-MA is not due to increased protein synthesis, and that mutant SOD1 is degraded by macroautophagy in these cells. To test the role of macroautophagy on SOD1 degradation in differentiated neuronal cells or neurons, we also used differentiated Neuro2a cells. In differentiated Neuro2a cells, 3-MA increased mutant SOD1 protein levels in the presence of cycloheximide. For further confirmation of the clearance of SOD1 by macroautophagy, we used Beclin 1 or Atg7 siRNA to inhibit macroautophagy. We observed inhibited degradation of mutant SOD1 in cells with Beclin 1 or Atg7 siRNA compared to cells with control siRNA.

We then assessed the relative contributions of the proteasome and macroautophagy to the clearance of mutant SOD1. The SOD1 level in 3-MA-treated cells was comparable to that of epoxomicin-treated cells. An increased level of mutant SOD1 was detected in cells co-treated with both inhibitors compared to that of 3-MA-treated cells or epoxomicin-treated cells. These data indicate that, in these cells, the contribution of macroautophagy to mutant SOD1 clearance is approximately equal to that of the proteasome pathway.

We examined whether inhibition of the macroautophagy-mediated degradation of mutant SOD1 could induce cell death in Neuro2a cells (Kabuta et al., 2006). In differentiated Neuro2a cells, there was no statistically significant difference in cell viability or cell death among control cells, WT SOD1-expressing cells, and mutant SOD1-expressing cells. In contrast, when cells were treated with 3-MA, mutant SOD1-expressing cells showed significantly increased cell death and significantly decreased cell viability compared to control cells or WT SOD1-expressing cells. When compared with cell death of 3-MA-untreated cells, cell death of 3-MA-treated cells was elevated in mutant SOD1-expressed cells, but not in cells with WT SOD1. These results suggest that macroautophagy reduces mutant SOD1-mediated toxicity in neurons.

Taken together, we showed that, for the first time, mutant SOD1 is degraded by macroautophagy as well as by the proteasome (Kabuta et al., 2006). Consistent with our report, macroautophagy has been reported to be increased in the G93A mutant SOD1-transgenic mice (Morimoto et al., 2007). Our data show that macroautophagy reduces mutant SOD1-mediated toxicity. Thus, macroautophagy inducers may have therapeutic potential for SOD1-linked ALS.

Roles of macroautophagy in sporadic ALS are less clear. It has been reported that transgenic mice with motor neuron-specific knockout of proteasomes, but not of macroautophagy, showed ALS-like phonotypes, and suggested that dysfunction of the proteasome may primarily contribute to the pathogenesis of sporadic ALS rather than that of macroautophagy (Tashiro et al., 2012). However, the cause of sporadic ALS is still unclear and remains to be elucidated.

INTERACTION BETWEEN PARKINSON'S DISEASE-ASSOCIATED UCH-L1 AND CHAPERONE-MEDIATED AUTOPHAGY

Parkinson's disease (PD) is the most common neurodegenerative movement disorder. It is characterized by progressive cell loss confined mostly to dopaminergic neurons in the substantia nigra pars compacta. Although the majority of PD cases occur sporadically, 5–10% of all cases are familial. Several missense mutations, and duplication and triplication of the α-synuclein gene are linked to dominant-inherited PD or parkinsonism, indicating that increases in the levels of α-synuclein could constitute a cause of PD, and that α-synuclein causes neurodegeneration by toxic gain of functions. α-Synuclein is also thought to be involved in the pathogenesis of sporadic PD. Thus, studies of the degradation mechanisms of α-synuclein proteins are important.

A missense mutation in the ubiquitin C-terminal hydrolase L1 (UCH-L1) gene, resulting in an I93M substitution at the protein level, has been reported in a German family with dominantly inherited PD (Leroy et al., 1998). We generated I93M UCH-L1-transgenic mice, and showed that these mice exhibit progressive dopaminergic cell loss (Setsuie et al., 2007). In addition, we showed that, compared with WT UCH-L1, I93M UCH-L1 exhibits increased insolubility and levels of interactions with other cellular proteins – features that are characteristic of several neurodegenerative disease-linked mutants (Kabuta et al., 2008a). These findings indicate that the I93M mutation in UCH-L1 contributes to the pathogenesis of PD.

Oxidative/carbonyl stresses are elevated in PD brains, and are thought to be involved in the pathogenesis of PD. In the brains of sporadic PD patients, UCH-L1 is a major target of carbonyl formation (Choi et al., 2004). We have also reported that I93M UCH-L1 and carbonyl-modified UCH-L1 display shared aberrant properties (Kabuta et al., 2008a), suggesting that carbonyl-modified UCH-L1 may constitute one of the causes of sporadic PD.

Alpha-synuclein has been reported to be degraded by the proteasome, and by macroautophagy and chaperone-mediated autophagy (CMA) (Cuervo et al., 2004; Webb et al., 2003). In CMA, cytosolic substrate proteins containing the KFERQ-like motif are selectively transported into lysosomes via Hsc70 and LAMP-2A and degraded (Cuervo and Dice, 1996; Dice 1990; Dice, 2007). LAMP-2A forms a complex with chaperones such as Hsc70, and functions as a receptor for CMA at the lysosomal membrane. α-Synuclein interacts with LAMP-2A. α-Synuclein contains a CMA recognition motif, VKKDQ, and it has been reported that WT α-synuclein is a CMA substrate (Cuervo et al., 2004). Pathogenic mutant A30P and A53T α-synuclein inhibit CMA by tight binding to LAMP-2A.

Using co-immunoprecipitation assays, we found that UCH-L1 also interacts with both LAMP-2A and Hsc70 (Kabuta et al., 2008b). The levels of LAMP-2A and Hsc70 interacting with I93M UCH-L1 were higher than the levels interacting with WT UCH-L1. We hypothesized that I93M UCH-L1, which exhibits elevated interactions with LAMP-2A and Hsc70, may also inhibit CMA. To examine this possibility, we assessed the effects of I93M UCH-L1 on the protein level of GAPDH, an established substrate of CMA, in the lysosomal fraction and whole-cell lysate. The GAPDH level in whole-cell lysate was elevated in cells expressing I93M UCH-L1 compared with that in cells expressing WT UCH-L1, while the GAPDH level in the lysosomal fraction was decreased in cells expressing I93M UCH-L1, supporting the idea that the aberrant interaction of I93M UCH-L1 with CMA machinery inhibits CMA function. The inhibition of CMA also results in the accumulation of other CMA substrates, including α-synuclein. We found that the amount of WT α-synuclein was increased in cells expressing I93M UCH-L1 compared with cells expressing WT UCH-L1 or control mock cells. These results suggest that the accumulation of α-synuclein in cells expressing I93M UCH-L1 is due to the inhibition of CMA-dependent degradation of α-synuclein. Mutant ΔDQ α-synuclein, in which DQ in the CMA recognition motif is replaced by AA, is not degraded by CMA (Cuervo et al., 2004). To confirm that the accumulation of α-synuclein in cells expressing I93M UCH-L1 is associated with CMA-dependent degradation of α-synuclein, we used mutant ΔDQ α-synuclein, and found that the I93M mutation does not affect the ΔDQ α-synuclein level (Kabuta *et al.*, 2008b). We propose that inhibition of CMA by I93M UCH-L1 is one of the mechanisms underlying toxic gain of functions by UCH-L1.

Whether UCH-L1 is a substrate of CMA or not is currently unknown. UCH-L1 physically interacts with LAMP-2A and Hsc70, but does not contain a typical KFERQ-like motif. According to the rule of the KFERQ-like motif (Dice, 1990), UCH-L1 is not a presumable substrate for CMA. However, MEF2D, which contains no typical KFERQ-like motif, has been reported to be a substrate of CMA (Yang et al., 2009). Multiple imperfect KFERQ-like motifs at the MEF2D N-terminus mediate its interaction with Hsc70 and degradation by CMA (Yang et al., 2009). Because UCH-L1 also contains several imperfect KFERQ-like motifs, it is possible that UCH-L1 is a substrate of CMA.

In the brains of sporadic PD patients, UCH-L1 is a major target of carbonyl formation (Choi *et al.*, 2004). We observed that the interactions of UCH-L1 with LAMP-2A and Hsc70 were also abnormally enhanced by carbonyl modification of UCH-L1 (Kabuta and Wada, 2008). In conclusion, aberrant interactions of UCH-L1 with CMA machinery may underlie the pathogenesis of I93M UCH-L1-associated PD, and possibly of sporadic PD. Carbonyl modification of UCH-L1 could be a therapeutic target for the treatment of sporadic PD.

DEGRADATION OF RNA BY RNAUTOPHAGY: ITS POSSIBLE ROLES IN NEURODEGENERATIVE DISORDERS

Lysosomes contain various enzymes that can degrade proteins, nucleic acids, lipids, and carbohydrates, and regulated degradation of these molecules by lysosomes is essential for biological homeostasis. In addition to various types of autophagy we have recently discovered a novel type of autophagy, which we term "RNautophagy" (Fujiwara *et al.*, 2013). In this pathway, RNA is directly taken up by lysosomes in an ATP-dependent manner and degraded. We found that a lysosomal membrane protein, LAMP-2C, functions as a receptor for this pathway.

To test whether RNA is directly taken up by lysosomes, a cell-free system using isolated lysosomes was employed (Fujiwara *et al.*, 2013). Freshly isolated lysosomes were incubated with purified total RNA, in the presence or absence of ATP. After incubation, lysosomes and the solution outside the lysosomes were separated by centrifugation, and the level of RNA outside the lysosomes was analyzed. The level of RNA outside the lysosomes was reduced only in the presence of ATP. In parallel, to assess the presence of RNA taken up inside the lysosomes, we degraded RNA outside the lysosomes with exogenous RNase A after incubation, and then analyzed the levels of RNase A-resistant RNA. As a result, RNA resistant to RNase A was detected only in lysosomes incubated in the presence of ATP. Immunoelectron microscopy of the lysosomes incubated with or without RNA in the presence of ATP also showed the presence of RNA taken up by lysosomes. These results indicate that RNA is taken up directly by lysosomes in a process that is dependent on ATP. The overall level of RNA incubated with isolated lysosomes was markedly reduced only in the presence of ATP, indicating ATP-dependent degradation of RNA by isolated lysosomes. Taken together, these results revealed a novel autophagic pathway that directly takes up RNA into lysosomes for degradation. We termed this pathway "RNautophagy" (Fujiwara *et al.*, 2013).

LAMP-2C is one of three splice variants of LAMP-2, a major lysosomal membrane protein with one transmembrane region (Eskelinen *et al.*, 2005). The three isoforms of LAMP-2 (LAMP-2A, B, and C) share identical luminal regions, but have different C-terminal cytosolic tails. LAMP-2A is known as a receptor for CMA, but the precise functions of LAMP-2B and C remain unknown. We found that the cytosolic sequence of LAMP-2C directly binds to almost all total RNA (Fujiwara *et al.*, 2013). Considering the relationship between LAMP-2A and CMA, we speculated that LAMP-2C functions as a receptor for RNA in RNautophagy. In CMA, LAMP-2A serves as a receptor through its interaction with substrate proteins on the surface of the lysosomal membrane (Cuervo and Dice, 1996; Dice, 2007). Cells transfected with LAMP-2C showed significant enhancement in the overall levels of RNA degradation, and lysosomes isolated from LAMP-2C-overexpressing cells showed increased levels of RNautophagy. The levels of RNautophagy were decreased significantly in lysosomes isolated from LAMP-2-deficient mice. In addition, a significant accumulation of total RNA was observed in the brains of LAMP-2 knockout mice. Collectively, these results indicate that LAMP-2C functions as a receptor for RNautophagy (Fujiwara *et al.*, 2013).

In CMA, substrate proteins are unfolded by Hsc70, and then directly imported into the lysosomal lumen (Dice, 2007). In contrast, RNautophagy is independent of Hsc70, because Hsc70 had no effect on the uptake of RNA by isolated lysosomes (Fujiwara *et al.*, 2013). Thus, RNautophagy is a distinct pathway from CMA. Yet precise mechanisms underlying RNautophagy still remain elusive. We cannot rule out the possibility of a LAMP-2-independent process in this pathway, because RNautophagy activity was not completely abolished in lysosomes isolated from LAMP-2-deficient mice (Fujiwara *et al.*, 2013).

RNautophagy likely contributes to the metabolism and homeostasis of RNA in cells and tissues, especially in those expressing LAMP-2C at high levels. Interestingly, the expression level of LAMP-2C is particularly high in brain. The expression level of LAMP-2C is high in neurons compared with that of glial cells (Fujiwara *et al.*, 2013). RNautophagy may play an important role in the maintenance and quality control of neurons. Recently, aberrant expression, function, and accumulation of RNA have been considered as key factors in the pathogenesis of some neurodegenerative disorders. A number of studies have revealed that aberrant expansions of nucleotide repeats in the introns are the cause of various neurodegenerative disorders, and strongly suggest that RNAs containing aberrant expansions of repeats exert toxicity in these diseases. In both familial and sporadic ALS, expansion of the GGGGCC repeat in the intron 1 of the *C9ORF72* gene has been reported (DeJesus-Hernandez *et al.*, 2011; Renton *et al.*, 2011). Expansions of intronic nucleotide repeats have also been reported in spinocerebellar ataxia (SCA), such as SCA10, 31, and 36 (Kobayashi *et al.*, 2011; Wojciechowska and Krzyzosiak, 2011). RNautophagy is possibly involved in degradation of such RNAs containing aberrant expansions of repeats. It is also possible that dysfunction of RNautophagy is related to the onset and progression of sporadic cases of neurodegenerative diseases. Induction and upregulation of RNautophagy may have therapeutic potential for diseases caused by aberrant RNAs.

References

Choi, J., Levey, A.I., Weintraub, S.T., et al., 2004. Oxidative modifications and down-regulation of ubiquitin carboxyl-terminal hydrolase L1 associated with idiopathic Parkinson's and Alzheimer's diseases. J. Biol. Chem. 279, 13256–13264.

Cuervo, A.M., Dice, J.F., 1996. A receptor for the selective uptake and degradation of proteins by lysosomes. Science 273, 501–503.

Cuervo, A.M., Stefanis, L., Fredenburg, R., et al., 2004. Impaired degradation of mutant alpha-synuclein by chaperone-mediated autophagy. Science 305, 1292–1295.

DeJesus-Hernandez, M., Mackenzie, I.R., Boeve, B.F., et al., 2011. Expanded GGGGCC hexanucleotide repeat in noncoding region of C9ORF72 causes chromosome 9p-linked FTD and ALS. Neuron 72, 245–256.

Dice, J.F., 1990. Peptide sequences that target cytosolic proteins for lysosomal proteolysis. Trends Biochem. Sci. 15, 305–309.

Dice, J.F., 2007. Chaperone-mediated autophagy. Autophagy 3, 295–299.

Di Noto, L., Whitson, L.J., Cao, X., et al., 2005. Proteasomal degradation of mutant superoxide dismutases linked to amyotrophic lateral sclerosis. J. Biol. Chem. 280, 39907–39913.

Eskelinen, E.L., Cuervo, A.M., Taylor, M.R., et al., 2005. Unifying nomenclature for the isoforms of the lysosomal membrane protein LAMP-2. Traffic 6, 1058–1061.

Fujiwara, Y., Furuta, A., Kikuchi, H., et al., 2013. Discovery of a novel type of autophagy targeting RNA. Autophagy 9, 403–409. <http://dx.doi.org/10.4161/auto.23002>.

Gurney, M.E., Pu, H., Chiu, A.Y., et al., 1994. Motor neuron degeneration in mice that express a human Cu,Zn superoxide dismutase mutation. Science 264, 1772–1775.

Hara, T., Nakamura, K., Matsui, M., et al., 2006. Suppression of basal autophagy in neural cells causes neurodegenerative disease in mice. Nature 441, 885–889.

Hoffman, E.K., Wilcox, H.M., Scott, R.W., et al., 1996. Proteasome inhibition enhances the stability of mouse Cu/Zn superoxide dismutase with mutations linked to familial amyotrophic lateral sclerosis. J. Neurol. Sci. 139, 15–20.

Johnston, J.A., Dalton, M.J., Gurney, M.E., 2000. Formation of high molecular weight complexes of mutant Cu, Zn-superoxide dismutase in a mouse model for familial amyotrophic lateral sclerosis. Proc. Natl. Acad. Sci. U.S.A. 97, 12571–12576.

Kabuta, T., Wada, K., 2008. Insights into links between familial and sporadic Parkinson's disease: physical relationship between UCH-L1 variants and chaperone-mediated autophagy. Autophagy 4, 827–829.

Kabuta, T., Suzuki, Y., Wada, K., 2006. Degradation of amyotrophic lateral sclerosis-linked mutant Cu,Zn-superoxide dismutase proteins by macroautophagy and the proteasome. J. Biol. Chem. 281, 30524–30533.

Kabuta, T., Setsuie, R., Mitsui, T., et al., 2008a. Aberrant molecular properties shared by familial Parkinson's disease-associated mutant UCH-L1 and carbonyl-modified UCH-L1. Hum. Mol. Genet. 17, 1482–1496.

Kabuta, T., Furuta, A., Aoki, S., et al., 2008b. Aberrant interaction between Parkinson's disease-associated mutant UCH-L1 and the lysosomal receptor for chaperone-mediated autophagy. J. Biol. Chem. 283, 23731–23738.

Kobayashi, H., Abe, K., Matsuura, T., et al., 2011. Expansion of intronic GGCCTG hexanucleotide repeat in NOP56 causes SCA36, a type of spinocerebellar ataxia accompanied by motor neuron involvement. Am. J. Hum. Genet. 89, 121–130.

Komatsu, M., Waguri, S., Chiba, T., et al., 2006. Loss of autophagy in the central nervous system causes neurodegeneration in mice. Nature 441, 880–884.

Leroy, E., Boyer, R., Auburger, G., et al., 1998. The ubiquitin pathway in Parkinson's disease. Nature 395, 451–452.

Miyazaki, K., Fujita, T., Ozaki, T., et al., 2004. NEDL1, a novel ubiquitin-protein isopeptide ligase for dishevelled-1, targets mutant superoxide dismutase-1. J. Biol. Chem. 279, 11327–11335.

Mizushima, N., Komatsu, M., 2011. Autophagy: renovation of cells and tissues. Cell 147, 728–741.

Morimoto, N., Nagai, M., Ohta, Y., et al., 2007. Increased autophagy in transgenic mice with a G93A mutant SOD1 gene. Brain Res. 1167, 112–117.

Niwa, J., Ishigaki, S., Hishikawa, N., et al., 2002. Dorfin ubiquitylates mutant SOD1 and prevents mutant SOD1-mediated neurotoxicity. J. Biol. Chem. 277, 36793–36798.

Reaume, A.G., Elliott, J.L., Hoffman, E.K., et al., 1996. Motor neurons in Cu/Zn superoxide dismutase-deficient mice develop normally but exhibit enhanced cell death after axonal injury. Nat. Genet. 13, 43–47.

Renton, A.E., Majounie, E., Waite, A., et al., 2011. A hexanucleotide repeat expansion in C9ORF72 is the cause of chromosome 9p21-linked ALS-FTD. Neuron 72, 257–268.

Setsuie, R., Wang, Y.L., Mochizuki, H., et al., 2007. Dopaminergic neuronal loss in transgenic mice expressing the Parkinson's disease-associated UCH-L1 I93M mutant. Neurochem. Int. 50, 119–129.

Tashiro, Y., Urushitani, M., Inoue, H., et al., 2012. Motor neuron-specific disruption of proteasomes, but not autophagy, replicates amyotrophic lateral sclerosis. J. Biol. Chem. 287, 42984–42994.

Traynor, B.J., Codd, M.B., Corr, B., et al., 1999. Incidence and prevalence of ALS in Ireland, 1995-1997: a population-based study. Neurology 52, 504–509.

Webb, J.L., Ravikumar, B., Atkins, J., et al., 2003. Alpha-Synuclein is degraded by both autophagy and the proteasome. J. Biol. Chem. 278, 25009–25013.

Wojciechowska, M., Krzyzosiak, W.J., 2011. Cellular toxicity of expanded RNA repeats: focus on RNA foci. Hum. Mol. Genet. 20, 3811–3821.

Yang, Q., She, H., Gearing, M., et al., 2009. Regulation of neuronal survival factor MEF2D by chaperone-mediated autophagy. Science 323, 124–127.

Autophagy and Crohn's Disease: Towards New Therapeutic Connections

Kris Nys, Séverine Vermeire, and Patrizia Agostinis

Abstract

In recent years strong progress has been made in understanding the molecular basis of Crohn's disease, a multifactorial chronic inflammatory disease of the gastrointestinal tract. Recent data suggest that if autophagy, the major lysosomal pathway for recycling of cytoplasmic material, is inhibited, this may significantly contribute to an increased susceptibility for Crohn's disease. Consequently, intense investigations have started to evaluate the potential value of autophagy as a druggable therapeutic target, and as a very necessary diagnostic tool. Interestingly, as well as the promising introduction of direct autophagic modulators, several other drugs already used clinically in the treatment of Crohn's disease may exert at least part of their effect through the regulation of autophagy. However, whether this phenomenon contributes to or counteracts their therapeutic use remains to be determined, and it may prove to be highly compound-specific. Here we review the complex and emerging role of autophagy modulation in the battle against Crohn's disease. Moreover, we discuss the potential benefits and deleterious effects of autophagic regulation by both new and clinically employed drugs.

M.A. Hayat (ed): Autophagy, Volume 1
DOI: http://dx.doi.org/10.1016/B978-0-12-405530-8.00005-4

© 2014 Elsevier Inc. All rights reserved.

INTRODUCTION: CROHN'S DISEASE AND FAULTY AUTOPHAGY GO HAND IN HAND

Crohn's disease (CD) is a multifactorial chronic inflammatory disease of the gastrointestinal tract (inflammatory bowel disease or IBD) for which the exact causative mechanism is still unknown. Moreover, current treatment options (conventionally consisting of corticosteroids, immunosuppressive compounds (e.g., thiopurines or anti-TNF-α therapy), and antibiotics in case of septic complications) are far from successful in all patients, showing a slow therapeutic onset and significant side effects, requiring surgery as the unfavorable last resort. Consequently, there is an urgent and constant need for new and more efficient diagnostic and therapeutic strategies.

Defects in microbial sensing have been indicated as a key pathogenic mechanism (Fritz et al., 2011), and in recent years strong progress has been made in understanding the genetic basis, using genome-wide association studies (Fritz et al., 2011). Interestingly, as well as genes important for innate immunity (e.g., CARD15), these genetic studies have identified several important unfolded protein response (UPR; e.g., XBP1, ORMDL3) and autophagy (e.g., Atg16L1, IRGM)-related genes to be primarily associated with Crohn's disease (Fritz et al., 2011). Additionally, a cohort study (Nys, Hoefkens et al., unpublished data) could confirm the genetic association of CD with genes of these pathways. From these premises, it can be assumed that maintenance of cellular homeostasis and immune response (i.e., through correct autophagy induction) is essential for safeguarding normal cellular functions. As a consequence, we hypothesize that events causing imbalances in normal autophagy are important drivers of human inflammatory diseases such as CD.

In this chapter we discuss the emerging role of autophagy as a regulator of immune/inflammatory responses and as a stress-responsive mechanism, and we analyze its value as a diagnostic and/or therapeutic target. Moreover, we highlight how several drugs used in the treatment of Crohn's disease have already been shown to affect autophagic induction as part of their method of action or as a side effect, and how these drug-specific effects may be manipulated to our advantage.

AUTOPHAGY: A HOT NOVEL TARGET OR AN OLD FRIEND?

Autophagy Regulates Immunity

Autophagy is generally known to act as a supplier of nutrients (e.g., lipids, amino acids, …) in order to preserve energy metabolism during stressful times of starvation and/or growth factor deprivation, and as an important quality control mechanism in order to maintain cellular integrity and homeostasis. Interestingly, recently its role has been expanded to include unique immunological functions, thereby interacting with many essential steps in the innate and adaptive immune responses (as discussed below and illustrated in Figure 5.1).

Direct recognition and consecutive elimination of invading intracellular pathogens is considered to be the principal manifestation of autophagy's role in innate immunity. This process is governed by specific autophagic adaptors or sequestosome 1/p62-like receptors (SLRs; Deretic, 2012), which have been shown to interact with LC3 (an important autophagic

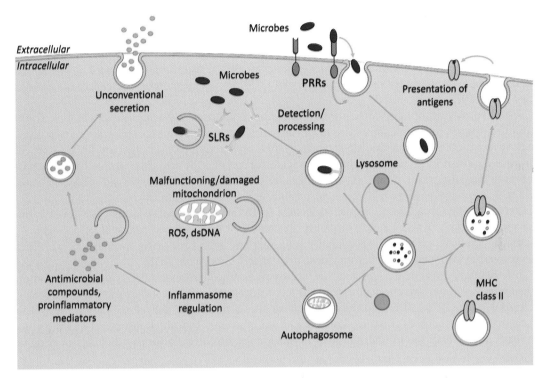

FIGURE 5.1 **Immunological regulation by autophagy.** Autophagy regulates several key steps of the immune response. First of all, in the innate immune response autophagy aids in direct microbial pattern detection and processing. Upon recognition by membrane-bound pattern recognition receptors (PRRs) and intracellular seques-tome1/p62-like receptors (SLRs), microbes will be degraded through autophagy. Moreover, autophagy-mediated removal of malfunctioning/damaged mitochondria suppresses inflammasome activation, since these organelles tend to release reactive oxygen species (ROS) and double-stranded (ds) DNA, which would otherwise stimulate inflammasome activation and the subsequent production of inflammatory initiators. Additionally, autophagy may also aid in the unconventional secretion of cytoplasmic components like antimicrobial compounds and/or pro-inflammatory mediators. The autophagosomal content (microbes, cytoplasmic components) will be degraded after fusion with lysosomes. The generated peptides may be subsequently presented by MHC class II heterodimers at the cell membrane, leading to regulation/activation of adaptive immune responses. See text for further details.

protein) on one side and cargo tags (such as ubiquitin) on the other. Depending on the tar-geted intracellular pathogen, different SLRs will be recruited – for example, removal of Sindbis virus, *Mycobacteria*, *Shigella*, and *Listeria* is mediated through SLRs p62 and/or nuclear domain 10 protein/Ag nuclear dot 52 kDa protein (NDP52), whereas *Salmonella* requires addi-tional factors such as intracellular galectin 3/8. Alternatively, SLRs also gather cytoplasmic cargo which is converted into antimicrobial compounds and delivered to infected cytoplasmic vesicles (Deretic, 2012).

Next, in the regulation of innate immunity autophagy has been shown to interact with pat-tern recognition receptors (PRRs) such as Toll-like receptors (TLRs), Nod-like receptors (NLRs), and RIG-I-like receptors (RLRs). Engagement of these receptors could induce autophagy in several cell types, including macrophages, DCs, and neutrophils (Deretic, 2012). On the one hand autophagy is induced as an effector mechanism downstream of PRRs when exposed to pathogen-associated molecular patterns (PAMPs); for example, Nod1/2 are known to interact and recruit Atg16L1 (Deretic, 2012), which is of particular importance for Crohn's disease since NOD2 and Atg16L1 are known risk loci (Fritz *et al.*, 2011). Alternatively, autophagy may also guide the activation of PRRs via the delivery of PAMPs to the lumen of intracellular organelles (Lee *et al.*, 2007).

Another way autophagy affects innate immune responses is through interaction with the inflammasomes. Inflammasomes are important inflammatory activation complexes that, upon exposure to, for example, double-stranded DNA or reactive oxygen species (ROS), activate caspase-1, which in its turn converts cytokines (e.g. pro-IL-1β) into their active form, thereby representing important initiators/sustainers of the inflammatory responses (Strowig *et al.*, 2012). Autophagy is known to play an inhibiting role in inflammasome activation, as illustrated by the fact that loss of Atg16L1 elevates IL-1β levels in a mouse model for Crohn's disease (Saitoh *et al.*, 2008). This is probably the result of the constant removal of endogenous damage signals (such as damaged/malfunctioning and ROS producing mitochondria), which decreases the basal level of inflammasome activation (Zhou *et al.*, 2011).

Interestingly, autophagy has also been shown, as first demonstrated in yeast, to promote the unconventional secretion of cytoplasmic components such as inflammatory modulators (Dupont *et al.*, 2011). Thus, autophagy aids in the extracellular delivery of inflammasome-activated factors such as IL-1β. It should be noted, however, that the latter effect quickly fades in time, after which the inhibiting effect of autophagy on the inflammasome takes over again (Shi *et al.*, 2012).

Finally, several reports indicate that autophagy has an important function in the adaptive immune system as well. Apart from capturing and sequestering invading pathogens, endogenous and microbial antigens are shuttled for MHCII-based presentation by autophagy, thereby playing a major role in antigen presentation for both pathogenic recognition and tolerance versus auto/commensal antigens. Next to its contribution to normal T lymphocyte homeostasis (McLeod *et al.*, 2012), autophagy has been shown to shape the T cell repertoire/tolerance (Nedjic *et al.*, 2008) by controlling their survival in the thymus. Moreover, proper functioning of antigen-presenting dendritic cells has been suggested to be at least partially autophagy dependent. Aberrant autophagic machinery in dendritic cells (DCs), key players in the regulation of the adaptive immunity, led to disregulated processing of antigens and increased DC maturation, inducing proinflammatory DCs (Strisciuglio *et al.*, 2012). Furthermore, autophagy deficiency could destabilize the immunologic synapse between DCs and T cells, potentially leading to increased T cell activation (Wildenberg *et al.*, 2012).

In organs such as the intestine, inflammatory mechanisms should direct the immune response to either a tolerogenic phenotype when responding to commensals or an immunogenic phenotype against potential pathogens. Aberrations in these mechanisms (e.g., exaggerated inflammatory responses and/or faulty autophagy) may inappropriately increase the immunogenic response against commensal bacteria. Consequently, the increased inflammatory status of the intestine leads to destabilization of the intestinal epithelial barrier, increased DC antigen exposure and activation, alteration of the intestinal microbial population, chronic self-amplification of both innate and adaptive immune responses, and manifestation of Crohn's disease.

Finally, given the importance of autophagy in regulating immune/inflammatory responses (i.e., immune "quality control"), modulation of this signaling pathway (for example, through the use of known inhibitors/stimulators) may be an appealing approach to restore and normalize the imbalanced inflammatory responses in CD patients. Interestingly, recent studies indicate that several drugs currently used in the treatment of IBD/CD appear to already (in) directly affect autophagy as part of their *modus operandi*, or may particularly benefit from combined autophagy manipulation.

Anti-TNF-α

Targeting TNF-α in order to block inflammation is a common strategy used in the treatment of Crohn's disease. Interestingly, autophagy has been identified as one of the TNF-α-activated pathways. For example, TNF-α was shown to stimulate autophagy in the synovial fibroblasts from patients with rheumatoid arthritis (Connor *et al.*, 2012) and atherosclerotic vascular smooth cells (Jia *et al.*, 2006). Concomitantly, anti-TNF-α therapeutics such as infliximab, adalimumab, certolizumab pegol, and etanercept, have been shown to induce the reactivation of tuberculosis – a process that has been suggested to, at least partially, depend on suppression of the autophagic machinery (Harris and Keane, 2010). Autophagy is known to protect epithelial cells against *M. tuberculosis* by performing an antibacterial and anti-inflammatory role (Castillo *et al.*, 2012). Furthermore, autophagy-deficient intestinal epithelial cells were shown to lose their adhesive capacity in the presence of TNF-α (Saito *et al.*, 2012), again illustrating the link between autophagy regulation and TNF-α signaling.

Although so far no studies have been performed linking anti-TNF-α agents to inhibition of autophagy in the context of Crohn's disease, the above-mentioned studies indicate that suppression of autophagy could be considered as a side effect of anti-TNF-α therapy. Hence, it would be interesting to investigate whether anti-TNF-α therapy could benefit from combined autophagy stimulation (e.g., rapamycin). This combinatorial treatment may upregulate the autophagy pathway, shown to be important for effectiveness of anti-TNF-α therapy (Wildenberg *et al.*, unpublished data).

Thiopurines

Thiopurines (e.g., azathioprine, 6-mercaptopurine) are useful in treatment of inflammatory diseases due to their immunosuppressive effect. However, their mode of action is still far from being understood. Interestingly, autophagy has been identified as a downstream activated pathway after thiopurine treatment (Guijarro *et al.*, 2012).

On the one hand, this may indicate that autophagy acts as one of the effector mechanisms by which thiopurines induce their immunosuppressive effect, because autophagy activation has been shown (as explained above) to downregulate inflammatory signaling and balance immune activation. On the other hand, autophagy may also be activated in response to the reported adverse hepatotoxic effects induced by thiopurine therapy (Petit *et al.*, 2008). As well as its emerging role in immunity, autophagy is a vital mechanism that maintains cellular function under normal homeostasis, but also provides the means for a cell to adapt to and survive stressful conditions (e.g., oxidative stress, hypoxia, nutrient deprivation; Kroemer *et al.*, 2010). For example, in cancer research autophagy has been suggested to aid malignant cells in adapting to the harsh tumor environment (White, 2012). Moreover, autophagy stimulation following acute stress as induced by anticancer treatments has been suggested to render cancer cells more resistant to chemotherapy (White, 2012), illustrating the stress-mitigation capacity of this catabolic pathway.

In conclusion, regardless of whether autophagy is upregulated as a direct downstream effector pathway of thiopurines or is induced as a supportive mechanism in an attempt to cope with the hepatotoxic side effects of these drugs, autophagy seems to have a protective effect in hepatocytes during thiopurine treatment (Guijarro et al., 2012). These observations should stimulate investigations not only to determine the precise link between thiopurine treatment and the induction of autophagy, but also to define whether Crohn's patients may potentially benefit from a combinatorial treatment of thiopurines and autophagy modulators.

Curcumin

As mentioned, clinical efficacy of the existing therapies in the treatment of Crohn's disease is limited because of loss of response/remission and severe side effects. Next to conventional medicine, there is a growing interest in complementary and alternative medicine (CAM) (Hilsden et al., 2011). In accordance with this, several beneficial results have been described for curcumin, a yellow pigment commonly used in food (Ali et al., 2012). This CAM's pharmacological effects include antioxidant, anti-inflammatory, hepatoprotective, antibacterial, and antitumor abilities (Aggarwal and Harikumar, 2009). As a result, this compound is now being used modestly to treat patients suffering from chronic diseases such as CD (Hilsden et al., 2011).

Although the functional mechanism(s) responsible for the curcumin-induced effects in patients suffering from CD remain unclear, a recent study identified autophagy as a curcumin-activated pathway. Han and colleagues showed that curcumin could protect endothelial cells against oxidative stress through autophagy induction (Han et al., 2012). Moreover, curcumin has recently been demonstrated to increase protein aggregate degradation in a likely autophagy-dependent manner (Alavez et al., 2011). In conclusion, these data suggest that at least part of the beneficial pharmacological effects of curcumin can be attributed to upregulation of the autophagic process, reinforcing the case that autophagy induction is an old friend in therapy against CD and has been a functional treatment strategy without us knowing it.

Direct Autophagy Modulators

As well as the discovery of the autophagy modulating effect demonstrated by several drugs mentioned above, direct autophagy promoters/inhibitors could have significant value in the treatment of CD. Several autophagy modulating compounds are already in use or hold potential as treatment modalities for a variety of human diseases – for example, the autophagy inhibitor (hydro)chloroquine for prevention and/or treatment of malaria (Totino et al., 2008) or cancer (Solomon and Lee, 2009), and the autophagy inducer rapamycin as maintenance therapy to prevent rejection following organ transplantation (Ferrer et al., 2011).

Although older studies tested hydrochloroquine in the prevention of recurring Crohn's disease after curative surgery (Louis and Belaiche, 1995), knowledge of the role of autophagy as an important immune regulator and as a stress-responsive mechanism activated by several CD therapies suggests its inhibition should not be pursued. Conversely, autophagy stimulators like rapamycin may signify an exciting new strategy to treat CD, as illustrated by a case study where sirolimus (rapamycin) markedly improved disease symptoms in a patient with severe refractory CD (Massey *et al.*, 2008). Moreover, rapamycin may also hold potential as a combination treatment with, for example, anti-TNF-α therapy or thiopurines. However, questions remain regarding the extent to which genetic variations in the autophagic machinery may interfere with the therapeutic effect of autophagy promoters. Therefore, the development of innovative diagnostic tools is important in order to predict and track therapeutic efficacy.

DIAGNOSTIC VALUE OF THE AUTOPHAGIC STATUS

In the continuous search for more efficient and effective treatments, the importance of inter-individual differences (e.g., environmental, genetic) in therapeutic outcome is becoming increasingly clear. This is illustrated by, for example, the variation in efficacy and side effects of commonly used drugs in treatment of Crohn's disease (Vermeire, 2012). Interestingly, as the volume of known susceptibility genes is increasing tremendously, new insights are being generated regarding the array of disease phenotypes that are collectively being labeled as Crohn's disease, and potential target pathways and molecules are subsequently being investigated.

So far, genotyping for thiopurine S-methyltransferase (TPMT) is the only test currently being used in clinical practice. Genetic variations of this enzyme predict the degree of hematological/hepatological toxicity after thiopurine treatment, and are therefore indicative for/against the use of either azathioprine or 6-mercaptopurine (Dubinsky *et al.*, 2005). However, several other pathways, such as the inflammatory IL-23 pathway, the NOD2-related pattern recognition machinery, and certainly also the autophagic machinery, are under intense investigation and may be shown to be highly relevant in the future. Interestingly, the specific genotype of TPMT has already been linked with more/less efficient autophagy-dependent degradation of this enzyme, thereby potentially influencing thiopurine drug metabolism (Li *et al.*, 2008).

Theoretically, the presence/absence of certain risk-carrying SNPs – for example, in the autophagy pathway (Atg16L1, IRGM, ULK1) – may be indicative for/against the use of specific drugs as treatment for CD. Moreover, as well as genetic analysis for polymorphisms, differences in protein markers and activation of specific cellular stress responses like autophagy may also be shown to have significant diagnostic value. In this way, biomarkers for disease progression, or even a predictive patient-specific therapy, may be designed. For example, a patient harboring a genetic mutation that blocks the autophagy machinery may specifically not benefit from autophagy inducers, since these compounds try to stimulate exactly that faulty machinery. This type of screening (both genetic and functional) could not only allow us to predict the individual capacity to metabolize therapeutic agents, but also ideally lead to a highly optimized personal treatment regime to treat Crohn's disease as effectively as possible, maximizing the treatment response while avoiding unwanted side effects (Cuffari, 2010).

CONCLUDING REMARKS

Although many of the precise signaling modalities linking malfunctioning autophagy to the incidence of Crohn's disease are far from unraveled, and further investigations are required, autophagy may be shown to be a promising target for treatment of this inflammatory bowel disease. First, targeting this cellular process should directly affect inflammatory signaling. In this regard, stimulation of autophagy may be an attractive approach to suppress immune/inflammatory responses because, compared to targeting a major upstream inflammatory initiator like TNF-α, modulation of autophagy may be a more gentle method to control, correct, or normalize imbalanced immune/inflammatory responses instead of drastically suppressing them. For example, the immune-suppressing and autophagy-inducing effect of curcumin could be amplified by combined treatment with an autophagy stimulator like rapamycin, potentially lowering the effective drug dosage and thereby increasing treatment efficacy. Moreover, since autophagy suppression is likely to be just one of the many anti-TNF-α-induced effects, anti-TNF-α antibodies might also benefit from rapamycin treatment.

Secondly, one can also try to modulate autophagy because of its importance as an adaptation mechanism against stress harboring the potential to increase cellular survival. This capacity of autophagy is well illustrated in cancer-related research, as advanced stages of several cancers have been reported to (at least partially) depend on autophagy for surviving hostile tumor environments and cytotoxic chemotherapeutic treatments (White, 2012). Whereas this calls for inhibitory strategies in cancer treatment, in the context of Crohn's disease the induction of autophagy may be considered as a supportive therapy. For example, autophagy inducers may be used to reduce and/or overcome the adverse hepatotoxic side effects of thiopurines, thereby avoiding the necessity for a treatment break. In conclusion, in the battle against Crohn's disease, stimulation of autophagy is a promising therapeutic option, both as a new ally and as a recently unraveled old strategy.

References

Aggarwal, B.B., Harikumar, K.B., 2009. Potential therapeutic effects of curcumin, the anti-inflammatory agent, against neurodegenerative, cardiovascular, pulmonary, metabolic, autoimmune and neoplastic diseases. Int. J. Biochem. Cell Biol. 41, 40–59.

Alavez, S., Vantipalli, M.C., Zucker, D.J., et al., 2011. Amyloid-binding compounds maintain protein homeostasis during ageing and extend lifespan. Nature 472, 226–229.

Ali, T., Shakir, F., Morton, J., 2012. Curcumin and inflammatory bowel disease: biological mechanisms and clinical implication. Digestion 85, 249–255.

Castillo, E.F., Dekonenko, A., Arko-Mensah, J., et al., 2012. Autophagy protects against active tuberculosis by suppressing bacterial burden and inflammation. Proc. Natl. Acad. Sci. U.S.A. 109, E3168–E3176.

Connor, A.M., Mahomed, N., Gandhi, R., et al., 2012. TNFα modulates protein degradation pathways in rheumatoid arthritis synovial fibroblasts. Arthritis Res. Ther. 14, R62.

Cuffari, C., 2010. The genetics of inflammatory bowel disease: diagnostic and therapeutic implications. World J. Pediatr. 6, 203–209.

Deretic, V., 2012. Autophagy as an innate immunity paradigm: expanding the scope and repertoire of pattern recognition receptors. Curr. Opin. Immunol. 24, 21–31.

Dubinsky, M.C., Reyes, E., Ofman, J., et al., 2005. A cost-effectiveness analysis of alternative disease management strategies in patients with Crohn's disease treated with azathioprine or 6-mercaptopurine. Am. J. Gastroenterol. 100, 2239–2247.

Dupont, N., Jiang, S., Pilli, M., et al., 2011. Autophagy-based unconventional secretory pathway for extracellular delivery of IL-1β. EMBO J. 30, 4701–4711.

Ferrer, I.R., Araki, K., Ford, M.L., 2011. Paradoxical aspects of rapamycin immunobiology in transplantation. Am. J. Transplant. 11, 654–659.

Fritz, T., Niederreiter, L., Adolph, T., et al., 2011. Crohn's disease: NOD2, autophagy and ER stress converge. Gut 60, 1580–1588.

Guijarro, L.G., Roman, I.D., Fernandez-Moreno, D., et al., 2012. Is the autophagy induced by thiopurines beneficial or deleterious? Curr. Drug Metab. 13, 1267–1276.

Han, J., Pan, X.Y., Xu, Y., et al., 2012. Curcumin induces autophagy to protect vascular endothelial cell survival from oxidative stress damage. Autophagy 8, 812–825.

Harris, J., Keane, J., 2010. How tumour necrosis factor blockers interfere with tuberculosis immunity. Clin. Exp. Immunol. 161, 1–9.

Hilsden, R.J., Verhoef, M.J., Rasmussen, H., et al., 2011. Use of complementary and alternative medicine by patients with inflammatory bowel disease. Inflamm. Bowel. Dis. 17, 655–662.

Jia, G., Cheng, G., Gangahar, D.M., et al., 2006. Insulin-like growth factor-1 and TNF-α regulate autophagy through c-jun N-terminal kinase and Akt pathways in human atherosclerotic vascular smooth cells. Immunol. Cell Biol. 84, 448–454.

Kroemer, G., Marino, G., Levine, B., 2010. Autophagy and the integrated stress response. Mol. Cell 40, 280–293.

Lee, H.K., Lund, J.M., Ramanathan, B., et al., 2007. Autophagy-dependent viral recognition by plasmacytoid dendritic cells. Science 315, 1398–1401.

Li, F., Wang, L., Burgess, R.J., et al., 2008. Thiopurine S-methyltransferase pharmacogenetics: autophagy as a mechanism for variant allozyme degradation. Pharmacogenet. Genomics 18, 1083–1094.

Louis, E., Belaiche, J., 1995. Hydroxychloroquine (Plaquenil) for recurrence prevention of Crohn's disease after curative surgery. Gastroenterol. Clin. Biol. 19, 233–234.

Massey, D.C., Bredin, F., Parkes, M., 2008. Use of sirolimus (rapamycin) to treat refractory Crohn's disease. Gut 57, 1294–1296.

McLeod, I.X., Jia, W., He, Y.W., 2012. The contribution of autophagy to lymphocyte survival and homeostasis. Immunol. Rev. 249, 195–204.

Nedjic, J., Aichinger, M., Emmerich, J., et al., 2008. Autophagy in thymic epithelium shapes the T-cell repertoire and is essential for tolerance. Nature 455, 396–400.

Petit, E., Langouet, S., Akhdar, H., et al., 2008. Differential toxic effects of azathioprine, 6-mercaptopurine and 6-thioguanine on human hepatocytes. Toxicol. In Vitro 22, 632–642.

Saito, M., Katsuno, T., Nakagawa, T., et al., 2012. Intestinal epithelial cells with impaired autophagy lose their adhesive capacity in the presence of TNF-α. Dig. Dis. Sci. 57, 2022–2030.

Saitoh, T., Fujita, N., Jang, M.H., et al., 2008. Loss of the autophagy protein Atg16L1 enhances endotoxin-induced IL-1β production. Nature 456, 264–268.

Shi, C.S., Shenderov, K., Huang, N.N., et al., 2012. Activation of autophagy by inflammatory signals limits IL-1β production by targeting ubiquitinated inflammasomes for destruction. Nat. Immunol. 13, 255–263.

Solomon, V.R., Lee, H., 2009. Chloroquine and its analogs: a new promise of an old drug for effective and safe cancer therapies. Eur. J. Pharmacol. 625, 220–233.

Strisciuglio, C., Duijvestein M., Verhaar A.P., et al., 2012. Impaired autophagy leads to abnormal dendritic cell-epithelial cell interactions. J. Crohns. Colitis. September 13, doi: 10.1016/j.crohns.2012.08.009 (epub ahead of print).

Strowig, T., Henao-Mejia, J., Elinav, E., et al., 2012. Inflammasomes in health and disease. Nature 481, 278–286.

Totino, P.R., Daniel-Ribeiro, C.T., Corte-Real, S., et al., 2008. Plasmodium falciparum: erythrocytic stages die by autophagic-like cell death under drug pressure. Exp. Parasitol. 118, 478–486.

Vermeire, S., 2012. Towards a novel molecular classification of IBD. Dig. Dis. 30, 425–427.

White, E., 2012. Deconvoluting the context-dependent role for autophagy in cancer. Nat. Rev. Cancer 12, 401–410.

Wildenberg, M.E., Vos, A.C., Wolfkamp, S.C., et al., 2012. Autophagy attenuates the adaptive immune response by destabilizing the immunologic synapse. Gastroenterology 142, 1493–1503.

Zhou, R., Yazdi, A.S., Menu, P., et al., 2011. A role for mitochondria in NLRP3 inflammasome activation. Nature 469, 221–225.

The Role of Autophagy in Atherosclerosis

Cédéric F. Michiels, Dorien M. Schrijvers,
Guido R.Y. De Meyer, and Wim Martinet

OUTLINE

Abstract

Atherosclerosis is a chronic inflammatory disease of large and middle-sized blood vessels, and the leading cause of death among adults in the Western world. Recent evidence suggests that several molecular and cellular mechanisms play an important role in atherosclerosis and plaque progression. One of these mechanisms includes autophagy, a subcellular process for elimination of damaged organelles and protein aggregates via lysosomes. According to *in vitro* observations, the autophagic machinery is stimulated by several stress-related stimuli inside plaques, such as oxidized lipids, endoplasmic reticulum stress, hypoxia, nutrient deprivation, and inflammation. Although its role in atherosclerosis has not yet been fully established, a growing body of evidence indicates that autophagy has a protective function in atherosclerosis. It stimulates cholesterol efflux and reduces foam cell formation. Moreover, it prevents apoptosis by removing oxidatively

© 2014 Elsevier Inc. All rights reserved.

damaged hyperpolarized mitochondria before reactive oxygen species production and cytochrome c release. Another important recent finding is that macrophage autophagy plays an essential role in delaying lesion progression by suppressing inflammasome activation. Interestingly, excessive everolimus-induced autophagy leads to selective macrophage death, and is a promising plaque-stabilizing strategy. Overall, autophagy seems to be a major player in atherosclerosis, but further research has to be performed to fully clarify its role in this disease.

INTRODUCTION

Atherosclerosis is one of the main underlying causes of death in the Western world. It occurs as a chronic inflammatory disease of the vascular system that progressively leads to the formation of atherosclerotic plaques in the vessel wall (Weber and Noels, 2011). Plaques that are formed in an early stage of life can be considered as being stable. Such lesions contain very few macrophages and have a small necrotic core, which is separated from the lumen of the blood vessel by a thick fibrous cap, consisting of smooth muscle cells (SMCs) and collagen fibers. Stable plaques can progress over decades to a more unstable phenotype which is characterized by a thin fibrous cap with few SMCs and numerous macrophage-derived foam cells. Lesional macrophages produce matrix metalloproteinases, reactive oxygen species, and proinflammatory cytokines, and are responsible for progressive thinning of the fibrous cap. Eventually, there is a risk that plaques rupture, causing severe complications such as acute myocardial infarction and stroke. Fortunately, our insight into the progression of the disease has expanded in recent years, making atherogenesis a process that is adaptable instead of being unavoidable. Indeed, a healthy diet, physical exercise, and lipid-lowering drugs (statins) are known to improve atherosclerosis (Weber and Noels, 2011). However, despite preventive measures, morbidity and mortality remains considerable, increasing the need for new and more adequate therapies.

Recent evidence suggests that autophagy plays an important role in atherosclerosis (Martinet and De Meyer, 2009). Autophagy is a subcellular degradation mechanism that protects the cell against the accumulation of damaged organelles and misfolded proteins. Specific autophagy-related proteins (Atg proteins) are essential for autophagy initiation and formation of small autophagic vacuoles, known as autophagosomes. These structures engulf portions of the cytosol containing protein aggregates, lipid droplets, and even complete organelles when the cell is stressed, damaged, or needs to survive in unfavorable conditions. Processing of cytosolic microtubule-associated protein 1 light chain 3 (LC3-I) into the membrane bound LC3-II is a crucial step. LC3-II is localized on the autophagosomal membrane and recruits proteins that are ubiquitinated for degradation via the adaptor protein p62. Moreover, p62 is a selective substrate of autophagy that rapidly accumulates when autophagy is inhibited or defective. After fusion of an autophagosome with a lysosome, the encapsulated cytoplasmic cargo is degraded by lysosomal enzymes. Mammalian target of rapamycin (mTOR), a serine/threonine protein kinase and important nutrient sensor of the cell, plays a central role in the regulation of autophagy. In a normal environment with sufficient nutrient supply and growth factors, mTOR suppresses autophagy. However, inhibition of mTOR, which mainly occurs under conditions of cellular distress, leads to autophagy induction (Mizushima and Komatsu, 2011).

Transmission electron microscopy (TEM) has revealed that autophagy occurs in advanced atherosclerotic plaques (Martinet and De Meyer, 2009). Most likely, autophagy functions as a protective mechanism in atherosclerosis and guards plaque cells from various adverse stimuli (see below). However, overstimulating the autophagic process leads to entire self-digestion and, eventually, autophagy-mediated cell death that lacks the typical features of apoptosis or necrosis. In contrast, inhibition of autophagy results in accumulation of damaged mitochondria and other intracellular structures, evoking apoptosis. Interestingly, during plaque progression, basal autophagy becomes deficient as demonstrated by increased p62 levels in plaques of apolipoprotein E (ApoE)-deficient and low density lipoprotein (LDL) receptor knockout mice fed a Western-type diet (Liao et al., 2012; Razani et al., 2012). Despite the findings described above and the growing interest in autophagy in human pathologies, the process remains a poorly investigated phenomenon in atherosclerosis. Therefore, further research is needed to clarify conclusively the role of autophagy in atherosclerosis.

AUTOPHAGY-STIMULATING FACTORS IN ATHEROSCLEROSIS

Based on *in vitro* observations, it seems that certain atherosclerosis-related factors are responsible for the stimulation of autophagy in plaque cells (Figure 6.1), as described in more detail below.

Oxidized Lipids

During plaque development LDL infiltrates atherosclerosis-prone regions, where it is oxidized or enzymatically modified. Oxidized LDL (oxLDL) is taken up by macrophages via scavenger and lectin-like oxidized low-density lipoprotein-1 (LOX-1) receptors, and promotes further accumulation and differentiation of monocytes in the plaque (Frostegård et al., 1990). *In vitro* treatment of human umbilical vein endothelial cells (HUVECs) with oxLDL increases the amount of autophagosomes; this is a phenomenon that could be blocked by the class III phosphatidylinositol 3-kinase inhibitor 3-methyladenine and augmented by the autophagy inducer rapamycin (Zhang et al., 2010). Other studies demonstrated that treatment of human vascular endothelial cells and SMCs with oxLDL increases cytosolic calcium. Apart from activating the intrinsic mitochondrial apoptotic pathway, elevated cytosolic calcium concentrations are also able to induce autophagy through AMP-activated protein kinase (AMPK)/mTOR-dependent and -independent pathways (Grotemeier et al., 2010; Muller et al., 2011). Moreover, oxLDL contributes to its own degradation, because the autophagosome–lysosome pathway is involved in oxLDL breakdown (Zhang et al., 2010).

7-Ketocholesterol (7-KC), the main oxysterol in oxLDL and abundantly present in the atherosclerotic plaque, triggers autophagic features in SMCs, such as intense vacuolization, depletion of organelles, myelin figure formation, LC3 processing, and ubiquitination of cellular proteins (Martinet et al., 2004). Moreover, it is known that 7-KC treated primary

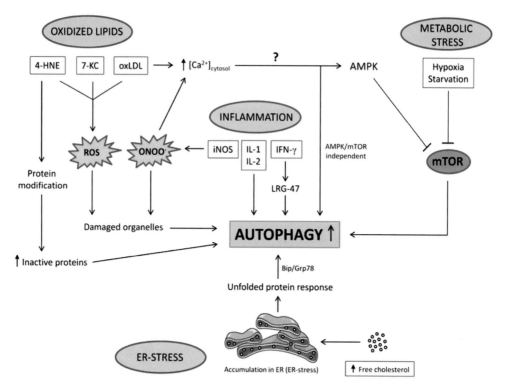

FIGURE 6.1 **Autophagy-stimulating factors in atherosclerosis.** Specific initiators of autophagy induction are indicated with a red border, the autophagy-inhibitor mTOR is marked in red, and oxidative damage is highlighted in yellow. ↑, increased; ?, still unknown; 4-HNE, 4-hydroxynonenal; 7-KC, 7-ketocholesterol; oxLDL, oxidized LDL; iNOS, inducible nitric oxide synthase; AMPK, adenosine monophosphate-activated protein kinase; mTOR, mammalian target of rapamycin; ROS, reactive oxygen species; ONOO⁻ peroxynitrite; ER, endoplasmic reticulum.

macrophages isolated from GFP-LC3 mice show an increased number of GFP-LC3-positive puncta as compared to control macrophages. Other autophagic phenomena such as autophagosome formation and LC3 processing were also obvious in 7-KC treated macrophages. In contrast, macrophages that lack the Atg5 gene, necessary for autophagy induction show neither autophagosome formation nor LC3 processing after 7-KC treatment (Liao *et al.*, 2012).

End products of oxidative degradation include lipid peroxidation-derived aldehydes, such as 4-hydroxynonenal (4-HNE). 4-HNE irreversibly modifies cytosolic proteins and interferes with their cellular function. Accumulation of multiple inactive proteins is harmful for the cell after long-term exposure. Therefore, removal of 4-HNE modified proteins is essential to prevent detrimental effects. Interestingly, autophagy is induced in SMCs exposed to 4-HNE, which confirms earlier findings showing that oxidative stress stimulates autophagy to get rid of the damaged intracellular material. However, the exact mechanism is unclear (Hill *et al.*, 2008). Possibly, 4-HNE or oxidized lipids in the plaque stimulate autophagy through the production of reactive oxygen species (ROS) and ROS-mediated organelle damage (Kiffin *et al.*, 2006). ROS induce mitochondrial membrane permeabilization by increasing the Bax/Bcl-2 or Bcl-x(L) ratio. As a consequence, mitochondria release cytochrome c, which triggers apoptosis. Autophagy might be induced in the plaque as an adaptive protection mechanism to prevent apoptosis by eliminating damaged mitochondria (Lemasters, 2005).

Endoplasmic Reticulum (ER) Stress and Metabolic Stress

Atherosclerotic plaques reveal changes in the ER due to the presence of oxidized lipids, inflammation and metabolic stress, leading to a condition known as ER stress (Muller *et al.*, 2011). Initially, ER stress is induced to protect macrophages against apoptotic cell death, albeit excessive induction has detrimental effects. Moreover, a direct link between lipid metabolism and ER exists. The ER chaperone molecule Bip/Grp78 has been found on the surface of lipid droplets, suggesting that the ER functions as a storage place for lipids (Prattes *et al.*, 2000). Indeed, the ER serves as a location where free fatty acids can be converted into triglycerides. Free intracellular cholesterol is present in both early and advanced atherosclerotic lesions, but the amount increases in macrophages during lesion progression (Tabas, 2002). Accumulation of free cholesterol in the ER induces ER stress and apoptotic cell death in peritoneal macrophages (Feng *et al.*, 2003). However, excessive concentrations of free cholesterol also induce autophagy, most likely to protect against free cholesterol-mediated cell death (Kedi *et al.*, 2010). Along these lines, it is worth mentioning that Bip/Grp78 is upregulated during ER stress and is necessary to induce autophagy in mammalian cells. Inhibition of Bip/Grp78 leads to the expansion of the ER and prevents autophagosome formation (Li *et al.*, 2008). Because apoptotic cell death of macrophages only occurs in advanced atherosclerotic lesions, it is plausible to assume that autophagy is initially able to protect macrophages against ER stress under mild circumstances but eventually fails after severe and prolonged ER stress exposure.

Metabolic stress is described as a combination of nutrient deprivation and hypoxia. Plaque cells that are located far away from the lumen are deprived of nutrients and oxygen, due to insufficient intraplaque vascularization. To compensate for this stressful condition, autophagy is induced, probably through inhibition of mTOR, to degrade cellular material, which in turn provides energy in the form of ATP and basic nutrients such as amino acids and fatty acids. The production of ATP is crucial, because the energy supply of the cell drastically decreases under conditions of metabolic stress (Lum *et al.*, 2005). Moreover, SMCs in the fibrous cap of advanced plaques are surrounded by a thick layer of basal lamina, strongly suggesting that autophagy in these cells is stimulated by starvation effects (Martinet and De Meyer, 2009). It is also noteworthy that SMCs and macrophages in culture activate autophagy upon nutrient deprivation (e.g., in amino acid-free Earle's balanced salt solution).

Inflammation

It has been reported that cytokines take part in the modulation of autophagy. Both IL-1 and IL-2 are strongly expressed in endarterectomy-derived plaque samples and are known to stimulate the autophagic process. Moreover, a large body of evidence suggests that there is an outspoken Th$_1$ response present in atherosclerotic lesions (Harris, 2011). Indeed, infiltrated T lymphocytes in early lesions produce IFN-γ and trigger autophagy in macrophages via LRG-47, a member of the interferon-inducible GTPase family. A Th2-dependent immune response, which is responsible for the production of IL-4 and IL-13, suppresses autophagy by indirect stimulation of mTOR through type I PI3 kinase. While the inhibition of autophagy by IL-4 and IL-13 depends on activation of Akt, autophagy stimulation by IFN-γ is Akt-independent. Furthermore, plaque T lymphocytes produce TNF-α, which induces autophagy in SMCs through an Akt/PKB and c-jun N-terminal signaling pathway (Harris, 2011).

Another important factor present in atherosclerotic plaques is inducible nitric oxide synthase (iNOS). Overexpression of iNOS is apparent in macrophage-derived foam cells, and may lead to cytotoxic amounts of nitric oxide that react with superoxide anion to form peroxynitrite. Peroxynitrite may induce oxidative damage to DNA and other cellular structures, thereby activating an autophagic response to remove the damaged material (Kiffin et al., 2006). Moreover, peroxynitrite damages the ER-dependent SERCA pump, redirecting calcium from the ER into the cytosol (Walia et al., 2003). An increased concentration of cytosolic calcium represents an additional mechanism for autophagy induction (Grotemeier et al., 2010).

PROTECTIVE EFFECTS OF AUTOPHAGY IN ATHEROSCLEROSIS

It has been demonstrated that the process of autophagy has beneficial effects in atherosclerosis (Figure 6.2), as outlined in this section.

Autophagy Protects Against Apoptosis

Autophagy is a basal housekeeping mechanism that prevents the accumulation of misfolded or damaged cytosolic material. In this way, it plays a protective anti-apoptotic role, as in atherosclerosis, where abundantly present oxidized lipids irreversibly modify proteins and other intracellular material. Indeed, autophagy-deficient macrophages exposed to stimuli that induce ER stress or oxidative stress undergo significantly more apoptotic cell death as compared to wild-type macrophages (Liao et al., 2012). Moreover, intravenous administration of the apoptosis inducer tunicamycin in autophagy-deficient mice induces significantly more apoptotic cell death of peritoneal macrophages as compared to wild-type mice. Apart from the removal of damaged cytosolic material, autophagy in atherosclerotic plaques protects against apoptosis because it prevents ROS production. ROS destabilizes mitochondria and ruptures the lysosomal membrane. Autophagy eliminates damaged polarized mitochondria before cytochrome c release and initiation of apoptosis (Kiffin et al., 2006). Similar protective effects were found in SMCs. For example, high concentrations of statins induce SMC apoptosis, but when 7-KC is given in combination with a statin, autophagy is induced and SMCs are protected against fluvastatin-induced apoptosis (Martinet et al., 2008). Overall, these results suggest that autophagy is critical for the structure and stability of atherosclerotic plaques. The protective autophagy-mediated effects, particularly against apoptosis, are lost when the autophagic pathway is defective.

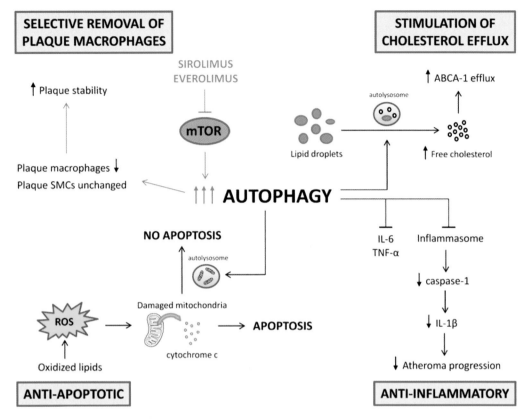

FIGURE 6.2 **Protective mechanisms of autophagy in atherosclerosis.** The sirolimus- and everolimus-dependent pathway for the removal of plaque macrophages is indicated in blue, the autophagy–inhibitor mTOR is marked in red, and oxidative damage is highlighted in yellow. ↑, increased; ↓, decreased; ↑↑↑, excessive induction; mTOR, mammalian target of rapamycin; SMCs, smooth muscle cells; ROS, reactive oxygen species; ABCA-1, ATP-binding cassette transporter A1.

Autophagy in Monocytes and Macrophages Suppresses Inflammation

Although it has been known for decades that monocytes and macrophages play a pivotal role in atherosclerosis, and that inflammation mediates atherosclerotic plaque progression, we are only beginning to understand the potential effects of autophagy on inflammation and inflammatory diseases such as atherosclerosis. Recently, it has been demonstrated that an autophagy haploinsufficiency in Beclin 1 heterozygous-deficient mice on ApoE-null background does not affect plaque progression (Razani *et al.*, 2012). However, a complete defect of macrophage autophagy in macrophage-specific Atg5-null mice on ApoE-null background is proinflammatory and results in accelerated plaque growth. A potential mechanism of lesion progression in macrophage-specific Atg5-null mice is over-activation of the pro-atherogenic inflammasome, leading to increased production of IL-1β via caspase-1 (Razani *et al.*, 2012). Indeed, excessive amounts of IL-1β are produced by autophagy-deficient macrophages, particularly when they are exposed to cholesterol crystals. Such crystals are abundantly present in advanced plaques. Other mechanisms that may activate the inflammasome include ROS production, lysosomal leakage, and defective removal of damaged mitochondria (Razani *et al.*, 2012).

Sirtuins (SIRTs) are NAD-dependent deacetylases that are strongly associated with cell survival. SIRT1 is well studied in cardiovascular research and is known to play an important role in autophagy regulation. It stimulates autophagy by direct deacetylation of Atg5, Atg7, and Atg8 (Lee *et al.*, 2008). A potent inhibitor of SIRT1, sirtinol, has been shown to induce inflammation in human acute monocytic leukemia cells. Sirtinol promotes NF-κB signaling, leading to overexpression of TNF-α and IL-6. The same inflammatory response is evident when cells are treated with the autophagy inhibitor 3-methyladenine. Interestingly, p62 accumulation is required for inflammation caused by autophagy suppression, as NF-κB phosphorylation is inhibited in p62 knockdown cells. Because SIRT1 inhibition is known to activate mTOR, and rapamycin abolishes sirtinol-mediated NF-κB signaling and inflammation induction, an mTOR-dependent pathway is most likely involved (Takeda-Watanabe *et al.*, 2012).

Autophagy Triggers Cholesterol Efflux

Reversed cholesterol transport (RCT), defined as the flux of accumulated cholesterol from macrophages back to the liver, is a protective factor in atherosclerosis. Therefore, affecting this mechanism would form an attractive strategy. In macrophages, cholesterol is esterified by acyl-coenzyme A cholesterol acyltransferase (ACAT) and stored in lipid droplets as cholesteryl esters (CE), which can be hydrolyzed by cholesterol esterases to generate free cholesterol. Unlike normal unloaded macrophages, in which cholesterol homeostasis is mainly managed by cytoplasmic neutral hydrolases, autophagy is induced in lipid-laden macrophages (Ouimet *et al.*, 2011). Lipid droplets are encapsulated by autophagosomes and, after fusion with a lysosome, the lysosomal acid lipase (LAL) hydrolyzes the cholesteryl esters, independent of neutral CE hydrolysis, thereby generating even more free cholesterol for ABCA1-efflux (Singh *et al.*, 2009). Consistent with this finding, upregulation of autophagy reduces the lipid load in macrophages. Indeed, stimulation of autophagy via oxLDL treatment inhibits lipid accumulation as compared to macrophages treated with VLDL (Ouimet *et al.*, 2011). Moreover, autophagy induction by deletion of wild-type p53-induced phosphatase 1 (WIP1) prevents accumulation of lipid droplets in macrophages, thereby suppressing their conversion into foam cells (Le Guezennec *et al.*, 2012). Autophagy-deficient macrophages have impaired cholesterol efflux due to a decrease in lysosomal CE hydrolysis. Overall, macrophage autophagy seems essential for RCT and has a beneficial impact on atherosclerosis.

Recently, the transient receptor potential cation channel subfamily V member 1 (TRPV1) was identified as a potential target to reduce the accumulation of lipids in vascular SMCs and to attenuate atherosclerosis (Ma *et al.*, 2011). Activation of TRPV1 leads to increased concentrations of cytosolic calcium. Although prolonged activation of TRPV1 in ApoE$^{-/-}$ mice stimulates cholesterol efflux and significantly reduces plaque size, the exact underlying mechanism is unclear. However, given that increased concentrations of cytosolic calcium lead to induction of autophagy (Grotemeier *et al.*, 2010), it is conceivable that autophagy is involved in TRPV1-stimulated cholesterol efflux.

Selective Removal of Plaque Macrophages by Autophagy

Although basal levels of autophagy are protective, excessive induction of autophagy can destroy major parts of the cytosol and eliminates functional organelles such as the ER, Golgi apparatus, and mitochondria. Eventually, all cellular functions will be lost and the cell will collapse due to complete self-digestion. Because macrophages are known to play a key role in the destabilization of atherosclerotic plaques, specific elimination of macrophages, without affecting the amount of SMCs and endothelial cells, could be an interesting strategy to stabilize rupture-prone lesions. Everolimus, a rapamycin derivative and potent inducer of autophagy through inhibition of mTOR, drastically reduces the amount of macrophages in plaques from cholesterol-fed rabbits via autophagy-mediated cell death without changing the SMC content (Verheye et al., 2007). Because cell viability is not affected when cultured macrophages are treated with tacrolimus, an mTOR-independent everolimus analogue, mTOR is clearly involved in everolimus-induced autophagy and macrophage depletion. Moreover, dephosphorylation of p70S6 kinase (an event downstream of mTOR) is evident in macrophages treated with everolimus (Verheye et al., 2007). Because autophagy-mediated cell death occurs as a suicidal process, production of metalloproteinases, deposition of necrotic "garbage," and activation of an inflammatory response are assumed to be limited. However, selective clearance of plaque macrophages by everolimus induces a proinflammatory reaction with increased production of TNF-α, IL-6, and chemokines. Although this is an mTOR-mediated phenomenon (as similar effects occur after treatment with sirolimus), activation of p38 MAP kinase, but not excessive autophagy itself, is responsible for this proinflammatory response. Co-treatment with a p38 MAP kinase inhibitor or clobetasol attenuates TNF-α expression both in vitro and in vivo, creating a potential role for anti-inflammatory agents in combination with everolimus for selective removal of macrophages (Martinet et al., 2012).

Besides mTOR inhibitors such as sirolimus and everolimus, mTOR-independent compounds have also been studied and found to induce autophagy. Although some seem promising regarding treatment of atherosclerosis, most of them induce off-target effects as well, which is unfavorable for plaque stability. For example, in vitro experiments showed that the Toll-like receptor 7 agonist imiquimod induces autophagy-mediated cell death of macrophages, but not of SMCs. However, local in vivo administration of imiquimod to atherosclerotic plaques in cholesterol fed rabbits promotes moderate induction of macrophage autophagy, resulting in macrophage survival instead of cell death. This is followed by macrophage accumulation, enhanced cytokine production through activation of NF-κB, infiltration of T lymphocytes, and plaque progression (De Meyer et al., 2012).

CONCLUDING REMARKS

Due to the high prevalence of atherosclerosis and the fact that current therapies are insufficient to prevent acute coronary syndromes, more adequate treatments are needed. In the past, research has mainly focused on anti-inflammatory therapies and mechanisms that directly or indirectly decrease cholesterol levels in plasma. Although this work has paid off, atherosclerosis-driven mortality and morbidity remains a significant problem. Therefore, it is important to investigate alternative mechanisms that could potentially function as new pharmacological targets. One of these promising mechanisms is autophagy. Despite the fact that the role of autophagy in atherosclerosis has not yet been fully clarified, a growing body of evidence indicates that autophagy has a protective function in atherosclerosis. It stimulates cholesterol efflux (Ouimet *et al.*, 2011), prevents inflammasome activation (Razani *et al.*, 2012), and has anti-apoptotic properties (Kiffin *et al.*, 2006). Thus, this mechanism seems to play a fundamental role in atherosclerotic plaque stability and/or development.

During mild oxidative stress conditions autophagy induction is responsible for the degradation of damaged mitochondria, and, in doing this, prevents the release of cytochrome c and production of ROS. Accordingly, autophagy protects against apoptosis. It is obvious that autophagy can only protect against apoptotic cell death to a certain extent. Under prolonged or intensive oxidative stress exposure, autophagy is no longer capable of eliminating all damaged mitochondria. In addition, severe oxidative stress will disrupt the lysosomal membrane structure and trigger the release of lysosomal enzymes into the cytosol. These enzymes can harm other cellular structures, and their release is associated with activation of the caspase pathway (Kiffin *et al.*, 2006). To promote plaque stability, macrophage apoptosis needs to be prevented. It might enhance the release of proinflammatory cytokines and other chemo-attractants that recruit phagocytic cells (Peter *et al.*, 2010). Furthermore, the capability to clear apoptotic cells by phagocytosis in advanced plaques is decreased (Schrijvers *et al.*, 2005), leading to secondary necrosis and enlargement of the necrotic core.

Due to the narrow margin between the cell survival and death aspects of autophagy, some important questions still need to be answered. How long can we stimulate autophagy and its beneficial effects before it becomes harmful and detrimental? Is an overall induction of autophagy in all plaque cells favorable? Indeed, pharmacological induction of autophagy also has its downsides, depending on the level of induction and the pharmacological compounds being used. Excessive autophagy stimulation might affect SMC viability and collagen production, leading to thinning of the fibrous cap and formation of a more vulnerable plaque phenotype. Thus, while autophagy has many functions that would suggest a positive effect on plaque stability and progression, overstimulation might occur, turning the beneficial process into a detrimental one. Another problem in the atherosclerotic context is the generation of iron as one of the end products of autolysosomal degradation. As mitochondria and ferritin contain iron, autophagic degradation of these ferruginous structures results in an iron-enriched autolysosomal compartment. Ferrous iron can react with hydrogen peroxide, which is produced by mitochondria. Hydrogen peroxide is membrane permeable and, in combination with reactive iron, may lead to the generation of hydroxyl radicals. These free radicals can induce lipid peroxidation and ultimately give rise to ceroid production. Ceroid is an insoluble complex of proteins and peroxidized polyunsaturated lipids, which cannot be degraded by autophagy. When these complexes pile up in the autolysosome, more and more lysosomal enzymes are redirected in an unsuccessful attempt to degrade them. As a consequence, these enzymes will neglect the degradation of other damaged proteins in the autolysosome, which in turn can induce apoptosis through impairment of autophagy. Furthermore, ongoing autophagy of iron-containing components together with hydrogen peroxide and the peroxidation of the lysosomal membrane by free hydroxyl radicals might lead to destruction of the lysosome. The membrane will rupture and lysosomal enzymes are released into the cytosol, thereby damaging other cell organelles and inducing apoptosis (Kurz *et al.*, 2007).

Given that basal autophagy becomes deficient in advanced plaques and that excessive autophagy induction by the mTOR inhibitor everolimus selectively eliminates plaque macrophages, pharmacological regulation of autophagy might be an innovative strategy to stabilize rupture-prone lesions. However, everolimus-mediated removal of macrophages is not inflammatory-silent, due to off-target effects. Co-treatment with anti-inflammatory drugs seems to be advised for *in vivo* administration. Both mTOR-dependent and independent inducers of autophagy that selectively deplete plaque macrophages with minimal side effects need to be tested. In conclusion, although more fundamental research is required to clarify the role and function of autophagy in atherosclerosis, autophagy seems to be a new big player in the underlying molecular mechanisms driving atherosclerotic plaque progression and stability.

Acknowledgments

This work was supported by the Fund for Scientific Research (FWO) – Flanders and the University of Antwerp (BOF). CFM is a doctoral fellow of the agency for Innovation by Science and Technology (IWT).

References

De Meyer, I., Martinet, W., Schrijvers, D.M., et al., 2012. Toll-like receptor 7 stimulation by imiquimod induces macrophage autophagy and inflammation in atherosclerotic plaques. Basic Res. Cardiol. 107 (3), 269.

Feng, B., Yao, P.M., Li, Y., et al., 2003. The endoplasmic reticulum is the site of cholesterol-induced cytotoxicity in macrophages. Nat. Cell Biol. 5, 781–792.

Frostegård, J., Nilsson, J., Haegerstrand, A., et al., 1990. Oxidized low density lipoprotein induces differentiation and adhesion of human monocytes and the monocytic cell line U937. Proc. Natl. Acad. Sci. U.S.A. 87 (3), 904–908.

Grotemeier, A., Alers, S., Pfisterer, S.G., et al., 2010. AMPK-independent induction of autophagy by cytosolic Ca^{2+} increase. Cell Signal. 22 (6), 914–925.

Harris, J., 2011. Autophagy and cytokines. Cytokine 56 (2), 140–144.

Hill, B.G., Haberzettl, P., Ahmed, Y., et al., 2008. Unsaturated lipid peroxidation-derived aldehydes activate autophagy in vascular smooth-muscle cells. Biochem. J. 410, 525–534.

Kedi, X., Yi, Y., Ming, Y., et al., 2010. Autophagy plays a protective role in free cholesterol overload-induced death of smooth muscle cells. J. Lipid Res. 51 (9), 2581–2590.

Kiffin, R., Bandyopadhyay, U., Cuervo, A.M., 2006. Oxidative stress and autophagy. Antioxid. Redox Signal. 8, 152–162.

Kurz, T., Terman, A., Brunk, U.T., 2007. Autophagy, ageing and apoptosis: the role of oxidative stress and lysosomal iron. Arch. Biochem. Biophys. 462, 220–230.

Lee, I.H., Cao, L., Mostoslavsky, R., et al., 2008. A role for the NAD-dependent deacetylase Sirt1 in the regulation of autophagy. Proc. Natl. Acad. Sci. U.S.A. 105 (9), 3374–3379.

Le Guezennec, X., Brichkina, A., Huang, Y.F., et al., 2012. Wip1-dependent regulation of autophagy, obesity, and atherosclerosis. Cell Metab. 16 (1), 68–80.

Lemasters, J.J., 2005. Selective mitochondrial autophagy, or mitophagy, as a targeted defense against oxidative stress, mitochondrial dysfunction, and aging. Rejuvenation Res. 8 (1), 3–5.

Li, J., Ni, M., Lee, B., et al., 2008. The unfolded protein response regulator GRP78/BiP is required for endoplasmic reticulum integrity and stress-induced autophagy in mammalian cells. Cell Death Differ. 15, 1460–1471.

Liao, X., Sluimer, J.C., Wang, Y., et al., 2012. Macrophage autophagy plays a protective role in advanced atherosclerosis. Cell Metab. 15 (4), 545–553.

Lum, J.J., Bauer, D.E., Kong, M., et al., 2005. Growth factor regulation of autophagy and cell survival in the absence of apoptosis. Cell. 120 (2), 237–248.

Ma, L., Zhong, J., Zhao, Z., et al., 2011. Activation of TRPV1 reduces vascular lipid accumulation and attenuates atherosclerosis. Cardiovasc. Res. 92 (3), 504–513.

Martinet, W., De Meyer, G.R.Y., 2009. Autophagy in atherosclerosis: a cell survival and deathphenomenon with therapeutic potential. Circ. Res. 104 (3), 304–317.

Martinet, W., De Bie, M., Schrijvers, D.M., et al., 2004. 7-ketocholesterol induces protein ubiquitination, myelin figure formation, and light chain 3 processing in vascular smooth muscle cells. Arterioscler. Thromb. Vasc. Biol. 24, 2296–2301.

Martinet, W., Schrijvers, D.M., Timmermans, J.P., et al., 2008. Interactions between cell death induced by statins and 7-ketocholesterol in rabbit aorta smooth muscle cells. Br. J. Pharmacol. 154, 1236–1246.

Martinet, W., Verheye, S., De Meyer, I., et al., 2012. Everolimus triggers cytokine release by macrophages: rationale for stents eluting everolimus and a glucocorticoid. Arterioscler. Thromb. Vasc. Biol. 32 (5), 1228–1235.

Mizushima, N., Komatsu, M., 2011. Autophagy: renovation of cells and tissues. Cell. 147 (4), 728–741.

Muller, C., Salvayre, R., Nègre-Salvayre, A., et al., 2011. Oxidized LDLs trigger endoplasmic reticulum stress and autophagy: prevention by HDLs. Autophagy. 7 (5), 541–543.

Ouimet, M., Franklin, V., Mak, E., et al., 2011. Autophagy regulates cholesterol efflux from macrophage foam cells via lysosomal acid lipase. Cell Metab. 13 (6), 655–667.

Peter, C., Wesselborg, S., Herrmann, M., et al., 2010. Dangerous attraction: phagocyte recruitment and danger signals of apoptotic and necrotic cells. Apoptosis 15, 1007–1028.

Prattes, S., Hörl, G., Hammer, A., et al., 2000. Intracellular distribution and mobilization of unesterified cholesterol in adipocytes: triglyceride droplets are surrounded by cholesterol-rich ER-like surface layer structures. J. Cell Sci. 113 (17), 2977–2989.

Razani, B., Feng, C., Coleman, T., et al., 2012. Autophagy links inflammasomes to atherosclerotic progression. Cell Metab. 15 (4), 534–544.

Schrijvers, D.M., De Meyer, G.R.Y., Kockx, M.M., et al., 2005. Phagocytosis of apoptotic cells by macrophages is impaired in atherosclerosis. Arterioscler. Thromb. Vasc. Biol. 25 (6), 1256–1261.

Singh, R., Kaushik, S., Wang, Y., et al., 2009. Autophagy regulates lipid metabolism. Nature 458 (7242), 1131–1135.

Tabas, I., 2002. Consequences of cellular cholesterol accumulation: basic concepts and physiological implications. J. Clin. Invest. 110 (7), 905–911.

Takeda-Watanabe, A., Kitada, M., Kanasaki, K., et al., 2012. SIRT1 inactivation induces inflammation through the dysregulation of autophagy in human THP-1 cells. Biochem. Biophys. Res. Commun. 427 (1), 191–196.

Verheye, S., Martinet, W., Kockx, M.M., et al., 2007. Selective clearance of macrophages in atherosclerotic plaques by autophagy. J. Am. Coll. Cardiol. 49 (6), 706–715.

Walia, M., Samson, S.E., Schmidt, T., et al., 2003. Peroxynitrite and nitric oxide differ in their effects on pig coronary artery smooth muscle. Am. J. Physiol. Cell Physiol. 284 (3), C649–C657.

Weber, C., Noels, H., 2011. Atherosclerosis: current pathogenesis and therapeutic options. Nat. Med. 17 (11), 1410–1422.

Zhang, Y.L., Cao, Y.J., Zhang, X., et al., 2010. The autophagy-lysosome pathway: a novel mechanism involved in the processing of oxidized LDL in human vascular endothelial cells. Biochem. Biophys. Res. Commun. 394 (2), 377–382.

Treatment of Diabetic Cardiomyopathy through Upregulating Autophagy by Stimulating AMP-Activated Protein Kinase

Yuran Xie and Zhonglin Xie

O U T L I N E

Abstract

Diabetic cardiomyopathy, which develops in diabetic patients in the absence of coronary artery disease and hypertension, is a major cause of heart failure. Despite the importance of this complication, the underlying mechanisms are poorly understood. Increasing evidence suggests that hyperglycemia is central to the pathogenesis of diabetic cardiomyopathy, which triggers a series of maladaptive events leading to cardiomyocyte apoptosis, collagen deposition, and cardiac fibrosis. Hyperglycemia inhibits AMP-activated protein kinase (AMPK) activity along with cardiac dysfunction and suppression of cardiac autophagy; chronic AMPK activation with metformin, one of the most used antidiabetic drugs and a well-characterized AMPK activator,

M.A. Hayat (ed): Autophagy, Volume 1
DOI: http://dx.doi.org/10.1016/B978-0-12-405530-8.00007-8

© 2014 Elsevier Inc. All rights reserved.

significantly enhances autophagic activity, preserves cardiac function, and prevents most of the primary characteristics of diabetic cardiomyopathy in diabetic mice. Thus, stimulation of autophagy by activation of AMPK may represent a novel approach to treating diabetic cardiomyopathy.

INTRODUCTION

Diabetic cardiomyopathy is a clinical condition characterized by ventricular dysfunction, which develops in patients with diabetes in the absence of coronary artery disease and hypertension. Diabetic cardiomyopathy was first reported by Rubler *et al.* (1972). Since then, many epidemiological and clinical studies have established the existence of diabetic cardiomyopathy in humans. The Framingham Heart Study demonstrates that, compared with age-matched control subjects, diabetic patients exhibit an increase in the incidence of heart failure (Kannel and McGee, 1979). This association is independent of other associated risk factors, including age, diabetic duration, hypertension, and ischemic heart disease.

In type 1 diabetes mellitus without known cardiac disease, echocardiography reveals diastolic dysfunction with a reduction in early diastolic filling, an increase in atrial filling, an extension of isovolumetric relaxation, and increased numbers of supraventricular premature beats. Carugo *et al.* (2001) reported that type 1 diabetic patients without micro- and macrovascular complications also exhibit early structural and functional cardiac abnormalities such as increased left ventricular wall thickness, declined ejection fraction, and increased diastolic diameter. Similarly, The UKPDS (UK Prospective Diabetes Study) found that, compared with matched controls, type 2 diabetic patients have an increased prevalence of heart failure, which is correlated with higher HbA1c (glycated hemoglobin) levels (Stratton *et al.*, 2000). These clinical studies suggest that diabetes may directly impair cardiac structure and function.

Hyperglycemia is central to the pathogenesis of diabetic cardiomyopathy, which triggers a series of maladaptive events leading to cardiomyocyte apoptosis, collagen deposition, and cardiac fibrosis. These processes are thought to be responsible for altered myocardial contractility, and manifest as diastolic dysfunction. The pathogenesis of diabetic cardiomyopathy is a chronic and complex process that is attributed to abnormal cellular metabolism and defects in organelles such as myofibrils, mitochondria, sarcoplasmic reticulum, and sarcolemma. Abnormal calcium handling in the diabetic heart is an early indicator of abnormal metabolism. This change leads to improper cardiac contraction and relaxation processes – and early diastolic and, later, systolic dysfunction – leading to heart failure. Diabetic cardiomyopathy has not only been attributed to hyperglycemia, but also is related to hyperlipidemia and inflammation. Although these pathogenic factors probably cause diabetic cardiomyopathy by different mechanisms, their major contribution to diabetic cardiomyopathy is oxidative stress. Increased mitochondrial reactive oxygen species (ROS) production has been documented in the development of diabetic cardiomyopathy. Kuo *et al.* (1983) first reported impaired mitochondrial function in diabetic hearts using the diabetic *db/db* mouse model. Subsequent studies showed reduced mitochondrial oxidative capacity in type 1 diabetes, and reduced levels of oxidative phosphorylation proteins and decreased mitochondrial respiration in type 2 diabetic mice. In addition to reduced oxidative phosphorylation, the mitochondria from diabetic hearts exhibit increased ROS production, which can alter the integrity of the inner mitochondrial membrane, facilitating further mitochondrial dysfunction. Thus, accumulation of dysfunctional mitochondria in cardiac myocytes may be an important source of ROS and proapoptotic factors (Green and Kroemer, 2004), which worsens the cardiac dysfunction in diabetic patients.

AUTOPHAGY IN THE HEART

Autophagy is a cellular degradation process responsible for the turnover of unnecessary or dysfunctional organelles and cytoplasmic proteins. It has been studied extensively in lower organisms such as yeast, *Caenorhabditis elegans*, and *Drosophila*. Autophagy involves sequestration of cytosolic constituents, including proteins and organelles, in autophagosomes. The autophagosomes fuse with lysosomes to form autolysosomes. Autophagy is controlled by autophagy-related genes (Atgs), many of which are involved in autophagosome formation. Both class I and class III phosphatidylinositol 3-kinases (PI3Ks) regulate autophagy by suppressing or activating the pathway through the production of phosphorylated phosphatidylinositol derivatives. Beclin 1 (Atg6) and class III PI3K are needed for the vesicle (called isolation membrane) nucleation step of autophagy (Kihara *et al.*, 2001).

The vesicle elongation process features two conjugation systems that are well conserved among eukaryotes. One pathway involves the conjugation of Atg12 to Atg5 with the help of Atg7 and Atg10. The second pathway involves the conjugation of phosphatidylethanolamine (PE) to Atg8 (microtubule-associated protein 1 light chain 3; LC3) by the sequential actions of Atg4, Atg7, and Atg3. LC3 is initially synthesized in an unprocessed form, pro-LC3, which is converted into a proteolytically processed form lacking amino acids from the C terminus, LC3-I, and is finally modified into the PE-conjugated form, LC3-II. Atg8–PE/LC3-II is the only protein marker that is reliably associated with completed autophagosomes, and is used as one of the autophagic markers. Class I PI3K, the mammalian target of the rapamycin (mTOR) pathway, acts to inhibit autophagy. Rapamycin induces autophagy by inactivating mTOR.

Several methods have been developed for monitoring autophagy in higher eukaryotes, including microscopy, biochemical methods, and detection of protein modifications through SDS-PAGE and western blotting. Because formation of autophagic vacuoles is by far the most important morphological feature of autophagic cells, demonstration of these structures by conventional electron microscopy remains currently the gold standard for assessing autophagy both in tissues and in cultured cells. LC3s are unique markers of the autophagic–lysosomal pathway, in that their lipidated forms (LC3-II in mammalian cells) appear to be predominantly associated with autophagic organelles (Kabeya *et al.*, 2000). Western blotting can easily be used to monitor changes in the amount of LC3. In mammalian cells, forced expression of GFP-conjugated LC3-II has been widely used to detect autophagic organelles in the microscope as fluorescent dots appearing, for example, upon amino acid starvation. One of the most useful alternative methods is the analysis of GFP-LC3 (e.g., in transgenic mice) via fluorescence microscopy (Klionsky *et al.*, 2007), although there are some practical limits – for example, a transgenic GFP-LC3 genetic background is needed. Importantly, investigators need to determine whether they are evaluating autophagosome levels or autophagic flux. If the question being asked is whether a particular condition changes autophagic flux (i.e., the rate of delivery of autophagy substrates to lysosomes, followed by degradation), it is also necessary to directly measure the flux of autophagosomes and/or autophagy cargo (e.g., in wild-type cells compared to autophagy-deficient cells, the latter generated by treatment with an autophagy inhibitor or resulting from *Atg* gene knockdowns).

Autophagy is essential in cell growth, development, and homeostasis. The process helps to maintain a balance between the synthesis, degradation, and subsequent recycling of cellular components. It allows the cell not only to recycle amino acids but also to remove damaged organelles, thereby eliminating oxidative stress and allowing cellular remodeling for survival. A low level of constitutive autophagy is important for maintaining the quality of protein and organelles, and cell functions, as recently reported in various organs, including the liver, brain, and heart. However, unrestrained stimulation of autophagy can induce a pathway for programmed cell death, known as type 2 cell death. Indeed, high autophagic activity may cause excessive degradation of cytosolic and organelle proteins, most noticeably the mitochondria and the endoplasmic reticulum (ER), leading to collapse of cellular functions (Levine and Yuan, 2005).

Autophagy plays an important role in the heart; under normal or mild stress conditions, autophagy degrades and recycles cytoplasmic components, such as long-lived proteins and organelles, and selectively removes damaged mitochondria as a cytoprotective mechanism for limiting mitochondria-derived oxidative stress (Kim *et al.*, 2007). As damaged mitochondria release pro-apoptotic factors such as cytochrome c, autophagy can also prevent activation of apoptosis. Ultrastructural analyses of Atg5-deficient hearts reveal a disorganized sarcomere structure, misalignment and aggregation of mitochondria, and aberrant concentric membranous structures. Inactivation of Atg5 also causes the accumulation of abnormal proteins and organelles, and promotes ER stress and apoptosis. These results indicate that constitutive cardiomyocyte autophagy is required for protein quality control and normal cellular structure and function under the basal state. Accumulation of abnormal proteins and organelles, especially mitochondria, may directly cause cardiac dysfunction. Autophagy is therefore essential for maintaining normal cardiac structure and function.

AUTOPHAGY IN HEART FAILURE

Autophagy has been demonstrated in heart failure caused by dilated cardiomyopathy, valvular disease, and ischemic heart disease. Kostin *et al.* (2003) reported that in human failing hearts with idiopathic dilated cardiomyopathy, in addition to apoptosis and necrosis, cardiac cells can also die through autophagy associated with ubiquitinated protein accumulation. In animal models of cardiomyopathy, dead and dying cardiomyocytes showing characteristics of aberrance/defects in autophagy have also been observed. Cardiomyocytes obtained from UM-7.1 hamsters, an animal model of human dilated cardiomyopathy, contain typical autophagic vacuoles, including degraded mitochondria, glycogen granules, and myelin-like figures (Miyata *et al.*, 2006). However, the precise role of autophagy in heart failure progression remains unclear. It is possible that autophagic activity performs different functions, depending on disease stage and severity.

A number of studies have implicated autophagy in cardioprotection. In a swine model, autophagy is upregulated in chronically ischemic myocardium and autophagosomes are seen in surviving cells, not apoptotic ones, suggesting that autophagy might play a beneficial role in chronic low-flow ischemia. Beta-adrenergic stimulation, which promotes apoptosis and induces cardiac hypertrophy and heart failure, has been reported to inhibit autophagy. Autophagy has also been shown to protect cells against β-adrenergic stimulation, where cardiac myocytes isolated from *Atg5*-deficient mice hearts have increased sensitivity to isoproterenol stimulation compared to wild-type cells (Nakai *et al.*, 2007). Moreover, isoproterenol treatment for 7 days leads to left ventricular dilation and cardiac dysfunction in autophagy-deficient mice but not in wild-type mice, suggesting that autophagy provides an important function in protecting cells against excessive β-adrenergic stimulation. In adult mice, cardiac-specific deficiency of Atg5 leads to cardiac hypertrophy, left ventricular dilatation, and contractile dysfunction, accompanied by increased levels of ubiquitinated proteins. On the other hand, cardiac-specific deficiency of Atg5 early in cardiogenesis show no such cardiac phenotypes under baseline conditions but developed cardiac dysfunction and left ventricular dilatation 1 week after treatment with pressure overload (Nakai *et al.*, 2007). These findings indicate that constitutive autophagy in the heart under basal conditions is a homeostatic mechanism for maintaining cardiomyocyte size and global cardiac structure and function, and upregulation of autophagy in failing hearts is an adaptive response that protects cells from hemodynamic stress (Nakai *et al.*, 2007).

In contrast, there is evidence that enhanced autophagy can contribute to heart failure. For instance, inhibition of autophagy through Beclin 1 downregulation is protective during ischemia/reperfusion *in vivo*, and inhibition of autophagy by Beclin 1 knockdown increases the cell viability in response to hydrogen peroxide in cultured cardiac myocytes *in vitro* (Matsui *et al.*, 2007). Moreover, Zhu *et al.* (2007) reported that, in a model of acute-onset hemodynamic stress, amplification of the autophagic response in *beclin 1* tansgenic mice leads to increased hypertrophic growth, decreased performance, and increased fibrosis, suggesting that enhanced autophagic activity has pathological consequences, potentially achieved by promoting autophagic cell death.

Several possibilities may explain why autophagy could be both protective and detrimental in the heart. First, the functional significance of autophagy may be determined by the level and duration of autophagy. For instance, low levels of autophagy induced by ischemia or mild sustained pressure overload inhibit apoptosis and play a protective role in wild-type mice. When autophagy is insufficient in cardiac-specific Atg5-deficient mice, apoptosis is promoted, leading to cell death. However, hyperactivation of autophagy could also cause cell death. For example, ischemia/reperfusion or severe constriction of the thoracic aorta (TAC) causes excessive mitochondrial damage that may exceed the cell's capacity for autophagy. Under these conditions of extreme stress, autophagic cell death may proceed in parallel with apoptotic cell death. In addition to autophagy and apoptosis, necrosis is also induced under such extreme conditions. Thus, inappropriate activation of autophagy, when the cell is dying by apoptosis, may be detrimental and even facilitate necrosis.

Second, Atg5 and Beclin 1 may have a molecule-specific function. Beclin 1 is a tumor suppressor gene. Beclin 1 heterozygous (Beclin 1$^{+/-}$) mice develop neoplastic mammary lesions and display an increased incidence of spontaneous malignancies (Qu *et al.*, 2003; Yue *et al.*, 2003). Autophagic cell death is reduced in Beclin 1$^{+/-}$ mice but promoted in Beclin 1 transgenic mice. Conventional Beclin 1-deficient mice die at 7.5–8.5 days of embryogenesis (Yue *et al.*, 2003), whereas conventional Atg5- and Atg7-deficient mice survive until birth (Kuma *et al.*, 2004). These results suggest that Beclin 1 may have additional functions beyond autophagy. As mentioned above, both Beclin 1 and Atg5 have functions that are related to apoptosis, which raises the possibility that autophagy and apoptosis could be interconnected by common mediators. It is possible that intervention to either stimulate or inhibit autophagy may secondarily affect other mechanisms of cell death, thereby affecting survival of cardiac myocytes during ischemia/reperfusion.

AMPK IN THE HEART

AMPK is a heterotrimeric protein consisting of a catalytic α and regulatory β and γ subunits. Each α and β subunit is encoded by two genes (α1 and α2 or β1 and β2), whereas the γ subunit is encoded by three genes (γ1, γ2, and γ3). The α subunit contains the catalytic site. However, all subunits are necessary for full activity. The α1 subunit is ubiquitously expressed, whereas α2-subunit is expressed in the heart, skeletal muscle, and liver. In the heart, α2-associated AMPK activity predominates over α1-activity (Li *et al.*, 2006). AMPK is activated in response to an increase in the ratio of AMP to ATP within the cell, and therefore acts as an efficient sensor for cellular energy state. Binding of AMP activates AMPK allosterically, and induces phosphorylation of a threonine residue (Thr-172) within the activation domain of the α subunit by an upstream kinase, the tumor suppressor LKB1. Furthermore, binding of AMP inhibits dephosphorylation of Thr-172 by protein phosphatase, whereas a high concentration of ATP inhibits the activation of AMPK. Recent studies identified calmodulin-dependent protein kinase kinase-β (CaMKK-β) as an additional upstream kinase of AMPK. Activation of AMPK by CaMKK-β is triggered by a rise in intracellular calcium ions, without detectable changes in the AMP/ATP ratio.

AMPK is ubiquitous in distribution, and its activity increases in a wide variety of cells in response to such stresses as hypoxia, oxidant stress, and hyperosmolarity, and in muscle exercise. AMPK activation appears to be a fundamental component of the response of many cells to stresses that threaten their viability. Activation of AMPK leads to phosphorylation of a number of target molecules, which results in increases in fatty acid oxidation and in muscle glucose transport (to generate more ATP) and inhibition of various synthetic processes (to conserve ATP). Thus, AMPK functions as a fuel gauge to sense the alternation of energy status within the cell. In addition to its action on cardiac energy metabolism, AMPK also has important actions on the activity of several essential physiological processes, including protein synthesis, apoptosis, and autophagy. Cardiac AMPK is rapidly activated during ischemia, which protects the heart against injury during myocardial ischemia. The earliest observation by Tian *et al.* (2001) has shown that activity of both AMPKα1 and -α2 is elevated in hypertrophic hearts subjected to chronic pressure overload. These hearts demonstrate energetic changes (increased AMP:ATP) and metabolic consequences (increased glucose uptake) consistent with AMPK activation. AMPK has been implicated in limiting hypertrophy in the heart. Treatment of neonatal rat cardiomyocytes with metformin, AICAR (5-aminoimidazole-4-carboxyamide ribonucleoside), or resveratrol activates AMPK and inhibits the development of hypertrophy during phenylephrine treatment.

AMPK AND AUTOPHAGY

Several studies have reported that the AMPK signaling pathway is involved in regulation of autophagy. AMPK is activated in cells treated with Ca^{2+}-mobilizing agents, and compound C, a specific AMPK inhibitor, effectively inhibited the increase in long-lived protein degradation triggered by Ca^{2+}-mobilizing drugs. These findings are in agreement with a recent study showing that compound C or a dominant-negative form of AMPK inhibits starvation-induced autophagy in various mammalian cells. Matsui *et al.* (2007) reported that glucose deprivation induces autophagy via activation of AMPK and inhibition of mTOR in isolated cardiac myocytes. mTOR is a negative regulator of autophagy and functions as a sensor for cellular energy and amino acid levels, and is negatively regulated by AMPK via a pathway involving the tuberous sclerosis complex (TSC1/2) and its substrate, Rheb, a Ras-related small GTPase. Moreover, induction of autophagy in response to myocardial ischemia is reduced in transgenic mice overexpressing a dominant-negative AMP. Recently, several groups reported that AMPK directly stimulates autophagy through phosphorylation and activation of ULK1 (the mammalian homologue of yeast autophagy-related gene 1 (Atg1)), a key initiator of the autophagic process. These data strongly suggest that AMPK serves as a positive regulator of autophagy in mammalian cells.

AMPK AND DIABETIC CARDIOMYOPATHY

Altered myocardial substrate and energy metabolism have emerged as an important mechanism underlying the development of diabetic cardiomyopathy. Since AMPK is an important enzyme in the regulation of cardiac energy metabolism, dysregulation of AMPK signaling may play an important role in this pathological process. Diabetes mellitus is characterized by reduced glucose and lactate metabolism, and enhanced fatty acid (FA) metabolism. Despite an increase in FA use in diabetic hearts, it is likely that FA uptake exceeds oxidation rates in the heart, thereby resulting in lipid accumulation in myocardium (Sharma *et al.*, 2004). Lipid intermediates such as ceramide promote cardiomyocyte apoptosis, thus representing a mechanism underlying cardiac dysfunction in diabetic patients. AMPK is activated when cellular energy is depleted. When activated, AMPK increases glucose uptake and FA oxidation to increase ATP production. AMPK regulates FA oxidation by phosphorylating enzymes related to malonyl CoA synthesis (acetyl CoA carboxylase, ACC) and degradation (malonyl coenzymeA decarboxylase, MCD). Malonyl CoA is a potent inhibitor of carnitine palmitoyl transferase (CPT-1), an enzyme that controls FA transport into the mitochondrion (Vavvas *et al.*, 1997). Inhibition of CPT-1 leads to accumulation of long chain fatty acid-CoA in the cytoplasm, and activates a series of intracellular metabolic events leading to cardiac hypertrophy and apoptosis.

Studies on mitochondria from diabetic patients demonstrate functional and structural abnormalities in mitochondria. Kuo *et al.* (1983) first reported impaired mitochondrial function in diabetic hearts by showing reduced state 3 respiration in heart mitochondria of *db/db* mice. This study was followed by others showing reduced mitochondrial oxidative capacity in type 1 diabetes. Ultrastructural analyses have revealed increased mitochondrial contents in models of type 1 and type 2 diabetes mellitus, and even in mouse models of the metabolic syndrome (Duncan *et al.*, 2007). Diabetic hearts exhibit a significantly increased mitochondrial area and number, as well as focal regions with severe damage to mitochondria; this may be attributed to defects in autophagy, because mitochondrial autophagy is the only cellular process that selectively removes abnormal mitochondria. AMPK is a major regulator of mitochondrial function and biogenesis in diabetes. Kukidome *et al.* (2006) reported that activation of AMPK reduces hyperglycemia-induced mitochondrial ROS production by induction of magnesium superoxide dismutase (Mn-SOD) and promotion of mitochondrial biogenesis through activation of the AMPK–peroxisome proliferator-activated receptor-γ coactivator-1α (PGC-1α) pathway in human umbilical vein endothelial cells. Intriguingly, young insulin-resistant and obese Zucker diabetic fatty rats display defects in AMPK phosphorylation and lower PGC-1α protein levels. Endurance exercise, which is known to lead to AMPK activation, prevents these abnormalities (Sriwijitkamol *et al.*, 2006).

Metformin is one of the most commonly prescribed antihyperglycemic agents for the treatment of type 2 diabetes (Davis *et al.*, 2006). Metformin lowers blood glucose levels through reducing hepatic glucose output and increasing insulin-dependent peripheral glucose utilization. The therapeutic effects of metformin, however, are not limited to its ability to lower blood glucose, as evidence supports that it also has direct vascular effects. Additionally, two large-scale clinical trials have reported that metformin improves vascular function and reduces mortality and cardiovascular end points of type 2 diabetic subjects, by actions that cannot be attributed entirely to its antihyperglycemic effects. Studies using the isolated perfused working heart model revealed that metformin provides cardioprotection in diabetic hearts against increasing preload, and in non-diabetic hearts against global ischemia (Gundewar *et al.*, 2009). Experimental studies suggest that the pleiotropic effects of metformin are mediated in part by activation of AMPK (Xie *et al.*, 2008, 2009). When activated, AMPK activates endothelial nitric oxide synthase and increases PGC1-α protein levels, both of which are important regulators of mitochondrial biogenesis and function. Thus, activation of AMPK by metformin may reduce cardiovascular disease risk and improve cardiac function in patients with type 2 diabetes.

AUTOPHAGY IN DIABETES AND ITS COMPLICATIONS

In cultured pancreatic β cells, chronic hyperglycemia induces the formation of ubiquitinated protein aggregates. Such ubiquitinated protein aggregates are also present in β cells (and other cell types) in the Zucker diabetic fatty rat during the development of diabetes (Kaniuk *et al.*, 2007). Treatment of pancreatic β cells with 3-methyladenine (an inhibitor of autophagy) induces the formation of ubiquitinated aggregates, suggesting that autophagy removes the misfolded or aggregated proteins under diabetic conditions. Impairment of autophagic machinery diminishes pancreatic β-cell mass and function, with resultant hyperglycemia, demonstrating that autophagy can act as a defense mechanism against diabetes-induced cellular damage (Kaniuk *et al.*, 2007) and play a role in the development of diabetes.

Deregulation of autophagy is also implicated in the development of diabetic cardiomyopathy. At 6 months of age, OVE26 mice, an established type 1 diabetic mouse model generated through targeted overexpression of calmodulin in β cells, exhibit very high blood glucose concentrations, reduced serum insulin values, and elevated serum triglyceride levels (Epstein *et al.*, 1989); they also exhibit cardiomyopathy, characterized by clear morphological abnormalities and impaired cardiac performance. Diabetes induces suppression of autophagic activity, as evidenced by decreased accumulation of lipidated microtubule-associated protein 1 light chain 3 (LC3-II) and autophagosome formation in the heart (Xie *et al.*, 2011a). Moreover, streptozotocin (STZ)-induced diabetes also suppresses cardiac autophagy and impairs cardiac function (Xie *et al.*, 2011a,b). Overall, these results suggest that basal levels of autophagy are important for protecting cardiomyocytes from hyperglycemic damage, and that suppression of autophagy in diabetes contributes to the development of cardiomyopathy. However, a recent study demonstrates that high glucose directly inhibits autophagic flux in neonatal rat cardiomyocytes, and in these cells the reduction of autophagy appears to be an adaptive response that functions to limit high glucose-induced cardiomyocyte injury. Neonatal cardiomyocytes have been reported to behave substantially differently from adult cardiomyocytes (Rothen-Rutishauser *et al.*, 1998). In particular, autophagy is upregulated in neonatal cardiac tissue during the perinatal period of relative starvation. Thus, autophagy could be either protective or detrimental, depending on the cell type and cellular environment.

Metabolic syndrome is a collection of medical disorders, including obesity, insulin resistance, and dyslipidemia, which can lead to diabetes and cardiovascular disease. Under these energy-rich conditions, the Akt signaling pathway is activated. In turn, Akt phosphorylates and activates the mTOR kinase, a negative regulator of autophagy. Inhibition of mTOR has been linked to autophagy induction in metabolic syndrome. For instance, obesity was reported to inhibit autophagy in the liver. In addition to activation of Akt–mTOR signaling, obesity also induces the calcium-dependent protease calpain, leading to cleavage and degradation of Atg7 and, ultimately, inhibition of autophagy. Similarly, a recent study in *Drosophila* demonstrates that high-fat diet-induced obesity and cardiac dysfunction through activation of the TOR signaling pathway and suppression of TOR signaling protected the heart against high-fat diet-induced cardiac dysfunction (Birse *et al.*, 2010). Because TOR is a primary inhibitor of the autophagic pathway, it is reasonable to propose that a high-fat diet may inhibit autophagy in this model. However, Mellor *et al.* reported that upregulation of autophagy is associated with decreased phosphorylation of Akt and S6 kinase, an mTOR downstream molecule, in a type 2 diabetic mouse model (Mellor *et al.*, 2011). In this animal model, 12 weeks of 60% fructose diet treatment induced systemic insulin resistance, as signified by impaired glucose tolerance and hyperglycemia. Concomitantly, downstream signaling of the class I phosphatidylinositol 3-kinase (PI3K) pathway is inactivated and the autophagic markers, lipidated LC3B (LC3B-II/LC3B-I) and p62, are upregulated. Activation of myocardial autophagy is accompanied by elevated production of ROS, fibrosis, and cardiomyocyte loss (without indication of apoptosis induction). These results suggest that, in insulin-resistant myocardium, suppression of Akt and S6 kinase as well as activation of autophagy has a detrimental impact on cardiomyocyte viability in the high fructose-induced diabetic mouse model. It is not yet clear how these contradictions may be explained. More investigations are warranted to determine how the PI3K–Akt signaling pathway can both promote and suppress autophagy in metabolic syndrome.

ACTIVATION OF AMPK ATTENUATES DIABETIC CARDIOMYOPATHY BY ACTIVATION OF AUTOPHAGY

In the heart, AMPK is responsible for activation of glucose uptake and glycolysis during low-flow ischemia, and plays an important role in limiting apoptotic activity associated with ischemia and reperfusion. Activation of AMPK by metformin has been shown to improve cardiac function and reduce the incidence of myocardial infarction in diabetic patients. Several studies have provided evidence linking the AMPK signaling pathway to autophagy. Compound C, a specific AMPK inhibitor, or a dominant-negative (DN) form of AMPK inhibits starvation-induced autophagy in various mammalian cells. Glucose deprivation induces autophagy via activation of AMPK and inhibition of mTOR in isolated cardiomyocytes (Matsui et al., 2007), whereas autophagy induced by myocardial ischemia is suppressed in transgenic mice overexpressing a DN-AMPK (Matsui et al., 2007). Interestingly, AMPK activity in diabetic OVE26 mice is significantly suppressed, and decreased cardiac AMPK activity is associated with lower Beclin 1 levels and defective autophagy; chronic metformin therapy restores Beclin 1 expression and autophagic activity in wild-type diabetic hearts, but this effect is abolished in mice deficient in AMPKα2, indicating that AMPK regulates cardiac autophagy in diabetic cardiomyopathy.

AMPK has been identified as a positive regulator of autophagy in response to energy depletion and ischemic injury. AMPK was thought to regulate autophagy through inhibition of mammalian target of rapamycin complex 1, a negative regulator of autophagy, either by phosphorylation of tuberous sclerosis complex 2, which in turn deactivates the Rheb GTPase, or by phosphorylation of Raptor. In the diabetic heart the TSC–mTOR signaling pathway is activated, as reflected by decreased phosphorylation of Raptor at both Ser722 and Ser792, and increased phosphorylation of mTOR at both Ser2448 and Thr2446, as well as its downstream effectors, 4E binding protein 1 (4EBP1) and p70 ribosomal protein S6 kinase 1 (p70 S6K1). Activation of AMPK by metformin inhibits the TSC–mTOR pathway and restores cardiac autophagy in diabetic mice (Xie et al., 2011b). It is likely that diabetes activates TSC–mTOR signaling through inactivation of AMPK, which inhibits the ULK1 kinase complex, preventing the initiation of autophagy.

In addition, AMPK can regulate the interaction of autophagy protein Beclin 1 with anti-apoptotic protein B-cell lymphoma 2 (Bcl-2), a switch between autophagy and apoptosis, in the development of diabetic cardiomyopathy. Beclin 1 is a part of the class III PI3K lipid complex, which is required for initiation of autophagy. Binding of Bcl-2 to Beclin 1 inhibits Beclin 1-mediated autophagy via sequestration of Beclin 1 away from class III PI3K. A strong interaction between Beclin 1 and Bcl-2 is observed in H9c2 cells treated with elevated glucose levels, and in hearts from diabetic animals. Treatment of cells or animals with metformin to activate AMPK resulted in disruption of the association between Beclin 1 and Bcl-2, and the free Beclin 1 bound to class III PI3K to form a kinase complex, leading to initiation of autophagy (He et al., 2012).

Mechanistically, AMPK can directly phosphorylate the c-Jun N-terminal kinases (JNK1); inhibition of AMPK in the presence of hyperglycemia decreases phosphorylation of JNK1 and Bcl-2, enhances the interaction between Beclin 1 and Bcl-2, and suppresses autophagic activity. Activation of AMPK by metformin or overexpression of constitutively active JNK1 stimulated the JNK1–Bcl-2 pathway, leading to dissociation of the Beclin 1–Bcl-2 complex and restoration of autophagy. These effects were blocked by inhibition of JNK1. More importantly, suppression of autophagy by inhibition of JNK1 prevented the apoptotic cell death induced by high glucose levels, indicating that JNK1–Bcl-2 signaling is a crucial pathway involved in AMPK promotion of cardiomyocyte survival under diabetic conditions (He et al., 2012).

Autophagy plays an essential role in cell growth, development, and homeostasis. Constitutive autophagy helps to maintain a balance between the synthesis, degradation, and subsequent recycling of cellular components. It allows degradation of misfolded proteins that may be toxic to the cell, and removal of damaged organelles such as mitochondria to reduce oxidative stress and promote remodeling for survival. In addition, phosphorylated Bcl-2 could preserve the integrity of the mitochondrial outer membrane and prevent pro-apoptotic proteins from escaping (or being released) into the cytoplasm, thus protecting against apoptosis. Therefore, activation of AMPK prevents diabetes-suppressed autophagy and protects against apoptotic cell death through disruption of the Bcl-2 and Beclin 1 complex under diabetic conditions.

In conclusion, activation of AMPK restores cardiac autophagy, protects against cardiac apoptosis, and ultimately improves cardiac structure and function through stimulation of JNK1–Bcl-2 signaling and subsequent dissociation of Beclin 1 and Bcl-2. These findings provide new insights into the role of autophagy in the development of diabetic cardiomyopathy, deepen our understanding of how AMPK regulates autophagy, and suggest that specific modulation of autophagy, perhaps by stimulation of AMPK, may represent a novel approach for the treatment of heart failure in diabetic patients.

References

Birse, R.T., Choi, J., Reardon, K., et al., 2010. High-fat-diet-induced obesity and heart dysfunction are regulated by the TOR pathway in. Drosophila. Cell. Metab. 12, 533–544.

Carugo, S., Giannattasio, C., Calchera, I., et al., 2001. Progression of functional and structural cardiac alterations in young normotensive uncomplicated patients with type 1 diabetes mellitus. J. Hypertens. 19, 1675–1680.

Davis, B.J., Xie, Z., Viollet, B., et al., 2006. Activation of the AMP-activated kinase by antidiabetes drug metformin stimulates nitric oxide synthesis in vivo by promoting the association of heat shock protein 90 and endothelial nitric oxide synthase. Diabetes 55, 496–505.

Duncan, J.G., Fong, J.L., Medeiros, D.M., et al., 2007. Insulin-resistant heart exhibits a mitochondrial biogenic response driven by the peroxisome proliferator-activated receptor-alpha/PGC-1alpha gene regulatory pathway. Circulation 115, 909–917.

Epstein, P.N., Overbeek, P.A., Means, A.R., 1989. Calmodulin-induced early-onset diabetes in transgenic mice. Cell 58, 1067–1073.

Green, D.R., Kroemer, G., 2004. The pathophysiology of mitochondrial cell death. Science 305, 626–629.

Gundewar, S., Calvert, J.W., Jha, S., et al., 2009. Activation of AMP-activated protein kinase by metformin improves left ventricular function and survival in heart failure. Circ. Res. 104, 403–411.

He, C., Zhu, H., Li, H., et al., 2012. Dissociation of Bcl-2-Beclin1 complex by activated AMPK enhances cardiac autophagy and protects against cardiomyocyte apoptosis in diabetes. Diabetes, doi: 10.2337/db12- 0533 (Epub ahead of print).

Kabeya, Y., Mizushima, N., Ueno, T., et al., 2000. LC3, a mammalian homologue of yeast Apg8p, is localized in autophagosome membranes after processing. EMBO J. 19, 5720–5728.

Kaniuk, N.A., Kiraly, M., Bates, H., et al., 2007. Ubiquitinated-protein aggregates form in pancreatic beta-cells during diabetes-induced oxidative stress and are regulated by autophagy. Diabetes 56, 930–939.

Kannel, W.B., McGee, D.L., 1979. Diabetes and cardiovascular disease. The Framingham study. JAMA 241, 2035–2038.

Kihara, A., Kabeya, Y., Ohsumi, Y., et al., 2001. Beclin-phosphatidylinositol 3-kinase complex functions at the trans-Golgi network. EMBO Rep. 2, 330–335.

Kim, I., Rodriguez-Enriquez, S., Lemasters, J.J., 2007. Selective degradation of mitochondria by mitophagy. Arch. Biochem. Biophys. 462, 245–253.

Klionsky, D.J., Cuervo, A.M., Seglen, P.O., 2007. Methods for monitoring autophagy from yeast to human. Autophagy 3, 181–206.

Kostin, S., Pool, L., Elsasser, A., et al., 2003. Myocytes die by multiple mechanisms in failing human hearts. Circ. Res. 92, 715–724.

Kukidome, D., Nishikawa, T., Sonoda, K., et al., 2006. Activation of AMP-activated protein kinase reduces hyperglycemia-induced mitochondrial reactive oxygen species production and promotes mitochondrial biogenesis in human umbilical vein endothelial cells. Diabetes 55, 120–127.

Kuma, A., Hatano, M., Matsui, M., et al., 2004. The role of autophagy during the early neonatal starvation period. Nature 432, 1032–1036.

Kuo, T.H., Moore, K.H., Giacomelli, F., et al., 1983. Defective oxidative metabolism of heart mitochondria from genetically diabetic mice. Diabetes 32, 781–787.

Levine, B., Yuan, J., 2005. Autophagy in cell death: an innocent convict? J. Clin. Invest. 115, 2679–2688.

Li, J., Coven, D.L., Miller, E.J., et al., 2006. Activation of AMPK alpha- and gamma-isoform complexes in the intact ischemic rat heart. Am. J. Physiol. Heart Circ. Physiol. 291, H1927–H1934.

Matsui, Y., Takagi, H., Qu, X., et al., 2007. Distinct roles of autophagy in the heart during ischemia and reperfusion: roles of AMP-activated protein kinase and Beclin 1 in mediating autophagy. Circ. Res. 100, 914–922.

Mellor, K.M., Bell, J.R., Young, M.J., et al., 2011. Myocardial autophagy activation and suppressed survival signaling is associated with insulin resistance in fructose-fed mice. J. Mol. Cell Cardiol. 50, 1035–1043.

Miyata, S., Takemura, G., Kawase, Y., et al., 2006. Autophagic cardiomyocyte death in cardiomyopathic hamsters and its prevention by granulocyte colony-stimulating factor. Am. J. Pathol. 168, 386–397.

Nakai, A., Yamaguchi, O., Takeda, T., et al., 2007. The role of autophagy in cardiomyocytes in the basal state and in response to hemodynamic stress. Nat. Med. 13, 619–624.

Qu, X., Yu, J., Bhagat, G., et al., 2003. Promotion of tumorigenesis by heterozygous disruption of the beclin 1 autophagy gene. J. Clin. Invest. 112, 1809–1820.

Rothen-Rutishauser, B.M., Ehler, E., Perriard, E., et al., 1998. Different behaviour of the non-sarcomeric cytoskeleton in neonatal and adult rat cardiomyocytes. J. Mol. Cell Cardiol. 30, 19–31.

Rubler, S., Dlugash, J., Yuceoglu, Y.Z., et al., 1972. New type of cardiomyopathy associated with diabetic glomerulosclerosis. Am. J. Cardiol. 30, 595–602.

Sharma, S., Adrogue, J.V., Golfman, L., et al., 2004. Intramyocardial lipid accumulation in the failing human heart resembles the lipotoxic rat heart. FASEB J 18, 1692–1700.

Sriwijitkamol, A., Ivy, J.L., Christ-Roberts, C., et al., 2006. LKB1-AMPK signaling in muscle from obese insulin-resistant Zucker rats and effects of training. Am. J. Physiol. Endocrinol. Metab. 290, E925–E932.

Stratton, I.M., Adler, A.I., Neil, H.A., et al., 2000. Association of glycaemia with macrovascular and microvascular complications of type 2 diabetes (UKPDS 35): prospective observational study. BMJ 321, 405–412.

Tian, R., Musi, N., D'Agostino, J., et al., 2001. Increased adenosine monophosphate-activated protein kinase activity in rat hearts with pressure-overload hypertrophy. Circulation 104, 1664–1669.

Vavvas, D., Apazidis, A., Saha, A.K., et al., 1997. Contraction-induced changes in acetyl-CoA carboxylase and 5'-AMP-activated kinase in skeletal muscle. J. Biol. Chem. 272, 13255–13261.

Xie, Z., Dong, Y., Scholz, R., et al., 2008. Phosphorylation of LKB1 at serine 428 by protein kinase C-zeta is required for metformin-enhanced activation of the AMP-activated protein kinase in endothelial cells. Circulation 117, 952–962.

Xie, Z., Dong, Y., Zhang, J., et al., 2009. Identification of the serine 307 of LKB1 as a novel phosphorylation site essential for its nucleocytoplasmic transport and endothelial cell angiogenesis. Mol. Cell Biol. 29, 3582–3596.

Xie, Z., Lau, K., Eby, B., et al., 2011a. Improvement of cardiac functions by chronic metformin treatment is associated with enhanced cardiac autophagy in diabetic OVE26 mice. Diabetes 60, 1770–1778.

Xie, Z., He, C., Zou, M.H., 2011b. AMP-activated protein kinase modulates cardiac autophagy in diabetic cardiomyopathy. Autophagy 7, 1254–1255.

Yue, Z., Jin, S., Yang, C., et al., 2003. Beclin 1, an autophagy gene essential for early embryonic development, is a haploinsufficient tumor suppressor. Proc. Natl. Acad. Sci. U.S.A. 100, 15077–15082.

Zhu, H., Tannous, P., Johnstone, J.L., et al., 2007. Cardiac autophagy is a maladaptive response to hemodynamic stress. J. Clin. Invest. 117, 1782–1793.

Hyperglycemia-Associated Oxidative Stress Induces Autophagy: Involvement of the ROS-ERK/JNK-p53 Pathway

Ying Tang, Jiangang Long, and Jiankang Liu

Abstract

Hyperglycemia refers to a condition in which an excessive amount of glucose circulates in the blood plasma. A wide range of evidence has proved hyperglycemia to be a great inducer of reactive oxygen species (ROS), through which various processes and signaling transduction cascades are activated or inhibited. Bursts of ROS can be produced by mitochondria, NADPH oxidase, and xanthine oxidase under hyperglycemia. These excessive ROS will further cause oxidative stress and contribute to the development of hyperglycemia complications. One of the downstream processes affected by redox imbalance is autophagy. Increasing evidence

© 2014 Elsevier Inc. All rights reserved.

shows disturbed autophagy in cell lines treated with high glucose or in animals under hyperglycemia. The signaling pathways involved in are quite controversial, however. Here, we focus on the ROS-ERK/JNK-p53 pathway and discuss its potential role in activating autophagy in the condition of hyperglycemia.

INTRODUCTION

The term "hyperglycemia" has a Greek origin, with "hyper" meaning excessive, "glyc" meaning sweet, and "emia" meaning blood. The blood glucose level varies in the course of a day. In general, the normal range of fasting glucose concentration is about 3.98–5.6 mmol/L, and a concentration higher than 7 mmol/L is defined as hyperglycemia. Besides an excessive glucose circulating level, hyperglycemia is also accompanied by abnormal plasma lipoprotein metabolism and an elevation in circulating nucleotide levels. Temporary hyperglycemia is often benign and asymptomatic, but acute hyperglycemia involving extremely high glucose levels can rapidly raise serious complications. It has been reported that postprandial hyperglycemia impairs vascular endothelial function in healthy men by inducing lipid peroxidation and reducing NO biosynthesis (Mah et al., 2011), and facilitates development of cardiovascular disease in subjects with impaired glucose tolerance (Ceriello, 2004). In type 1 diabetic patients, a few hours of hyperglycemia leads to a reduction of isometric muscle performance, which plays a role in the development of fatigue in diabetes (Andersen et al., 2005). Chronic hyperglycemia in diabetes is a major cause of various diabetic complications, including nephropathy, retinopathy, and neuropathy.

Blood glucose is strictly regulated in health, while homoeostasis of fasting and post-load glucose becomes abnormal during diseases. Fasting blood glucose is determined by endogenous glucose production, which depends mostly on the liver, while changes in glucose concentration after a meal are caused by suppression of endogenous glucose production and upregulation of total glucose uptake, which are regulated by insulin and affected by the insulin sensitivity of the main insulin target tissues. Secretion and biosynthesis of insulin by β cells increase rapidly in response to elevated blood glucose. However, when insulin fails to dispose of excessive blood glucose, in cases such as insulin resistance, the resulted chronic hyperglycemia will cause impaired insulin biosynthesis and secretion, which further leads to apparent hyperglycemia and hyperglycemic damages in organs.

During treatment for hyperglycemia or high glucose, both activated and inhibited autophagy has been reported in varies tissues and cell lines, suggesting a complicated regulation of autophagy in this condition. However, the regulatory mechanism has not yet been well clarified. Four pathways – the polyol pathway, hexosamine pathway, diacylglycerol–protein kinase C pathway, and advanced glycation end-products pathway – are activated and mediate the deleterious effect of hyperglycemia. They are evidenced to potentially induce oxidative stress, which further has an influence on autophagy. Previously, our study in diabetic Goto–Kakizaki rats found excessive autophagy in skeletal muscle that was accompanied by overproduction of ROS and activation of the ERK/JNK-p53 pathway (Yan et al., 2012), indicating a potential role of an upregulated ROS-ERK/JNK-p53 pathway in the activation of autophagy in hyperglycemia.

OXIDATIVE STRESS IN HYPERGLYCEMIA

In organisms, ROS form as a natural byproduct of numerous endogenous enzymatic and biological processes. At a proper level ROS have important beneficial roles in the physiological condition, as they induce apoptosis of effete or defective cells and killing of microorganisms and cancer cells by macrophages and cytotoxic lymphocytes (Devasagayam *et al.*, 2004). However, excessive ROS can cause damage by adversely altering lipids, proteins, and DNA, which will lead to loss of enzyme activity and to mutagenesis and carcinogenesis (Devasagayam *et al.*, 2004). When the antioxidant system fails to detoxify reactive intermediates or repair the resulting damage, oxidative stress is induced.

It is now widely accepted that deleterious effects of hyperglycemia observed in disease are partly associated with an overproduction of reactive oxygen species and the subsequently induced oxidative stress.

Sources of ROS in Hyperglycemia

ROS are formed from the reduction of molecular oxygen or by oxidation of water to yield products such as superoxide ($O_2 \cdot^-$), hydrogen oxide (H_2O_2), and hydroxyl radicals ($\cdot OH$). The sources discussed below are considered to be main contributors to ROS generation in hyperglycemia.

1 Electron Transport Chain in Mitochondria

Mitochondria are thought to be responsible for most ROS production in both physiological and pathological conditions. Inside mitochondria, electrons from NADH and $FADH_2$ that are generated by the tricarboxylic acid (TCA) cycle move from complexes I and II through complexes III and IV to oxygen, forming water and causing protons to be pumped across the mitochondrial inner membrane. This drives protons back through the ATP synthase, forming ATP and phosphate. In this scenario, electrons leaking from the respiratory chain may react with oxygen to generate superoxide. Superoxide radicals are normally removed by manganese superoxide dismutase (MnSOD) located in the mitochondrial matrix to generate hydrogen peroxide, which is further converted to oxygen and water in the matrix by catalase and glutathione peroxidase. However, when the rate of hydrogen peroxide generation exceeds that of its removal, heavy metals (Fe^{2+}) can produce highly reactive hydroxyl radicals via the Fenton reaction with hydrogen peroxide.

Hyperglycemia is hypothesized to increase ROS generation through providing excessive glucose to accelerate glycolysis, TCA, and oxidative phosphorylation. Consequently, there is an increase in the ATP/ADP ratio and hyperpolarization of the mitochondrial membrane potential, which results in partial inhibition of electron transport in complex III and accumulation of electrons to coenzyme Q. This in turn leads to partial reduction of oxygen to generate superoxide and other free radicals.

2 NADPH Oxidases

NADPH oxidase (NOX) is a transmembrane enzyme that is located in intracellular organelles and comprises several isoforms, including NOX1–5, NOX oxidase 1 and 2, NOX organizer 1, and NOX activator 1. NOX is activated when it is translocated to the membrane and co-localized with p22^{phox}, p67^{phox}, p47^{phox}, and p40^{phox}. NADPH oxidase is currently the only enzyme family known to produce ROS as its sole function. The electron transfer system in NOX is composed of the C-terminal cytoplasmic region homologous to the prokaryotic enzyme ferredoxin reductase, and the N-terminal six-transmembrane segments containing two hemes, a structure similar to that of cytochrome b of the mitochondrial bc1 complex. NOX mediates the transfer of electrons from cytosolic NADPH, through FAD to penetrate the membrane, via hemes, to oxygen, leading to superoxide generation in the cytoplasm.

Multiple evidences show that activation of NOX contributes to ROS overproduction in hyperglycemia. Monocytes of patients with type 2 diabetes presented higher p22^{phox} expression, p47^{phox} translocation, and oxidative stress (Huang et al., 2011). p22^{phox} and p47^{phox} were found to have increased membrane translocation in tissues of streptozotocin (STZ)-induced diabetic rats (Lei et al., 2012).

3 Xanthine Oxidase

Xanthine oxidase is a form of xanthine oxidoreductase, an enzyme that generates reactive oxygen species such as superoxide radicals and hydrogen peroxide when it catalyzes the oxidation of hypoxanthine to xanthine, and can further catalyze the oxidation of xanthine to uric acid. This enzyme plays an important role in the catabolism of purines in some species, including humans.

The participation of xanthine oxidase in oxidative stress in hyperglycemia is suggested by increased oxidative stress in the muscle of hyperglycemic STZ-induced diabetic mice, which is associated with an increase of xanthine oxidase expression and activity (Bravard et al., 2011). Consistently, increased xanthine oxidase enzyme activity was also found accompanied by increased oxidative stress in the heart of alloxan (ALX)-induced diabetic rats (Das et al., 2011).

Evidence for Excessive Production of ROS in Hyperglycemia

A large amount of clinical evidence has proved the overproduction of ROS and induction of oxidative stress in hyperglycemia, especially in the disease of diabetes. Studies show that plasma and urinary malondialdehyde (MDA, an index of lipid peroxidation) levels were raised whereas plasma total antioxidant activity was reduced in type 2 diabetes patients (Maharjan et al., 2008). Two other biomarkers of oxidative stress, 8-hydroxy-2′-deoxyguanosine (8-OHdG) and acrolein-lysine, were found to be higher in patients with type 1 diabetes (Castilho et al., 2012). Hyperglycemia also tends to induce oxidative stress in patients with non-alcoholic fatty liver disease, as indicated by a significant increase in the leukocyte level of hydrogen peroxide and serum concentration of MDA (Shams et al., 2011).

Increased oxidative stress biomarkers such as MDA (Modak et al., 2011), 8-OHdG (Modak et al., 2011), protein carbonyls (Das et al., 2011; Palsamy and Subramanian, 2011; Yan et al., 2012), and hydroperoxides (Palsamy and Subramanian, 2011) were also found in tissues of various animal models that exhibit hyperglycemia, seemingly resulting from decreased antioxidative enzymes such as catalase (CAT), superoxide dismutase (SOD), glutathione reductase (GR), glutathione peroxidase (GPx), and glutathione-S-transferase (GST) (Das *et al.*, 2011; Modak *et al.*, 2011; Palsamy and Subramanian, 2011), and decreased anti-oxidative molecules such glutathione, uric acid, Vitamin C, and Vitamin E (Das *et al.*, 2011; Modak *et al.*, 2011). However, antioxidant enzymes can sometimes show increased activation in oxidative stress as a resultant compensatory mechanism.

AUTOPHAGY IN HYPERGLYCEMIA

According to present studies, regulation of autophagy is quite complicated in the presence of high glucose. Activated autophagy was found in myocardial tissue of fructose-fed hyperglycemic mice (Mellor *et al.*, 2011), while an opposing result was showed in isolated cardiomyocytes from type 2 diabetic db/db mice (Marsh *et al.*, 2012). Consistently, both upregulated and inhibited autophagy were found in high-glucose treated H9c2 cardiomyoblasts (Younce *et al.*, 2010) and neonatal rat cardiomyocytes (Kobayashi *et al.*, 2012; Younce *et al.*, 2010). Furthermore, enhanced autophagy presented in the adipocytes from type 2 diabetic patients (Öst *et al.*, 2010) and the skeletal muscle of diabetic GK rats (Yan *et al.*, 2012), whereas the liver tissue of both genetic and dietary-induced obesity mice exhibited decreased autophagy (Yang *et al.*, 2010).

To date, autophagy has been shown to be regulated by several signaling pathways, including nutrient signaling, insulin/growth factor pathways, energy sensing, stress response, and pathogen infection. Indeed, in the condition of hyperglycemia, some molecules involved in these signaling pathways are affected. What's more, oxidative stress and endoplasmic reticulum stress have been observed in hyperglycemia, indicating a potential role of these effectors in regulating autophagy in response to high glucose.

ROS-ERK/JNK-p53 PATHWAY ACTIVATES AUTOPHAGY IN HYPERGLYCEMIA

Previously, we reported that autophagy was enhanced in the skeletal muscle of diabetic GK rats, accompanied by oxidative stress, ERK/JNK activation, and p53 upregulation. Supported by further evidence, which will be discussed below, we speculate about a potential role of the activated ROS-ERK/JNK-p53 pathway in enhancing autophagy in hyperglycemia.

The MAPK Signaling Pathway

The MAPK signaling pathway refers to a family of signaling cascades that consists of the ERK (extracellular regulated kinase), JNK (Jun N-terminal kinase), p38 kinase, ERK3/4, and the big mitogen-activated protein kinase 1 (BMK1) pathways. ERKs, JNKs, p38, and BMK1 are all serine/threonine kinases that are directed by a proline residue sharing the same cascade of activation; that is, a MAP kinase kinase kinase (MAPKKK) phosphorylates and activates a MAP kinase kinase, which then phosphorylates and activates a MAP kinase.

ERK/JNK Responds to Oxidative Stress

1   Activation of ERKs by Oxidative Stress

The ERK proteins – which generally refers to ERK1 and ERK2 – reside downstream of the Ras/Raf/MEK/ERK cascade, which is the most studied pathway leading to the activation of the ERK proteins. This cascade is activated following the triggering of cell surface receptors, and involves the regulation of transcription factors and apoptosis related proteins.

ROS are well known activators of ERKs. Mechanisms of ROS-induced ERK activation can be sorted into two types: ligand-independent receptor activation and receptor activation-independent pathways. In the former, ROS can act through growth receptors to induce phosphorylation and activation of ERK. Hydrogen peroxide has been demonstrated to lead to tyrosine phosphorylation of epidermal growth factor (EGF) receptor in the absence of EGF, leading to activation of Ras and subsequent activation of the Raf/MEK/ERK cascade. Although it is still unclear how receptors are activated by ROS at present, some studies suggest that certain Src kinases, reported to be activated by hydrogen peroxide, may be involved. Src was reported to associate with and then phosphorylate the EGF receptor (Haas *et al.*, 2000), then downstream molecules, such as PLC (phospholipase C)-gamma, may participate in the final activation of ERK in various mechanisms (Wang *et al.*, 2001).

Receptor activation is not the only mechanism by which oxygen radicals activate ERK. The second type of activation may occur as a result of inhibition of phosphatase activity. Hydrogen peroxide was found to inhibit protein phosphatases such as protein tyrosine phosphatase (PTP) and protein phosphatase 2A (PP2A) (Whisler *et al.*, 1995), which enabled activation of the ERK signaling pathway.

2   Activation of JNK by Oxidative Stress

c-Jun N-terminal kinases (JNKs), also known as stress activated protein kinases (SAPKs), form an important subgroup of the MAPK family. The JNK pathway has been widely suggested to participate in controlling diverse cellular functions. Similar to the ERK signaling pathway, activation of JNK comprises MAPKKK and MAPKK. JNK is phosphorylated by two cascades – JNNK1/MKK4 and JNKK2/MKK7 – which possess dual specificity on critical threonine and tyrosine residues and result in JNK activation. Upstream of JNKK1 and JNKK2, several MAPKKK have been identified. It has been well established that ROS are potent inducers of JNK. Either adding exogenous or inducing endogenous ROS stimulates JNK activation. At present, both MKK4/MKK7-dependent and -independent signaling have been found to serve as molecular links between ROS and JNK.

ASK1 is a ubiquitously expressed MAPKKK that activates both JNK and p38 by phosphorylation and activation of respective MAPKKs. Activity of ASK1 regulated by redox is controlled by thioredoxin and glutaredoxin, two cellular redox regulatory proteins. Binding of ASK1 to the reduced forms of thioredoxin (Saitoh *et al.*, 1998) and glutaredoxin (Song *et al.*, 2002) results in inhibition of its kinase activity. In the presence of ROS, thioredoxin and glutaredoxin are oxidized and then dissociate from ASK1, leading to its activation (Saitoh *et al.*, 1998; Song *et al.*, 2002). Other proteins, such as 14-3-3 and protein phosphatase 5, are also identified as regulating ASK1 activity by sharing the same pattern.

The MKK4/MKK7-independent regulatory mechanism involves the association of JNK with other proteins, including glutathione S-transferase pi (GST-π), receptor-interacting protein (RIP), and tumor necrosis factor receptor-associated factor 2 (TRAF2). In the presence of hydrogen peroxide, oligomerized GST-π dissociated from JNK, leading to JNK activation (Adler *et al.*, 1999). In contrast, hydrogen peroxide treatment resulted in the binding of JNK to RIP and TRAF2, which also activated JNK (Shen *et al.*, 2004).

ERK/JNK Involved in p53 Pathway

p53 plays a critical role in the cellular response to acute stress, and thereby possesses prominent tumor-suppressing function. In physiological conditions, p53 is strictly controlled by Mdm2 mediated ubiquitination and proteasomal degradation. In response to damage, p53 undergoes reversible post-translational modifications such as phosphorylation, acetylization, ubiquitinoylation, and sumoylation, which allows for its dissociation from the suppressor. Phosphorylation of p53 is classically regarded as the first essential step of p53 stabilization. The MAPK proteins have been proved to be involved in this process, as evidenced by observations that p53 activation in response to cell death inducers is mediated by ERK and/or JNK, and the main action of ERK and JNK on p53 is thought to be through their phosphorylation activity.

JNK will phosphorylate p53 at various residues in response to different stimuli, such as UVB radiation, oxidative stress, and DNA damage. The direct role of JNK on p53 phosphorylation is evidenced by observing interaction between JNK and p53 (She *et al.*, 2002), while JNK deficiency resulted in inhibition of p53 (She *et al.*, 2002).

The involvement of ERK in p53 activation is also suggested by numerous studies. Activation of p53, and of p53-mediated growth inhibition and apoptosis, was observed in cells exposed to benzo-(α)-pyrene, while inhibiting ERK reversed p53 phosphorylation and cell death (Lin *et al.*, 2008). Similarly, ERK is also found to interact with and phosphorylate p53 at serine 15 under other conditions that potentially lead to oxidative stress. Additionally, phosphorylation of p53 at this site is inhibited by the MEK1 inhibitor, indicating an upstream role of ERK in inducing phosphorylation and the resultant activation of p53 in response to stress.

Regulation of Autophagy via ERK/JNK-p53 Pathway

p53 controls autophagy in an ambiguous fashion, depending on its subcellular localization and involving transcriptional and transcription-independent mechanisms. To date, the cytoplasmic pool of p53 has been found to play a role in autophagy suppression, but the mechanisms are poorly characterized. On the contrary, the function of nuclear p53 in activating autophagy is better clarified, and is attributed to its ability to transactivate pro-autophagic genes. As evidenced by previous studies, p53 is able to transactivate proteins that participate in autophagy or positively regulate the autophagic signaling axis.

As upstream molecules, the roles of ERK and JNK in mediating autophagy via p53 have been illustrated. In autophagic cell death, both ERK and JNK are responsible for the activation of p53 and the resultant increase of Beclin 1 and LC3 (Cheng *et al.*, 2008). JNK activation can also decrease the association of Beclin 1 and Bcl-2 with induced autophagy, while either p53 deficiency or JNK inhibition blocks autophagy induced by JNK (Hong *et al.*, 2012; Park *et al.*, 2009). Exposure of cells to oridonin upregulates autophagic flux, as evidenced by increased

Beclin 1 and conversion of LC3I to LC3II, which is accompanied by ERK-p53 activation and reversed by ERK and p53 inhibition or deficiency (Ye *et al.*, 2012). These all suggest that the ERK/JNK-p53 pathway positively regulates autophagy in response to various stimulations.

Hyperglycemia Tends to Enhance Autophagy via ROS-ERK/JNK-p53 Pathway

Autophagy has been reported to be ambiguously regulated in hyperglycemia, as discussed previously in this chapter. Distinct outcomes may result from complicated signaling pathways that can compete or cooperate to activate or suppress autophagy. In addition, the measurement of autophagy itself is a great challenge. However, it has been widely suggested that autophagy is activated to function against ROS production in conditions of oxidative stress – a major characteristic in hyperglycemia. Here, without taking other signaling pathways into consideration, we speculate that hyperglycemia-associated oxidative stress tends to increase autophagy via the ROS-ERK/JNK-p53 pathway.

It has been reported that ROS can regulate autophagy directly through modulating the modification of autophagy-related proteins. Another study reported that SOD2 deficiency tends to aggravate oxidative stress but suppress autophagy in the brain of hyperglycemic mice (Mehta *et al.*, 2011), suggesting that hydrogen peroxide may play a significant role in hyperglycemia-associated autophagy, since the generation of hydrogen peroxide maybe inhibited by SOD2 deficiency.

As discussed above, hydrogen peroxide is able to induce activation of both ERK and JNK *in vitro* via different mechanisms. In the condition of hyperglycemia, activated ERK and JNK have also been reported (Nagai *et al.*, 2012; Yan *et al.*, 2012), and this hyperglycemia-promoted activation is abrogated by ROS inhibitors (Singh *et al.*, 2012). As well as inducing oxidative stress and ERK/JNK activation, high glucose can also promote nuclear accumulation of p53 (Liu *et al.*, 2011) – an indispensable process for p53 to activate autophagy. All these evidences together indicate a scheme in which high glucose-induced oxidative stress causes autophagy upregulation through activation of ERK/JNK and resultant p53 stabilization and nuclear translocation. Indeed, this mechanism has been well verified in other conditions discussed previously in this review.

DISCUSSION

Hyperglycemia has been shown to be a deleterious condition leading to development of serious diabetic complications in various organs. It also presents as a risk factor for other diseases. In the hyperglycemic condition, cells undergo homeostatic disturbances such as oxidative stress and autophagy perturbation. Since autophagy plays such an important role in cellular function, regulation of autophagy in hyperglycemia has received great attention. However, as reported by different studies, autophagy can be either activated or inhibited in response to high glucose. Another difficult issue of significant importance is how autophagy is modulated. Herein, based on our previous study in skeletal muscle of diabetic GK rats, we suggest that hyperglycemia-associated oxidative stress tends to induce autophagy via the ROS-ERK/JNK-p53 signaling cascade, a pathway through which autophagy was also enhanced in response to other stimulations. However, to our knowledge, there is still no direct evidence showing that autophagy can be inhibited by disturbing the ROS-ERK/JNK-p53 pathway in hyperglycemia at present.

Further, another question that remains to be solved is whether JNK and ERK play different roles in the scenario of hyperglycemia. ERK and JNK are considered to process opposing functions; that is JNK activation promotes whereas ERK activation inhibits superoxide-induced cell death. These results suggest that ERK and JNK are probably activated to develop different responses to high glucose-induced oxidative stress. However, both ERK and JNK have been shown to promote activation of autophagy and autophagic cell death. Thus, identification of the respective functions of ERK and JNK in oxidative stress-induced autophagy may provide targets for intervening and treating diseases caused by autophagy perturbation.

What's more, activation of both ERK and JNK by ROS needs triggering by a series of upstream factors, as discussed previously in this chapter. However, only a limited number of studies have reported mechanisms of how ERK and JNK are activated in hyperglycemia. A previous study showed that acute hyperglycemia led to activation of Ras and ERK in peripheral blood mononuclear cells (Schiekofer et al., 2003). Recently, hyperglycemia has been found to enhance Src activation via increasing Nox-4 derived ROS in vascular smooth muscle cells (Xi et al., 2012). Since the Src–Ras cascade has been identified to result in both ERK and JNK triggering, this suggests that high glucose-associated oxidative stress may also promote ERK and JNK activation via the Src–Ras signaling pathway. In addition, hyperglycemia is widely reported to be associated with a proinflammatory state, as indicated by increased secretion of cytokines such as TNF-α. Coincidently, it is well established that activation of TNF receptors triggers the activation of JNK signaling, and is thought to be mediated in part by ROS since superoxide and lipid peroxide scavengers inhibit JNK activation. Thus TNF receptor signaling may also serve as a regulatory mechanism that promotes oxidative stress-associated JNK activation in hyperglycemia.

Another unknown is how p53 activates autophagy in the high-glucose state. As suggested by present studies, the induction of autophagy by p53 involves several pathways including AMPK/TSC2/mTOR signaling, pro-apoptotic members of the Bcl-2 protein family, and other molecules responsive to damage. Actually, improper regulation of mTOR and AMPK has been observed in hyperglycemia (Kobayashi et al., 2012; Towler and Hardie 2007), indicating a role of the p53-dependent AMPK/TSC2/mTOR pathway in modulating autophagy in this scenario. The pro-apoptotic members of the Bcl-2 protein family may also play a potential role, as high glucose exposure is always found to result in apoptosis.

However, since more factors that may participate in autophagy regulation have not yet been assessed in conditions of hyperglycemia or oxidative stress, and there is still a lack of direct evidence showing that the ROS-ERK/JNK pathway induces autophagy (at least partly) through a p53-dependent mechanism in response to high glucose, we can't exclude the contribution of other signaling downstream of ROS-ERK/JNK to regulated autophagy in hyperglycemia.

References

Adler, V., Yin, Z., Fuchs, S.Y., et al., 1999. Regulation of JNK signaling by GSTp. EMBO J. 18, 1321–1334.

Andersen, H., Schmitz, O., Nielsen, S., 2005. Decreased isometric muscle strength after acute hyperglycaemia in type 1 diabetic patients. Diabet. Med. 22, 1401–1407.

Bravard, A., Bonnard, C., Durand, A., et al., 2011. Inhibition of xanthine oxidase reduces hyperglycemia-induced oxidative stress and improves mitochondrial alterations in skeletal muscle of diabetic mice. Am. J. Physiol. Endocrinol. Metab. 300, E581–E591.

Castilho, Á.F., Aveleira, C.A., Leal, E.C., et al., 2012. Heme oxygenase-1 protects retinal endothelial cells against high glucose-and oxidative/nitrosative stress-induced toxicity. PloS ONE 7, e42428.

Ceriello, A., 2004. Impaired glucose tolerance and cardiovascular disease: the possible role of post-prandial hyperglycemia. Am. Heart J. 147, 803–807.

Cheng, Y., Qiu, F., Tashiro, S., et al., 2008. ERK and JNK mediate TNFα-induced p53 activation in apoptotic and autophagic L929 cell death. Biochem. Biophys. Res. Commun. 376, 483–488.

Das, J., Vasan, V., Sil, P.C., 2011. Taurine exerts hypoglycemic effect in alloxan-induced diabetic rats, improves insulin-mediated glucose transport signaling pathway in heart and ameliorates cardiac oxidative stress and apoptosis. Toxicol. Appl. Pharmacol. 258, 296–308.

Devasagayam, T., Tilak, J., Boloor, K., et al., 2004. Free radicals and antioxidants in human health: current status and future prospects. J. Assoc. Physicians. India 52, 794–804.

Haas, M., Askari, A., Xie, Z., 2000. Involvement of Src and epidermal growth factor receptor in the signal-transducing function of Na+/K+-ATPase. J. Biol. Chem. 275, 27832–27837.

Hong, M., Gao, J., Cui, J., et al., 2012. Effect of c-Jun NH2-terminal kinase-mediated p53 expression on neuron autophagy following traumatic brain injury in rats. Chin. Med. J. 125, 2019–2024.

Huang, X., Sun, M., Li, D., et al., 2011. Augmented NADPH oxidase activity and p22phox expression in monocytes underlie oxidative stress of patients with type 2 diabetes mellitus. Diabetes Res. Clin. Pract. 91, 371–380.

Kobayashi, S., Xu, X., Chen, K., et al., 2012. Suppression of autophagy is protective in high glucose-induced cardiomyocyte injury. Autophagy 8, 577–592.

Lei, S., Liu, Y., Liu, H., et al., 2012. Effects of N-acetylcysteine on nicotinamide dinucleotide phosphate oxidase activation and antioxidant status in heart, lung, liver and kidney in streptozotocin-induced diabetic rats. Yonsei. Med. J. 53, 294–303.

Lin, T., Mak, N., Yang, M., 2008. MAPK regulate p53-dependent cell death induced by benzo [a] pyrene: involvement of p53 phosphorylation and acetylation. Toxicology 247, 145–153.

Liu, S., Yuan, Q., Zhao, S., et al., 2011. High glucose induces apoptosis in embryonic neural progenitor cells by a pathway involving protein PKCδ. Cell. Signal. 23, 1366–1374.

Mah, E., Noh, S.K., Ballard, K.D., et al., 2011. Postprandial hyperglycemia impairs vascular endothelial function in healthy men by inducing lipid peroxidation and increasing asymmetric dimethylarginine: arginine. J. Nutr. 141, 1961–1968.

Maharjan, B., Jha, J., Adhikari, D., et al., 2008. A study of oxidative stress, antioxidant status and lipid profile in diabetic patient in the western region of Nepal. Kathmandu Univ. Med. J. 6, 16–22.

Marsh, S.A., Powell, P.C., Dell'Italia, L.J., et al., 2012. Cardiac O-GlcNAcylation blunts autophagic signaling in the diabetic heart. Life Sci. (Epub ahead of print).

Mehta, S.L., Lin, Y., Chen, W., et al., 2011. Manganese superoxide dismutase deficiency exacerbates ischemic brain damage under hyperglycemic conditions by altering autophagy. Transl. Stroke Res. 2, 42–50.

Mellor, K.M., Bell, J.R., Young, M.J., et al., 2011. Myocardial autophagy activation and suppressed survival signaling is associated with insulin resistance in fructose-fed mice. J. Mol. Cell Cardiol. 50, 1035–1043.

Modak, M.A., Parab, P.B., Ghaskadbi, S.S., 2011. Control of hyperglycemia significantly improves oxidative stress profile of pancreatic islets. Islets 3, 234–240.

Nagai, K., Fukushima, T., Oike, H., et al., 2012. High glucose increases the expression of proinflammatory cytokines and secretion of TNFα and β-hexosaminidase in human mast cells. Eur. J. Pharmacol. 687, 39–45.

Öst, A., Svensson, K., Ruishalme, I., et al., 2010. Attenuated mTOR signaling and enhanced autophagy in adipocytes from obese patients with type 2 diabetes. Mol. Med. 16, 235–246.

Palsamy, P., Subramanian, S., 2011. Resveratrol protects diabetic kidney by attenuating hyperglycemia-mediated oxidative stress and renal inflammatory cytokines via Nrf2–Keap1 signaling. Biochim. Biophys. Acta 1812, 719–731.

Park, K.J., Lee, S.H., Lee, C.H., et al., 2009. Upregulation of Beclin-1 expression and phosphorylation of Bcl-2 and p53 are involved in the JNK-mediated autophagic cell death. Biochem. Biophys. Res. Commun. 382, 726–729.

Saitoh, M., Nishitoh, H., Fujii, M., et al., 1998. Mammalian thioredoxin is a direct inhibitor of apoptosis signal-regulating kinase (ASK) 1. EMBO J. 17, 2596–2606.

Schiekofer, S., Andrassy, M., Chen, J., et al., 2003. Acute hyperglycemia causes intracellular formation of CML and activation of ras, p42/44 MAPK, and nuclear factor κB in PBMCs. Diabetes 52, 621–633.

Shams, M.E.E., Al-Gayyar, M.M.H., Barakat, E.A.M.E., 2011. Type 2 diabetes mellitus-induced hyperglycemia in patients with NAFLD and normal LFTs: relationship to lipid profile, oxidative stress and pro-inflammatory cytokines. Sci. Pharm. 79, 623–634.

She, Q.B., Ma, W.Y., Dong, Z., 2002. Role of MAP kinases in UVB-induced phosphorylation of p53 at serine 20. Oncogene 21, 1580–1589.

Shen, H.M., Lin, Y., Choksi, S., et al., 2004. Essential roles of receptor-interacting protein and TRAF2 in oxidative stress-induced cell death. Mol. Cell Biol. 24, 5914–5922.

Singh, A.B., Guleria, R.S., Nizamutdinova, I.T., et al., 2012. High Glucose-induced repression of RAR/RXR in cardiomyocytes is mediated through oxidative stress/JNK signaling. J. Cell Physiol. 227, 2632–2644.

Song, J.J., Rhee, J.G., Suntharalingam, M., et al., 2002. Role of glutaredoxin in metabolic oxidative stress glutaredoxin as a sensor of oxidative stress mediated by H2O2. J. Biol. Chem. 277, 46566–46575.

Towler, M.C., Hardie, D.G., 2007. AMP-activated protein kinase in metabolic control and insulin signaling. Circ. Res. 100, 328–341.

Wang, X.T., McCullough, K.D., Wang, X.J., et al., 2001. Oxidative stress-induced phospholipase C-γ1 activation enhances cell survival. J. Biol. Chem. 276, 28364–28371.

Whisler, R.L., Goyette, M.A., Grants, I.S., et al., 1995. Sublethal levels of oxidant stress stimulate multiple serine/threonine kinases and suppress protein phosphatases in Jurkat T cells. Arch. Biochem. Biophys. 319, 23–25.

Xi, G., Shen, X., Maile, L.A., et al., 2012. Hyperglycemia enhances IGF-I–stimulated Src activation via increasing Nox4-derived reactive oxygen species in a PKCζ-dependent manner in vascular smooth muscle cells. Diabetes 61, 104–113.

Yan, J., Feng, Z., Liu, J., et al., 2012. Enhanced autophagy plays a cardinal role in mitochondrial dysfunction in type 2 diabetic Goto–Kakizaki (GK) rats: ameliorating effects of (−)-epigallocatechin-3-gallate. J. Nutr. Biochem. 23, 716–724.

Yang, L., Li, P., Fu, S., et al., 2010. Defective hepatic autophagy in obesity promotes ER stress and causes insulin resistance. Cell Metab. 11, 467–478.

Ye, Y., Wang, H., Xu, L., et al., 2012. Oridonin induces apoptosis and autophagy in murine fibrosarcoma L929 cells partly via NO-ERK-p53 positive-feedback loop signaling pathway. Acta Pharmacol. Sin. 33, 1055–1061.

Younce, C.W., Wang, K., Kolattukudy, P.E., 2010. Hyperglycaemia-induced cardiomyocyte death is mediated via MCP-1 production and induction of a novel zinc-finger protein MCPIP. Cardiovasc. Res. 87, 665–674.

Role of Autophagy in Cellular Defense Against Inflammation

Eun-Kyeong Jo, Dong-Min Shin, and Jae-Min Yuk

Abstract

Innate immune responses provide the first line of defense against invading pathogens or damaged self-molecules. However, both dysregulation and hyperactivation of immune responses are linked to inflammatory or autoimmune diseases. Autophagy is a component of primary host defense that mediates elimination of pathogens, particularly intracellular microbes. Recent advances have shown that autophagy plays an important role in the regulation of inflammation, thus providing new insights into the relationship between autophagy and inflammation. During innate immune responses, nuclear factor-κB signaling plays an important role in regulation of the autophagy pathway. Two key energy/growth sensors, the AMP-activated protein kinase and the mammalian target of rapamycin, play important roles in the autophagy-regulated signaling network connected with inflammation. Abnormalities or defects in autophagy appear

© 2014 Elsevier Inc. All rights reserved.

to lead to pathologic inflammatory status with defective microbial killing, as in cases of immunopathologic responses in Crohn's disease, lung inflammation, sepsis, or other inflammatory diseases. Furthermore, basal autophagy can play an important dual role in the regulation of inflammasome activation, thus shaping overall immune homeostasis, and in the unconventional secretion of a leaderless cytokine interleukin-1β. Numerous human pathologies and diseases related to inflammasome activation are impacted by defective or dysregulated autophagy. In this overview, we describe recent advances in the roles of autophagy in the regulation of chronic inflammatory conditions and pathological reactions in autoimmune diseases.

INTRODUCTION

As frontline cells in immune defense, innate immune cells, including neutrophils, macrophages, and dendritic cells (DCs), receive important input messages from extracellular and intracellular environments. These messages are recognized and integrated by pattern-recognition receptors (PRRs), and, in turn, the appropriate immune responses destroy or eliminate invading pathogens or limit damaging signals. This coordinated signaling network is generated by specialized molecular mechanisms that are synchronized and maintain the fine balance between protective immune responses and pathologic inflammation. The antagonistic regulatory pathways against hyper- and chronic inflammation appear to be important in dampening unwanted immunopathologic host responses (Hajishengallis and Lambris, 2011).

Fundamentally, the autophagy process is a stress response to harsh conditions, and integrates other multiple forms of cellular stress responses, including nutrient deprivation as well as hypoxic and oxidative stresses. The autophagy pathway is known to function in inflammatory stress as a crucial biological component of homeostatic regulation against proinflammatory responses when the host encounters a variety of microbial and other hazardous insults from the environment (Levine *et al.*, 2011). The autophagy pathway has a profound influence on communication with the immune system.

Inflammation is involved in the pathology of many major human diseases, including cardiovascular diseases, rheumatoid arthritis, diabetes, obesity, and cancer. Recent genome-wide and animal studies have revealed the intersection between autophagy and human inflammatory diseases. For example, autophagy (atg)-related genes that encode essential components of autophagic machinery, including Atg16L1 and immunity-related GTPase family M protein (IRGM), were found to be major genetic risk factors for Crohn's disease. Additionally, an innate cytosolic receptor, nucleotide-binding oligomerization domain containing proteins 2 (NOD2), is involved in the induction of antibacterial autophagosomes, and NOD2 mutation is linked to Crohn's disease (Saitoh and Akira, 2010). Accumulating evidence suggests that the involvement of autophagy in the pathogenesis of multiple human diseases is mediated through the regulation of autophagy in inflammatory responses.

Activation of the "inflammasome," a large intracellular protein complex that activates caspase-1 and synthesis of mature interleukin (IL)-1β, is a key mechanism in the inflammatory circuit. Mitochondria play a key role in the activation of inflammasomes and other inflammatory responses, and damaged mitochondria can be targeted by autophagy (mitophagy). The autophagy pathway plays a dominant role in cytoprotective and anti-inflammatory effects against a variety of inflammatory pathologies. In human diseases related to inflammasome activation, autophagy is partially responsible for the removal of dysfunctional mitochondria (Green *et al.*, 2011). Reactive oxygen species (ROS) are highly reactive small molecules that are potentially harmful due to their ability to oxidize proteins, lipids, and DNA. However, ROS are being recognized as important signaling molecules that control diverse biological responses – including autophagy pathways – to the presence of bacteria. Notably, recent works point to the role of ROS of mitochondrial origin in the reduction–oxidation regulation of autophagy and mitophagy (Scherz-Shouval and Elazar, 2011). The molecular mechanisms underlying autophagy in inflammatory responses are mediated through the mammalian target of rapamycin (mTOR) kinase and the AMP-activated protein kinase (AMPK), both key energy sensors important in cellular metabolism regulation (Figure 9.1).

Although further studies are required to elucidate the mechanisms by which host autophagy regulates inflammatory responses, potential therapeutic strategies for the prevention and treatment of inflammation-related human diseases might include the control of autophagy. Here, we focus on the roles of and mechanisms by which autophagy regulates inflammation and autophagy-based strategies for controlling human diseases associated with inflammation. The human diseases discussed in this chapter have been summarized in Table 9.1.

INNATE IMMUNITY, INFLAMMATION AND AUTOPHAGY

Cross-talk between Innate Immunity and Autophagy Suppresses Excessive Inflammation

After initial recognition of invading microorganisms, the innate immune system plays a pivotal role in defense through germline-encoded PRRs. Within the past decade remarkable progress in elucidating this new immunological system has been made, which has provided an improved understanding of the immunopathogenesis of infectious and inflammatory diseases.

Toll-like receptors (TLRs) are among the most important discoveries in infection and immunity in recent years, and are the best characterized innate immune receptors. The initial engagement of TLRs by microbial and damaged motifs affects the ultimate outcome of immune reactions through a delicate host–pathogen interaction. Upon exposure to these ligands, innate immune system receptors initiate complicated intracellular signaling cascades. These culminate in the expression of a variety of mediators involved in the inflammatory and immune responses through the activation of specific transcriptional factors, such as nuclear factor (NF)-κB.

Various mechanisms and key factors, including anti-inflammatory molecules and cytokines, limit the TLR-induced inflammatory signaling cascade. If these limitations fail, uncontrolled and high-level production of inflammatory mediators results in excessive inflammatory responses and tissue damage through the effects of both inflammatory mediators and systemic inflammation – for example, septic shock, acute lung injury, and dysfunction of other organs (Heumann *et al.*, 1998).

Macroautophagy or autophagocytosis is a type of autophagy in which cellular components and organelles are wrapped by typical double-membrane autophagosomal structures,

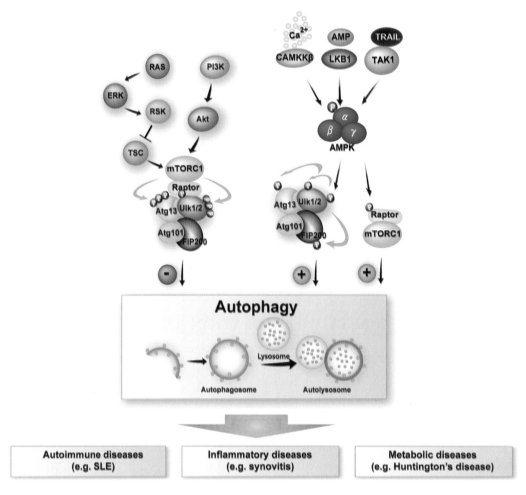

FIGURE 9.1   **Autophagy is regulated by the mTOR and AMPK signaling.** The AMPK and mTORC1 protein complexes have opposing roles for regulating autophagy through activation of Ulk1/2–Atg13/Atg/101/FIP200. Under sufficient nutrient conditions, the mTORC1 activated by the PI3K–AKT pathway or TSC inhibition through the RAS–ERK–RSK pathway interacts with the Ulk1/2–Atg13–FIP200 complex through direct association between Raptor and Ulk1/2, and thereby induces hyperphosphorylation of Atg13 and Ulk1/2 to inhibit autophagy. In response to nutrient deprivation or rapamaycin treatment, mTORC1 is inactivated and in turn leads to rapid Ulk1/2 dephosphorylation in several residues. The activated Ulk1/2-induced autophosphorylation of itself and phosphorylation of Atg13 and FIP200 results in autophagy induction. AMPK is activated by diverse upstream mediators, such as LKB1, CAMKKβ, and TAK1, under low energy conditions. The activated AMPK indirectly induces autophagy by regulating mTORC1 activity through phosphorylation of Raptor. Alternatively, AMPK leads to phosphorylation of Ulk1/2 through direct interaction between AMPK and Ulk1/2. Activation of the autophagy pathway contributes to improvement of several autoimmune, inflammatory, and metabolic diseases.

TABLE 9.1 Summary of Human Diseases Discussed in this Chapter

Human Diseases		Autophagy Pathway Molecules Related to Diseases	References
Autoinflammatory diseases	Crohn's disease	Atg16L1, NOD2, IRGM, XBP1, ORMDL3	Hampe et al., 2007; Kaser and Blumberg, 2009; Kaser et al., 2008; Waterman et al., 2011
	Vitiligo	UVRAG	Jeong et al., 2010
Pulmonary diseases	Cystic fibrosis	CFTR	Luciani et al., 2010; O'Sullivan and Freedman, 2009
	Chronic obstructive pulmonary disease	LC3B, Atg4, Atg5/12, Atg7	Chen et al., 2008, 2010; Lee et al., 2011; Ryter et al., 2012
Inflammatory disease	Sepsis	HO-1, depletion of autophagic proteins	Carchman et al., 2011; Nakahira et al., 2011

digested, and degraded by the lysosomal system. Other types of autophagy are microautophagy and chaperone-mediated autophagy, by which cytoplasmic materials can be delivered directly into lysosomes without the formation of autophagosomes. The autophagic process coordinates overall intracellular homeostasis to prevent cellular damage.

Accumulating data suggest the roles of Atg proteins and the mechanisms underlying their involvement in autophagosome formation. It is thought that the NF-κB signaling system and autophagic process interact closely in many contexts. The NF-κB pathway generally inhibits autophagy activation; however, this regulation is strongly associated with the cellular context. Distinct lines of evidence suggest that NF-κB directly regulates Beclin 1 transactivation and other members of the Beclin 1 interactome, and that the Beclin 1 interactome is a key initiator of autophagy activation. Additionally, NF-κB signaling can regulate oxidative stress and ROS generation; induction of the expression of major antioxidants is a potent activator of autophagy. Furthermore, NF-κB signaling stimulates the generation of ROS by inducing expression of many ROS-producing enzymes, including NADPH oxidase 2. Thus, the NF-κB signaling pathways and autophagy system likely cross-talk intimately and play crucial roles in host defense, in cooperation with other major cellular signaling pathways, such as those associated with ROS (Salminen et al., 2012).

Autophagy is increasingly recognized as a key cellular event in the fine-tuning of signal regulation, in which selective autophagy degrades aggregated signaling proteins, such as MyD88 and toll/IL-1 receptor domain-containing adaptor inducing IFN-β (TRIF), in a process called aggrephagy. Increasing data related to critical inflammatory diseases, including sepsis and ischemia reperfusion injury, demonstrate an important role for autophagy in the regulation of inflammation (Levine et al., 2011).

Mechanisms of Autophagy-Mediated Regulation of Inflammation

Among the signaling pathways that control both autophagy and inflammation, we will focus on the roles of those mediated by the mTOR, AMPK, and AMPK pathways upon autophagy cross-talk with inflammatory responses.

mTOR: A Negative Regulator of Autophagy

The mTOR signaling pathway is an important serine/threonine kinase involved in multiple biological functions, including cell metabolism, growth, proliferation, survival, and autophagy. It is a master regulator of the autophagy pathway, which it regulates negatively. mTOR, a central regulator of various cell functions, forms two distinct complexes: mTORC1 and mTORC2. Activated through the PI3K–AKT pathway, mTORC1 is involved mainly in negative regulation of autophagy. In addition, mTOR plays a role in the termination of autophagy and restoration of the full complement of lysosomes, thus contributing to lysosome homeostasis during nutrient deprivation (Yu *et al.*, 2010). Rapamycin is an immunosuppressant widely used for autophagy activation, since it is a potent inhibitor of mTORC1. The RAS–ERK–RSK pathway is also known to activate mTORC1 through phosphorylation and inhibition of tuberous sclerosis complex (TSC) 2. TSC is a genetic disease resulting from mutations in either the TSC1 or TSC2 tumor suppressor genes, which encode hamartin and tuberin, respectively. TSC inhibits mTOR signaling by targeting the Ras-related small G protein Rheb, which is a critical mediator of the nutrient signaling input to mTOR (Roux *et al.*, 2004).

mTOR is a major stress-related signal known to be involved in the pathogenesis of a variety of human diseases, including cancer, aging, inflammation, autoimmunity, metabolic disorders, neurologic inflammation, and transplantation rejection. Accumulating evidence shows that activation of mTOR is key in the pathogenesis of these autoimmune and inflammatory diseases. During the immune response, mTOR plays a pleiotropic role in innate and adaptive immunity – i.e., the proper activation and proliferation of effector T cells, production of cytokines, limitation of proinflammatory responses, and migration of neutrophils and mast cells (Dazert and Hall, 2011; Weichhart and Säemann, 2009). The roles of mTOR are dependent on cell type: mTOR plays an anti-inflammatory role in monocytes/macrophages and peripheral myeloid dendritic cells, whereas it promotes high-level type I interferon production in plasmacytoid dendritic cells (Dazert and Hall, 2011; Weichhart and Säemann, 2009). In terms of autophagy-related immune disorders, recent studies have reported the potential involvement of mTOR in the pathogenesis of systemic lupus erythematosus (SLE), a chronic autoimmune disease with a wide range of manifestations that lead to significant morbidity and, potentially, mortality. Recent genome-wide association studies have suggested that certain single-nucleotide polymorphisms (SNPs) in the autophagy-related gene *Atg5* are linked to SLE susceptibility. Additionally, activation of mTOR has been suggested to be involved in T cell dysfunction and the pathogenesis of SLE (Pierdominici *et al.*, 2012). Earlier studies reported that autophagy activation by mTOR inhibition promotes the mutant huntingtin fragment clearance pathway and attenuates cell death in cell-based models, and improves clinical parameters in mouse models of Huntington's disease (Ravikumar *et al.*, 2004). The contribution of the mTOR pathway to joint inflammation and bone damage has been reported; the mTOR inhibitor rapamycin significantly reduces the severity of cartilage degradation and synovitis (Caramés *et al.*, 2012). Altogether, these data suggest a close relationship between dysregulation of the autophagy pathway and the pathogenesis of several autoimmune diseases. Targeting the autophagy pathway may thus provide innovative therapeutic approaches to many autoimmune diseases.

AMPK: A Positive Regulator of Autophagy

AMPK acts as an energy sensor in cellular metabolism, and inhibits energy-consuming functions. It plays an important role not only in the maintenance of cellular energy homeostasis, but also in activation of autophagy. AMPK is a heterotrimeric protein complex, and phosphorylation of a conserved threonine residue (T172) in the catalytic α subunit is required for activation. There are several upstream kinases for AMPK: the ubiquitously expressed and constitutively active kinase LKB1, Ca^{2+}-activated Ca^{2+}/calmodulin-dependent kinase kinase β (CaMKKβ), and transforming growth factor β-activated kinase-1 (TAK1). In turn, activated AMPK activates the TSC1–TSC2 complex, resulting in the inhibition of mTORC1 and enhancement of autophagy (Alers *et al.*, 2012). Additionally, various Ca^{2+} mobilizing agents (Vitamin D compounds, ATP and ionomycin) and ER stress (thapsigargin) are associated with the AMPK pathway via CaMKKβ activation (Høyer-Hansen and Jäättelä, 2007). Because Ca^{2+}-mediated signaling pathways play a key regulatory role in diverse innate responses, including those mediated by the TLR or C-type lectins (Connolly and Kusner, 2007), AMPK might function as a general regulator of autophagy and innate immunity. Moreover, cytokine or TLR-mediated TAK1 activation – as an upstream signal of AMPK – phosphorylates and activates AMPK, leading to autophagy activation in various innate and inflammatory conditions in an LKB1- or CaMKKβ-independent manner (Into *et al.*, 2012). Collectively, these data provide new insights into the mechanisms that link innate immunity and autophagy, suggesting potential targets for treatment of infectious, inflammatory, and autoimmune diseases.

DISEASES RELATED TO INFLAMMATION AND AUTOPHAGY

Autophagy and Autoinflammatory Diseases (Crohn's Disease and Vitiligo)

Crohn's disease is a chronic inflammatory bowel disease that results from inappropriate inflammatory responses caused by both genetic and environmental factors. Genome-wide association studies of the pathophysiology of Crohn's disease have defined SNPs in autophagy genes such as Atg16L1, and other genes related to autophagic processing (i.e., NOD2 and IRGM), to be associated with susceptibility to Crohn's disease (Hampe *et al.*, 2007; Waterman *et al.*, 2011). Autophagy induction is defective in Crohn's disease patients with NOD2 or Atg16L1 risk variants. Dendritic cells from these patients have defects in bacterial trafficking and antigen presentation, which leads to impaired bacterial clearance from gut epithelia and gastrointestinal inflammation (Cooney *et al.*, 2010). Moreover, gene variants (XBP1, ORMDL3) in the unfolded protein response (UPR) have been reported to be susceptibility factors for both Crohn's disease and ulcerative colitis (Kaser and Blumberg, 2009; Kaser *et al.*, 2008). The genetic convergence of these intracellular pathways has important implications for the intersection among autophagy, inflammation, and UPR (Fritz *et al.*, 2011).

Vitiligo is a cutaneous depigmentary disorder characterized by the appearance of white macules of varying size and distribution. Recent studies of genetic, immune, and oxidative stress factors have suggested that the pathogenesis of vitiligo is associated with autophagy and immunity, and the association of neuropeptides from peripheral nerve endings with new cytokines. In Korean patients with non-segmental vitiligo, several susceptibility-associated SNPs were found in the ultraviolet radiation resistance-associated gene (UVRAG), which induces autophagy by activating the Beclin 1–PI3K complex (Jeong et al., 2010). These studies provide new insights into the roles of autophagy in autoimmune and autoinflammatory diseases.

Autophagy and Lung Diseases

Autophagy-dependent mechanisms are thought be involved in the pathogenesis of several pulmonary inflammatory diseases, including cystic fibrosis (CF) and pulmonary hypertension. CF is the most common inherited disorder in Caucasians, and is characterized by increased inflammation and aberrant accumulation of viscous mucous in the airways. The gene responsible for CF, cystic fibrosis transmembrane conductance regulator (CFTR), encodes a chloride channel that is expressed in epithelial cells. Recent studies demonstrated that human airway epithelial cells from CF patients have an impaired autophagic function, with reduced clearance of aggresomes and accumulation of p62 (also known as SQSTM1). CFTR mutation or knockdown results in impaired autophagy processing through ROS–tissue transglutaminase-mediated aggresome formation and lung inflammation (Luciani et al., 2010). Rescue of autophagy activation may promote clearance of aggresomes and CFTR trafficking, suggesting a promising new target for CF treatment (O'Sullivan and Freedman, 2009).

Recent studies have revealed the role of autophagy in the etiology of various pulmonary diseases (Ryter et al., 2012). Increased autophagy and autophagic proteins (microtubule-associated protein 1 light chain 3B (LC3B), Atg4, Atg5/12, Atg7) were identified in lung specimens from patients with chronic obstructive pulmonary disease (COPD). Similarly, the lungs of mice after chronic inhalation of cigarette smoke displayed increased autophagy (Chen et al., 2010). Furthermore, increased levels of the autophagic protein LC3B were required for the activation of cigarette smoke-induced apoptosis and emphysema development through a mechanism involving caveolin-1. These studies indicate that autophagy modulation may represent a novel target for treatment of COPD-associated airway obstruction and emphysema (Chen et al., 2010). In clinical samples from patients with pulmonary arterial hypertension (PAH) the expression of LC3B was increased, presumably as a protective mechanism during chronic hypoxia. Increased autophagy was observed in small pulmonary vessels of the lungs from mice with chronic hypoxia, and in cultured human pulmonary vascular cells under hypoxic conditions. Furthermore, mice defective in LC3B ($LC3B^{-/-}$) exhibited increased patterns of pulmonary hypertension, indicating a protective role for autophagic protein LC3B (Lee et al., 2011). In conclusion, selectively targeting the autophagic pathway may be a promising strategy for the design of novel therapeutics for the treatment of CF and other lung diseases.

Autophagy and Sepsis

Sepsis is a systemic inflammatory response to bacterial, fungal, parasitic, or viral infection, which results in fever, hypertension, cachexia, hypermetabolism, and multiple organ failure (Sprung et al., 2008). Despite a multitude of clinical trials of various agents, sepsis remains a serious problem, with intensive care unit mortality rates of 30–60% (Sprung *et al.*, 2008). It is unclear whether extensive autophagy has a beneficial or detrimental influence on sepsis progression. Autophagosome structures accumulate in the liver tissue in septic patients, and also accumulated in mice that underwent surgical sepsis in both clinical and laboratory-based studies (Watanabe *et al.*, 2009). Additionally, recent studies have shown that TLR4-mediated autophagy is related to induction of assembly of aggresome-like structures, in which p62 is involved (Fujita and Srinivasula, 2011). Moreover, a key function of heme oxygenase-1 (HO-1) was reported by Carchman *et al.*, 2011). HO-1 levels were increased in liver tissues from cecal ligation and puncture (CLP)-treated mice or lipopolysaccharides (LPS)-stimulated hepatocytes, and induction of autophagy protected septic animals from hepatocellular injury and cell death (Carchman *et al.*, 2011). Thus, HO-1 may be an important link between autophagy and apoptosis in the experimental sepsis model. The genetic deletion of autophagic proteins results in increased susceptibility of mice subjected to CLP or challenged with LPS (Nakahira *et al.*, 2011). Therefore, autophagy induction in septic conditions may play protective and anti-inflammatory roles, ameliorating the pathology of systemic inflammation. Further studies are needed to elucidate whether autophagy affects disease severity during sepsis, and how its induction prevents inflammation and cell death during sepsis.

INFLAMMASOMES AND AUTOPHAGY

The inflammasome is an intracellular multiprotein complex responsible for caspase-1 activation, proteolytic maturation, and secretion of IL-1β and IL-18, both of which are importantly involved in systemic inflammatory circuits. The NLRP3 inflammasome is the most extensively characterized, and can be activated by various infectious/damage signals in the host. To avoid excessive proinflammatory and pyrogenic production of IL-1β and IL-18, inflammasome activity must be tightly regulated (Leemans *et al.*, 2011).

Numerous previous studies on the effects of autophagy on inflammasomes have obviously indicated that autophagy plays a negative role in inflammasome activation (Cadwell *et al.*, 2008; Harris *et al.*, 2011; Saitoh *et al.*, 2008; Shi *et al.*, 2012). Harris *et al.* (2011) reported that blockage of autophagy by pharmacological inhibitors, such as 3-methyladenine and wortmannin, induce the processing and secretion of IL-1β by macrophages in an NLRP3- and TRIF-dependent manner. The same study also demonstrated that induction of autophagy by the classical autophagy inducer rapamycin reduces IL-1β secretion by targeting intracellular IL-1β for lysosomal degradation. An additional recent report showed that activation of AIM2 or NLRP3 inflammasomes leads to the polyubiquitination of ASC, which is dependent on the cargo receptor p62 (Shi *et al.*, 2012). The ubiquitnated p62-associated ASC degraded through autophagosome/lysosomal maturation, which is negative feedback in response to AIM2 or NLRP3 inflammasome activation.

Although numerous studies have demonstrated the negative regulation of autophagy in inflammasome activation (Harris *et al.*, 2011; Shi *et al.*, 2012), it should be noted that the autophagy pathway is required for secretion of IL-1β, a leaderless cytosolic protein secreted via membranous organelles. Moreover, several inflammasome activators, including mitochondrial DNA and ROS, may accumulate in autophagy-defective conditions (Nakahira *et al.*, 2011; Zhou *et al.*, 2011). Thus, maintenance of basal autophagy facilitates preservation of a clean intracellular environment by removing endogenous, potentially harmful factors that could induce inflammasome activation. With regard to uncontrolled release of inflammatory mediators, the induced autophagy levels are important for the unconventional trafficking and release of IL-1β (Deretic *et al.*, 2012).

Autophagy-Related Genes and Inflammasomes

Autophagy plays an important role in the regulation of inflammasome activities and the resulting inflammation. Earlier studies showed that deficiency in the autophagy-related gene Atg16L1 in macrophages is linked to high-level production of the proinflammatory cytokines IL-1β and IL-18 through TRIF-dependent activation of caspase-1. Moreover, mice with Atg16L1-deficient hematopoietic cells have an increased susceptibility to dextran sulfate sodium-induced acute colitis, suggesting an essential role for Atg16L1 in the regulation of intestinal inflammatory responses (Saitoh *et al.*, 2008). Paneth cells from patients with Crohn's disease who carry the Atg16L1 risk allele had increased patterns of disorganized or diminished granules, similar to those found in autophagy-protein-deficient mice (Cadwell *et al.*, 2008). Thus, autophagy may play an important role in controlling inflammasome activation and regulating injury responses in the intestines of mice and patients with Crohn's disease.

Recent studies showed that defective autophagic proteins LC3B and Beclin 1 enhanced inflammasome activation, increased production of caspase-1-dependent proinflammatory cytokines, and increased the susceptibility to LPS-induced sepsis. Defective autophagy leads to the accumulation of dysfunctional mitochondria and release of mitochondrial DNA into the cytosol through a mechanism dependent on activation of the NLRP3 inflammasome and mitochondrial ROS (Nakahira *et al.*, 2011; Zhou *et al.*, 2011).

Therapeutic Autophagy Against Inflammasome-Related Diseases

Several recent reports have revealed that aberrations in the clearance of insoluble protein deposits (amyloid) or UPRs initiate inflammatory cascades through the inflammasome protein complex. In the experimental settings of neurodegenerative diseases and hepatic damage, enhanced autophagy is essential for the clearance of infection-related particles, which are sensed by the inflammasome, resulting in production of IL-1β (Masters and O'Neill, 2011). The aggregating and misfolding propensities of the amyloidogenic proteins amyloid-β (Aβ) peptides and islet amyloid polypeptide (IAPP) may contribute to the development of common degenerative diseases, including Alzheimer's disease and type 2 diabetes. Thus, autophagy activation might decrease the incidence of these protein-misfolding degenerative diseases, both of which are initiated by amyloidogenic and non-amyloidogenic protein aggregates (Masters and O'Neill, 2011).

Accumulating data suggest that inflammasome activation is a causative factor of a variety of metabolic disorders, including type 2 diabetes and obesity. Indeed, chronic low-grade inflammation is strongly associated with obesity, and termed "metainflammation." In addition, type 2 diabetes patients often exhibit an elevated IL-1β level, supporting a rationale for IL-1β-targeted therapy using Anakinra for treatment of this disease (Wen *et al.*, 2012). Our recent study demonstrated that type 2 diabetes patients exhibit elevated levels of mature IL-1β in sera, peripheral blood mononuclear cells, and monocyte-derived macrophages after stimulation of NLRP3 inflammasome activation (Lee *et al.*, 2013).

Similar to IAPP, the saturated fatty acid palmitate induces activation of the NLRP3 inflammasome, leading to insulin resistance and type 2 diabetes. Interestingly, this inflammasome-inducing pathway is regulated through autophagy signaling, i.e., the AMPK- and unc-51-like kinase-1 (ULK1)-dependent pathways (Wen *et al.*, 2011). These findings strongly suggest an association between inflammasome activation, autophagy dysregulation, and many human inflammatory diseases.

DISCUSSION

Discovery of the autophagy system has shed new light on cellular biological control; continuous communication and signaling via autophagy pathways and other cellular processes are necessary for clean-up of the intracellular environment and protection from harmful injury due to both extracellular and endogenous factors. Current evidence supports an important role for autophagy as an innate effector through cooperation with cellular factors that participate in the host defense against infectious (exogenous) and potentially damaging (endogenous) threats. From the disposal of protein aggregates to the supply of energy for essential anabolic processes, the fundamental function of autophagy is related to a variety of health-related issues, including aging, infections, neurodegeneration, and cancer (Deretic *et al.*, 2012; Levine *et al.*, 2011). In this chapter, we have described the dedicated function of autophagy in controlling inflammation, and suggest various pathophysiologic factors to be important in the initiation and development of many human diseases.

Here, we have described the essential aspects of autophagy-related signaling networks that control the inflammatory process, including NF-κB- and mTOR/AMPK-dependent pathways. Accumulating evidence suggests that many other intracellular signaling mechanisms are involved, representing a mechanism of autophagy regulation. Clearly, autophagy communicates with other fundamental biological machineries/organelles, including mitochondria, UPRs, and ROS. Through this communication, autophagy may regulate the well-organized cellular environment that protects against pathogenic microbes and inflammation. Besides the indirect role of autophagy-mediated control of inflammation mediated by degradation of protein aggregates and harmful materials, direct modulation of inflammatory responses by autophagy can also be involved, as revealed by both genetic and clinical studies. However, many questions remain: for example, how do autophagy-related genes modulate the inflammatory response? Do autophagy-related genes interact directly with innate molecules, or do they signal other proteins which then affect innate and inflammatory pathways? Although genome-wide studies have revealed the roles of several autophagy- and innate immunity-associated genes in susceptibility to human inflammatory disorders, the roles of many other genes in host defense/risk in a variety of diseases related to inflammation remain unknown.

Additional complexities exist in autophagy induction, fine-tuning, and regulation of communication with inflammatory pathways. Besides the inhibitory function of autophagy in inflammatory responses, it is increasingly clear that autophagy plays a positive role in protein trafficking and secretion of biologically active proteins, such as IL-1β. It should be noted that the autophagy pathway is required for initial inflammatory responses in the early phase (Deretic *et al.*, 2012). The same inflammasome activation and inflammation signals, including mitochondrial sources of ROS and DNA, cellular ROS, and intracellular Ca^{2+} influx (Tschopp, 2011), also play roles in autophagy activation. Thus, we speculate that the initial alarmins activate both inflammatory and autophagic responses to cooperate in host defense against harmful and dangerous circumstances. When the threat has been eliminated, the cell must reset its intracellular biological environment to resting status in preparation for other stimuli. Overall, autophagy-dependent inhibition dominates the later phase of inflammation, through downregulation of endogenous sources of inflammasome activation (Deretic *et al.*, 2012), and other mechanisms that will be elucidated in future studies.

Anticancer drugs have been reported to modulate the mode of autophagy in various cancers. However, it is unclear whether an autophagy enhancer/modulator can influence infection and inflammatory diseases in the clinic. The effects of rapamycin inhibition of mTOR, especially in the neuroprotection of spinal cord injury, are mediated by the promotion of autophagy (Chen *et al.*, 2012).

A mutant protein, termed α_1-antitrypsin Z, a polymer in the endoplasmic reticulum of liver cells, is prone to polymerization and aggregate formation, leading to hepatic inflammation, fibrosis and carcinogenesis through a gain-of-toxicity mechanism. Using a mouse model of α_1-antitrypsin deficiency, the autophagy enhancer carbamazepine, an anticonvulsant and mood stabilizer, was shown to attenuate hepatotoxicity and exert beneficial effects in liver diseases (Hidvegi *et al.*, 2010). Therefore, it would be interesting to determine whether autophagy enhancers that act through mTOR-dependent or -independent pathways are effective in the treatment of aggregate-related inflammatory diseases.

Autophagy processing plays crucial roles in the regulation of cellular pathways, facilitating provision of an environment suitable for the maintenance of cytoplasmic homeostasis. Thus, autophagy likely impacts many cellular pathways that influence health and disease status. Advances in our knowledge of autophagy may lead to development of innovative therapeutic strategies for control of human inflammatory diseases.

Acknowledgments

This work was supported by the National Research Foundation of Korea (NRF) grant funded by the Korea government (MSIP) (No. 2007-0054932) at Chungnam National University, and by a grant of the Korea Healthcare Technology R&D Project, Ministry for Health, Welfare & Family Affairs, Republic of Korea (A100588).

References

Alers, S., Löffler, A.S., Wesselborg, S., et al., 2012. Role of AMPK–mTOR–Ulk1/2 in the regulation of autophagy: cross talk, shortcuts, and feedbacks. Mol. Cell. Biol. 32, 2–11.

Cadwell, K., Liu, J.Y., Brown, S.L., et al., 2008. A key role for autophagy and the autophagy gene Atg16L1 in mouse and human intestinal Paneth cells. Nature 456, 259–263.

Caramés, B., Hasegwa, A., Taniguchi, N., et al., 2012. Autophagy activation by rapamycin reduces severity of experimental osteoarthritis. Ann. Rheum. Dis. 71, 575–581.

Carchman, E.H., Rao, J., Loughran, P.A., et al., 2011. Heme oxygenase-1-mediated autophagy protects against hepatocyte cell death and hepatic injury from infection/sepsis in mice. Hepatology 53, 2053–2062.

Chen, H.C., Fong, T., Hsu, P.W., Chiu, W.T., 2012. Multifaceted effects of rapamycin on functional recovery after spinal cord injury in rats through autophagy promotion, anti-inflammation, and neuroprotection. J. Surg. Res. 179 (1), e203–e210.

Chen, Z.H., Kim, H.P., Sciurba, F.C., et al., 2008. Egr-1 regulates autophagy in cigarette smoke-induced chronic obstructive pulmonary disease. PLoS ONE 3, e3316.

Chen, Z.H., Lam, H.C., Jin, Y., et al., 2010. Autophagy protein microtubule-associated protein 1 light chain-3B (LC3B) activates extrinsic apoptosis during cigarette smoke-induced emphysema. Proc. Natl. Acad. Sci. U.S.A. 107, 18880–18885.

Connolly, S.F., Kusner, D.J., 2007. The regulation of dendritic cell function by calcium-signaling and its inhibition by microbial pathogens. Immunol. Res. 39, 115–127.

Cooney, R., Baker, J., Brain, O., et al., 2010. NOD2 stimulation induces autophagy in dendritic cells influencing bacterial handling and antigen presentation. Nat. Med. 16, 90–97.

Dazert, E., Hall, M.N., 2011. mTOR signaling in disease. Curr. Opin. Cell. Biol. 23, 744–755.

Deretic, V., Jiang, S., Dupont, N., 2012. Autophagy intersections with conventional and unconventional secretion in tissue development, remodeling and inflammation. Trends. Cell. Biol. 22, 397–406.

Fritz, T., Niederreiter, L., Adolph, T., Blumberg, R.S., Kaser, A., 2011. Crohn's disease: NOD2, autophagy and ER stress converge. Gut 60, 1580–1588.

Fujita, K., Srinivasula, S.M., 2011. TLR4-mediated autophagy in macrophages is a p62-dependent type of selective autophagy of aggresome-like induced structures (ALIS). Autophagy 7, 552–554.

Green, D.R., Gaulluzzi, L., Kroemer, G., 2011. Mitochondria and the autophagy-inflammation-cell death axis in organismal aging. Science 333, 1109–1112.

Hajishengallis, G., Lambris, J.D., 2011. Microbial manipulation of receptor crosstalk in innate immunity. Nat. Rev. Immunol. 11, 187–200.

Hampe, J., Franke, A., Rosenstiel, P., et al., 2007. A genome-wide association scan of nonsynonymous SNPs identifies a susceptibility variant for Crohn disease in Atg16L1. Nat. Genet. 39, 207–211.

Harris, J., Hartman, M., Roche, C., et al., 2011. Autophagy controls IL-1β secretion by targeting pro-IL-1β for degradation. J. Biol. Chem. 286, 9587–9597.

Heumann, D., Glauser, M.P., Calandra, T., 1998. Molecular basis of host–pathogen interaction in septic shock. Curr. Opin. Microbiol. 1, 49–55.

Hidvegi, T., Ewing, M., Hale, P., et al., 2010. An autophagy-enhancing drug promotes degradation of mutant alpha1-antitrypsin Z and reduces hepatic fibrosis. Science 329, 229–232.

Høyer-Hansen, M., Jäättelä, M., 2007. AMP-activated protein kinase: a universal regulator of autophagy? Autophagy 3, 381–383.

Into, T., Inomata, M., Takayama, E., et al., 2012. Autophagy in regulation of Toll-like receptor signaling. Cell. Signal. 24, 1150–1162.

Jeong, T.J., Shin, M.K., Uhm, Y.K., et al., 2010. Association of UVRAG polymorphisms with susceptibility to non-segmental vitiligo in a Korean sample. Exp. Dermatol. 19, e323–e325.

Kaser, A., Blumberg, R.S., 2009. Endoplasmic reticulum stress in the intestinal epithelium and inflammatory bowel disease. Semin. Immunol. 21, 156–163.

Kaser, A., Lee, A.H., Franke, A., et al., 2008. XBP1 links ER stress to intestinal inflammation and confers genetic risk for human inflammatory bowel disease. Cell 134, 743–756.

Lee, H.M., Kim, J.J., Kim, H.J., et al., 2013. Upregulated NLRP3 inflammasome activation in patients with type 2 diabetes. Diabetes 62, 194–204.

Lee, S.J., Smith, A., Guo, L., et al., 2011. Autophagic protein LC3B confers resistance against hypoxia-induced pulmonary hypertension. Am. J. Respir. Crit. Care. Med. 183, 649–658.

Leemans, J.C., Cassel, S.L., Sutterwala, F.S., 2011. Sensing damage by the NLRP3 inflammasome. Immunol. Rev. 243, 152–162.

Levine, B., Mizushima, N., Virgin, H.W., 2011. Autophagy in immunity and inflammation. Nature 469, 323–335.

Luciani, A., Villella, V.R., Esposito, S., et al., 2010. Defective CFTR induces aggresome formation and lung inflammation in cystic fibrosis through ROS-mediated autophagy inhibition. Nat. Cell. Biol. 12, 863–875.

Masters, S.L., O'Neill, L.N., 2011. Disease-associated amyloid and misfolded protein aggregates activate the inflammasome. Trends. Mol. Med. 17, 276–282.

Nakahira, K., Haspel, J.A., Rathinam, V.A., et al., 2011. Autophagy proteins regulate innate immune responses by inhibiting the release of mitochondrial DNA mediated by the NALP3 inflammasome. Nat. Immunol. 12, 222–230.

O'Sullivan, B.P., Freedman, S.D., 2009. Cystic fibrosis. Lancet 373, 1891–1904.

Pierdominici, M., Vomero, M., Barbati, C., et al., 2012. Role of autophagy in immunity and autoimmunity, with a special focus on systemic lupus erythematosus. FASEB J. 26, 1400–1412.

Ravikumar, B., Vacher, C., Berger, Z., et al., 2004. Inhibition of mTOR induces autophagy and reduces toxicity of polyglutamine expansions in fly and mouse models of Huntington disease. Nat. Genet. 36, 585–595.

Roux, P.P., Ballif, B.A., Anjum, R., et al., 2004. Tumor-promoting phorbol esters and activated Ras inactivate the tuberous sclerosis tumor suppressor complex via p90 ribosomal S6 kinase. Proc. Natl. Acad. Sci. U.S.A. 101, 13489–13494.

Ryter, S.W., Nakahira, K., Haspel, J.A., et al., 2012. Autophagy in pulmonary diseases. Annu. Rev. Physiol. 74, 377–401.

Saitoh, T., Akira, S., 2010. Regulation of innate immune responses by autophagy-related proteins. J. Cell. Biol. 189, 925–935.

Saitoh, T., Fujiyta, N., Jang, M.H., et al., 2008. Loss of the autophagy protein Atg16L1 enhances endotoxin-induced IL-1beta production. Nature 456, 264–268.

Salminen, A., Hyttinen, J.M., Kauppinen, A., et al., 2012. Context-dependent regulation of autophagy by IKK–NF-κB signaling: impact on the aging process. Int. J. Cell. Biol. 2012, 849541.

Scherz-Shouval, R., Elazar, Z., 2011. Regulation of autophagy by ROS: physiology and pathology. Trends. Biochem. Sci. 36, 30–38.

Shi, C.S., Shenderov, K., Huang, N.N., et al., 2012. Activation of autophagy by inflammatory signals limits IL-1beta production by targeting ubiquitinated inflammasomes for destruction. Nat. Immunol. 13, 255–263.

Sprung, C.L., Annane, D., Keh, D., et al., 2008. Hydrocortisone therapy for patients with septic shock. N. Engl. J. Med. 358, 111–124.

Tschopp, J., 2011. Mitochondria: sovereign of inflammation? Eur. J. Immunol. 41, 1196–1202.

Watanabe, E., Muenzer, J.T., Hawkins, W.G., et al., 2009. Sepsis induces extensive autophagic vacuolization in hepatocytes: a clinical and laboratory-based study. Lab. Invest. 89, 549–561.

Waterman, M., Xu, W., Stempak, J.M., et al., 2011. Distinct and overlapping genetic loci in Crohn's disease and ulcerative colitis: correlations with pathogenesis. Inflamm. Bowel. Dis. 17, 1936–1942.

Weichhart, T., Säemann, M.D., 2009. The multiple facets of mTOR in immunity. Trends. Immunol. 30, 218–226.

Wen, H., Gris, D., Lei, Y., et al., 2011. Fatty acid-induced NLRP3-ASC inflammasome activation interferes with insulin signaling. Nat. Immunol. 12, 408–415.

Wen, H., Ting, J.P., O'Neill, L.A., 2012. A role for the NLRP3 inflammasome in metabolic diseases–did Warburg miss inflammation? Nat. Immunol. 13, 352–357.

Yu, L., McPhee, C.K., Zheng, L., et al., 2010. Termination of autophagy and reformation of lysosomes regulated by mTOR. Nature 465, 942–946.

Zhou, R., Yazdi, A.S., Menu, P., et al., 2011. A role for mitochondria in NLRP3 inflammasome activation. Nature 469, 221–225.

Mitophagy Plays a Protective Role in Fibroblasts from Patients with Coenzyme Q_{10} Deficiency

David Cotán, Ángeles Rodríguez Hernández, Mario D. Cordero, Juan Garrido Maraver, Manuel Oropesa-Ávila, Mario de la Mata, Alejandro Fernández-Vega, Carmen Pérez Calero, Marina Villanueva Paz, Ana Delgado Pavón, Macarena Alanís Sánchez, and José A. Sánchez Alcázar

© 2014 Elsevier Inc. All rights reserved.

Abstract

Coenzyme Q_{10} (CoQ) deficiencies are clinically and genetically heterogeneous diseases that can occur due to defects of ubiquinone biosynthesis (primary deficiencies) or other causes (secondary deficiencies). Radical oxygen species (ROS) production and oxidative stress is a common consequence of dysfunctional mitochondria and CoQ deficiency. Mitochondrial damage induced by ROS can trigger mitochondrial permeability transition (MPT) by opening of non-specific high conductance permeability transition pores in the mitochondrial inner membrane. This, in turn, leads to a simultaneous collapse of mitochondrial membrane potential and the activation of selective elimination of depolarized and dysfunctional mitochondria by mitophagy. In this respect, mitophagy could be considered as a protective mechanism for elimination of potential harmful mitochondria. Mitophagy must be accompanied by mitochondrial biogenesis activation to compensate the mitochondrial loss. However, massive and persistent mitophagy may impair cell bioenergetics, autophagy flux, and mitochondrial biogenesis, and eventually may cause cell death.

INTRODUCTION

Mitochondria are essential organelles for every cell, as the powerhouse to provide ATP for a multitude of cellular processes. They are also at the center of metabolic pathways, primary sources of reactive oxygen species (ROS), and regulators of apoptosis, and participate in calcium homeostasis. Damage to the mitochondrial outer membrane leads to release of cytochrome c, triggering caspase activation and apoptosis. Thus, mitochondrial function is central to cellular life and death. With increasing lifespan, mitochondrial function has been reported to be impaired in humans, and mitochondrial dysfunction is well documented in a wide variety of human disorders (Schatz, 2007).

Coenzyme Q_{10} (CoQ) is an essential electron and proton carrier in the mitochondrial respiratory chain (MRC), transferring electrons from complexes I and II to complex III (Crane *et al.*, 1957) and contributing to ATP biosynthesis. Furthermore, CoQ is essential for the stability of complex III in the mitochondrial respiratory chain, functions as an antioxidant in cell membranes, and is involved in multiple aspects of cellular metabolism. In addition, CoQ is required for pyrimidine nucleoside biosynthesis, and may modulate apoptosis and mitochondrial uncoupling protein. CoQ is composed of a benzoquinone ring, synthesized from tyrosine, and a polyprenyl side chain, generated from acetyl-CoA through the mevalonate pathway.

COENZYME Q_{10} DEFICIENCY

In eukaryotes, biosynthesis of CoQ is a very complex process involving at least 10 genes (COQ genes) (Tran and Clarke, 2007). Mutations in these genes cause primary CoQ deficiency, a severe and often fatal multisystem disorder. However, affected patients respond well to oral CoQ supplementation. To date, mutations have been identified in the COQ2, PDSS1, and PDSS2 genes (Quinzii and Hirano, 2011). The first COQ2 mutation was found in two patients with encephalomyopathy and nephropathy. This gene encodes the para-hydroxybenzoate-polyprenyltransferase that condensates the 4-OH benzoate ring with the prenyl side chain. Mutations in the PDSS2 gene, encoding the small subunit of prenyldisphosphate synthase, have also been reported in a patient with Leigh syndrome and nephropathy, as well as a homozygous PDSS1 missense mutation in two patients with a less severe multisystem disease.

Some patients with cerebellar ataxia or isolated myopathies have secondary CoQ deficiencies due to mutations in APTX and ETFDH – genes not directly related to ubiquinone synthesis. Secondary CoQ deficiency with multisystemic infantile presentation has also been described in one patient with cardiofaciocutaneous syndrome due to a BRAF mutation. CoQ is frequently reduced in muscle of patients with mitochondrial myopathy due to mutation in nuclear or mitochondrial DNA, and CoQ is very widely used for treatment of primary mitochondrial disorders.

Fibromyalgia (FM) is a chronic pain syndrome with unknown etiology and a wide spectrum of symptoms, such as allodynia, debilitating fatigue, joint stiffness, and migraine. Recent studies have shown some evidence demonstrating that oxidative stress is associated with clinical symptoms in FM. Recent findings by our group have shown reduced levels of CoQ, decreased mitochondrial membrane potential, increased levels of mitochondrial superoxide, and increased levels of lipid peroxidation in blood mononuclear cells (BMCs) from FM patients. Mitochondrial dysfunction was also associated with increased expression of autophagic genes, and the elimination of dysfunctional mitochondria by mitophagy (Cordero et al., 2010).

MITOCHONDRIAL DYSFUNCTION IN COENZYME Q$_{10}$ DEFICIENCY

The hallmark of CoQ deficiency syndrome is a decrease in CoQ levels in muscle and/or fibroblasts. Patients exhibit variable degrees of CoQ deficiency in muscle and/or fibroblasts causing decreased of CoQ-dependent MRC activities, such as NADH:cytochrome c oxidoreductase (complex I + III) and succinate:cytochrome c oxidoreductase (complex II + III). However, the effects of CoQ deficiency on other MRC aspects, such as ATP synthesis, oxygen consumption, and mitochondrial membrane potential measurements, have scarcely been reported. Some authors have reported decreases in oxygen consumption (state 3 respiration) in muscle mitochondria for several substrates except ascorbate/TMDP (Rotig et al., 2000), suggesting a CoQ-level dependent impairment of oxidative phosphorylation. A reduction in the mitochondrial membrane potential of cultured fibroblasts from patients with CoQ deficiency has also been demonstrated (Artuch et al., 2006). These findings suggest that dysfunctional oxidative phosphorylation may be an important factor in CoQ deficiency syndromes. There have been few reports regarding antioxidant status and oxidative stress in CoQ deficiency, and even these few have yielded conflicting results. Recently, it has been demonstrated that CoQ levels seem to correlate with ROS production and that varying degrees of CoQ deficiency cause variable defects of ATP synthesis and oxidative stress (Quinzii et al., 2010). In light of these observations, a more exhaustive and complete assessment of the role of oxidative stress in CoQ deficiency syndrome appears necessary.

In addition, studies examining cell death, in the context of CoQ deficiency, have also been limited and somewhat contradictory. While an increase in apoptotic features has consistently been demonstrated in muscle biopsies of CoQ-deficient patients (Di Giovanni *et al.*, 2001), no evidence of apoptosis could be established in fibroblasts of CoQ-deficient patients in another study (Boitier *et al.*, 1998). Therefore, changes in cell death (apoptosis or autophagy) that are closely related to increased free radical damage merit further investigation with respect to CoQ deficiency syndromes.

MITOPHAGY

Autophagy is a process by which cytosol and organelles are sequestered within double-membrane vesicles that deliver the contents to the lysosome/vacuole for degradation and recycling of the resulting macromolecules. Autophagy is typically activated by fasting and nutrient deprivation to generate amino acids and metabolic intermediates to maintain ATP production. Both insufficient and excess autophagy can promote cell injury. Appropriate regulation of autophagy is thus essential for cellular homeostasis. The molecular mechanism underlying autophagy has been extensively researched in the past decade, and the genes participating in this process, denoted Atgs, were found to be conserved from yeast to humans. The selective removal of cellular components, including organelles such as mitochondria, occurs via selective (i.e., cargo-specific) autophagy. Damaged mitochondria are selectively degraded by a specialized form of autophagy called mitophagy, ensuring the maintenance of a functional mitochondria population. Therefore, clearance of damaged and aging mitochondria is a critical process for cell survival. Increasing mitophagy activity in the elderly may thus be beneficial in that it contributes to the maintenance of a functional mitochondrial population.

Today, many forms of selective autophagy are known. However, the molecular mechanisms for cargo recognition and transport into autophagolysosomes in the case of mitophagy are not yet completely clarified. In particular, how dysfunctional mitochondria are distinguished from functional ones on a molecular level is not understood. Mitophagy has been reported to be increased in mammalian and yeast cells harboring dysfunctional mitochondria. It is also induced by nutrient starvation, and depends on the general autophagy machinery. Although the presence of mitochondria in lysosomes was first demonstrated in mammalian cells, understanding of mitophagy at the molecular level was pioneered in yeast (Kanki and Klionsky, 2010). In particular, these studies identified genes that are required for mitophagy but not for other forms of autophagy, highlighting selective regulation of mitophagy.

In yeast, Uth1, a mitochondrial outer membrane protein, as well as Aup1, a mitochondrial phosphatase, were reported to be critical for mitophagy (Kanki and Klionsky, 2008). Recently, systematic screens for components involved in this process have revealed several additional components required for this selective type of autophagy, including Atg11, Atg20, Atg24, Atg32, and Atg33 (Kanki and Klionsky, 2008, 2009; Okamoto *et al.*, 2009). Atg32 is of particular interest, as it was reported to act as a mitophagy receptor. It is anchored to the outer membrane of mitochondria, and is involved in the local recruitment of Atg8, a component essential for autophagosome formation. Mitochondria-derived ROS, at low concentrations, may act as signaling molecules and trigger mitophagy through redox regulation of Atg4, an essential cysteine protease in the autophagic pathway (Scherz-Shouval *et al.*, 2007). The formation of autophagosomes depends on Atg4-mediated cleavage of Atg8 and its subsequent conjugation to phosphatidyl ethanolamine at autophagosomal membranes (Yorimitsu and Klionsky, 2005).

In mammalian cells, a critical role of mitochondrial permeability transition (MPT) in mitophagy has been proposed. Lemasters' group (Rodriguez-Enriquez *et al.*, 2006) demonstrated that induction of autophagy in rat hepatocytes by serum deprivation and glucagon causes an increase of spontaneously depolarizing mitochondria, and these mitochondria are sequestered by autophagosomes. The authors concluded that the MPT is responsible for mitochondrial depolarization, and that it leads to mitochondrial sequestration into autophagosomes. Different proteins, such as ULK1, NIX, BNIP3, PARKIN, PINK1, and Cisd2, have been recently reported to be involved in degradation of mitochondria at the molecular level.

Mitophagy has been carefully investigated during the process of erythroid differentiation. Erythroid differentiation involves the programmed clearance of organelles, including the nucleus, to eventually form the nascent reticulocyte. A considerable body of evidence suggests that mitochondrial degradation during this process is achieved by mitophagy. Ulk1, the mammalian orthologue of yeast Atg1, is a critical upstream regulator of macroautophagy, and is required for mitophagy during erythroid differentiation. Ulk1 knockout mice develop red blood cells that retain mitochondria (Kundu *et al.*, 2008).

In addition to ULK1, a Bcl-2 family member protein, NIX, is required for mitochondrial clearance during erythroid differentiation, as Nix knockout mice fail to target mitochondria to autophagosomes (Sandoval *et al.*, 2008).

Expression of BNIP3, another member of the BH3-only proteins, is critical for the induction of mitophagy, a survival adaptation to control ROS production and DNA damage under hypoxic conditions. There is evidence that BNIP3 functions as a mitochondrial sensor of oxidative stress where an increase in reactive oxygen species (ROS) induces the homodimerization and activation of BNIP3 via a conserved cysteine residue in the NH_2 terminus (Kubli *et al.*, 2008).

Removal of aberrant mitochondria has been shown to play a protective role in age-related neurodegenerative disorders such as Parkinson's disease. Specifically, the E3-like ubiquitin-ligase Parkin, the loss of function of which causes Parkinson's disease, is involved. Parkin is selectively recruited to dysfunctional mitochondria with a low membrane potential in mammalian cells and causes their autophagy-mediated degradation (Narendra *et al.*, 2008), suggesting that Parkinson's disease may be at least in part associated with failure to eliminate dysfunctional mitochondria. The translocation of Parkin to mitochondria requires PINK1, which is a protein kinase that is ubiquitously expressed in the human brain and localized to the intermembrane space, as well as in membranes of the mitochondria. Once recruited by PINK1, activated Parkin leads to the formation of polyubiquitin chains on certain protein(s) believed to reside on the mitochondrial outer membrane. This triggers recruitment of p62 to mitochondria; p62 has a LC3 binding domain, and is an adaptor protein for autophagic degradation of polyubiquinated proteins. VDAC1 is one of many proteins shown to be polyubiquitinated by Parkin, and its specific role in the recruitment of p62 has not been established and remains speculative; however, Parkin poly-ubiquitination of VDAC1, or more likely some other protein, initiates a process that culminates in mitochondrial degradation by mitophagy.

A recent study linked the mitochondrial protein Cisd2 to autophagy and aging. Cisd2 is a member of the gene family containing the CDGSH iron sulfur domain; its cellular function is unclear. Cisd2 knockout mice show phenotypes of premature aging, which appears to be a consequence of mitochondrial dysfunction accompanied by increased mitophagy and "autophagic cell death" (Chen et al., 2009).

Mitochondrial Dynamics Allows Differentiation of Functional from Dysfunctional Mitochondria

How dysfunctional mitochondria are distinguished from functional ones on a molecular level is not understood. Recent studies examining the molecular mechanisms that link mitochondrial dynamics to the functionality of mitochondria in yeast and mammalian cells have tried to clarify this question. Mitochondrial morphology is highly variable, and is known to be altered in many pathological situations. Normally, mitochondria form a large network of interconnected tubules which is maintained by a balance of fission and fusion events of mitochondria. When mitochondria are functional, fusion and fission of mitochondria occur in a constant and balanced manner.

As soon as individual parts of the mitochondrial network become dysfunctional (e.g., by oxidative damage), damaged mitochondria become spatially isolated and re-fusion with the intact network is blocked. Thus, dysfunctional mitochondria are distinguished, on a morphological basis, from the rest. Fission and fusion events permit the segregation of dysfunctional mitochondria, which are eventually degraded by autophagy. Work on the pro-fission protein Fis1 demonstrates that fission events trigger autophagy per se, but only when associated with mitochondrial dysfunction (Gomes and Scorrano, 2008).

This type of intracellular quality control mechanism is of particular importance for post-mitotic tissues such as neurons and muscle cells. Future studies will need to investigate whether impaired quality control of mitochondria indeed limits lifespan in eukaryotes.

Mitophagy and Mitochondrial Biogenesis

Removal of mitochondria usually needs to be compensated by mitochondrial biogenesis or it will become detrimental. For example, in the liver during subacute sepsis, mitochondrial function is impaired and mitochondria are removed by autophagy. In this model, clearance of mitochondria is followed by mitochondrial replenishment (Crouser et al., 2006). Mitochondrial biogenesis in the presence of defective mitochondrial function is also observed in type 1 diabetes (Shen et al., 2004). In hearts of OVE26 mice, a chronic model of type 1 diabetes, there is upregulation of mitochondrial proteins, and an increase in mitochondrial area and number and mitochondrial DNA. Despite the greater number of mitochondria, their function is impaired. It is possible that increased biogenesis is a compensatory mechanism for defective mitochondrial function. Biogenesis in the absence of balanced mitophagy to remove defective mitochondria may be maladaptive.

MITOPHAGY IN PRIMARY COENZYME Q_{10} DEFICIENCY

The molecular basis and pathogenic mechanisms of the various primary and secondary forms of CoQ deficiency remain largely unknown. In our work, we have studied the pathophysiology of CoQ deficiency in cultured fibroblasts derived from four patients with primary CoQ deficiency (Rodriguez-Hernandez *et al.*, 2009). First, we assessed mitochondrial function in cultured fibroblasts. As expected, CoQ-deficient fibroblasts showed reduced CoQ-dependent respiratory enzymatic activities (complex III and complex II + III). Interestingly, complex IV also showed reduced activity, while the activity of complex I was not affected. These data correlate with the reduced levels of subunits of complex III and IV seen on immunoblots, while the levels of complex I subunits were not affected. Thus, the expression of proteins of complexes III and IV were reduced, while the expression of proteins of complex I was not affected. These observations suggest that the primary effect of CoQ deficiency might be to affect the activity, organization, and assembly of complex III, as has been reported in yeast (Santos-Ocana *et al.*, 2002), with effects on complex IV being a secondary consequence. The respiratory chain consists of interconnected complex I_1–complex III_2–complex IV_4, and III_2–IV_4 supercomplexes, in a 2:1 ratio (Schagger and Pfeiffer, 2001). Therefore, complex III disorganization might affect complex IV association with complex III in these large supercomplexes, thus altering complex IV activity and composition.

Deficient mitochondrial protein expression levels and reduced respiratory enzyme activities may impair normal mitochondrial electron flow and proton pumping, inducing a drop in mitochondrial membrane potential. Our data have shown that CoQ-deficient fibroblasts possess reduced mitochondrial potential, which may contribute to impaired mitochondrial protein import and aggravate mitochondrial dysfunction. Similar results in fibroblasts harboring COQ2 or PDSS2 mutations have been shown (Quinzii *et al.*, 2008).

Production of ROS and oxidative stress is another common consequence of dysfunctional mitochondria. Our results show a significant increase in ROS generation in primary CoQ-deficient fibroblasts that was partially mitigated by CoQ supplementation. Generated ROS can be released into the cytosol and trigger Reactive Oxygen Species (ROS)-induced ROS release (RIRR) in neighboring mitochondria. This mitochondrion-to-mitochondrion ROS signaling constitutes a positive feedback mechanism for enhanced ROS production, potentially leading to significant mitochondrial injury (Zorov *et al.*, 2006). Recent studies by a number of groups have demonstrated that ROS can directly modify signaling proteins through different modifications – for example, via nitrosylation, carbonylation, disulfide bond formation, and glutathionylation. Moreover, redox modification of proteins permits further regulation of cell signaling pathways. Thus, it has been proposed that ROS damage can induce MPT by opening of non-specific high conductance permeability transition pores in the mitochondrial inner membrane. This in turn leads to a simultaneous collapse of mitochondrial membrane potential. Our results verify this hypothesis, showing the presence of MTP in CoQ-deficient fibroblasts. In MPT, the opening of PT pores causes mitochondria to become permeable to all solutes up to a molecular mass of about 1500 Da. After MPT, mitochondria undergo a dramatic swelling driven by colloid osmotic forces, which culminates in the rupture of the outer membrane and release of pro-apoptotic mitochondrial intermembrane proteins, such as cytochrome c, apoptosis inducing factor, Smac/Diablo, and others, into the cytosol. Cyclosporin A (CsA) and various of its analogues inhibit MPT through interaction with cyclophilin D (CypD). PT pores are composed of the voltage-dependent anion channel (VDAC) in the outer membrane, the adenine nucleotide translocator (ANT) in the inner membrane, and CypD in the matrix space. It has been reported that ROS can promote MPT by causing oxidation of thiol groups on adenine nucleotide translocase (ANT), which forms part of the MPT pore (Kanno *et al.*, 2004). Therefore, oxidative stress in CoQ-deficient fibroblasts might cause mitochondrial damage, MPT activation, and mitochondrial dysfunction. Elimination of these dysfunctional mitochondria would be critical to protect cells from the damage of altered mitochondrial function and release of potentially pro-apoptotic molecules. Mitochondrial turnover is predominantly autophagic sequestration and delivery to lysosomes for hydrolytic degradation, a process also called mitophagy. Our data suggest mitophagy could take place as a process that specifically targets dysfunctional mitochondria in primary CoQ-deficient fibroblasts. We have postulated that the structural composition of mitochondria might be affected by increased ROS production, which in turn determines their self-elimination. An example could be the presence of oxidized mitochondrial unsaturated fatty acids and/or proteins.

In primary CoQ-deficient fibroblasts we demonstrated increased expression of autophagic genes and proteins, suggesting activation of the autophagic machinery in these patients. Moreover, lysosomal/autophagic markers (β-galactosidase, LC3, cathepsin, LysoTracker) were enhanced in CoQ-deficient fibroblasts, indicating lysosomal proliferation. Such findings led to the assumption that autophagy was activated in primary CoQ-deficient fibroblasts. We confirmed these results by electron microscopy, which clearly showed the presence of laminar bodies and autophagosomes engulfing mitochondria (Figure 10.1). Immunofluorescence studies also verified that typical lysosomal enzymes, such as cathepsin D, co-localized with a mitochondrial marker, such as cytochrome c. These results suggest that autophagy in primary CoQ-deficient fibroblasts is characterized by selective degradation of dysfunctional mitochondria or mitophagy.

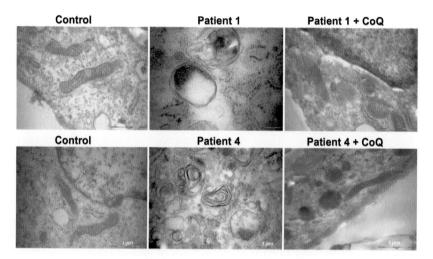

FIGURE 10.1   Ultrastructure of control and primary CoQ deficient fibroblasts from two patients in the absence or presence of CoQ supplementation (100 μm) for 72 h.

Are ROS and MPT essential for autophagy in primary CoQ deficiency? To address this question, we tested the effects of N-acetyl-cysteine (NAC) and BHA, two general anti-oxidants, and the MTP inhibitor cyclosporin on the formation of autophagosomes in CoQ-deficient fibroblasts, using β-galactosidase as a marker. Results showed that both anti-oxidants and MPT inhibitors reduced β-galactosidase staining. These data suggest that ROS generation and MPT are involved in CoQ-deficiency induced autophagy. Increasing evidence corroborates the fact that autophagy of mitochondria may occur selectively. Our work also strongly indicates that ROS/MPT-induced autophagy can show selectivity for mitochondria in primary CoQ deficiency.

Protective Role of Mitophagy in Primary Coenzyme Q_{10} Deficiency

There is controversy regarding whether autophagy promotes or prevents cell death. If autophagy removes damaged mitochondria that would otherwise activate caspases and apoptosis, then autophagy could be protective. In agreement with this hypothesis, we demonstrated that disruption of autophagic processing in CoQ-deficient fibroblasts by 3-MA or wortmannin promoted caspase-dependent cell death. To verify this hypothesis, we examined the effects of CoQ deficiency in a well-established genetic knockout of autophagy, Atg5$^{-/-}$ mouse embryonic fibroblasts (MEFs). The absence of autophagy in Atg5$^{-/-}$ cells sensitized them to apoptosis when coenzyme Q deficiency was induced by treatment with a specific inhibitor of CoQ biosynthesis (PABA). Together, these findings indicate that inhibition of autophagy in CoQ deficiency can promote cell death, suggesting a protective role of autophagy in this disease.

MITOPHAGY IN SECONDARY COENZYME Q_{10} DEFICIENCY

In our work, we have also studied the pathophysiology of secondary CoQ deficiency in primary cultured fibroblasts derived from two patients with MELAS (mitochondrial encephalomyopathy, lactic acidosis, and stroke-like episodes) syndrome harboring the A3243G mutation in mitochondrial DNA (Cotan *et al.*, 2011). First, we assessed mitochondrial proliferation and function in cultured fibroblasts. Mitochondrial proliferation is commonly observed in affected tissues of patients with mitochondrial disorders, and is believed to be a compensatory mechanism triggered by the OXPHOS defect. We found an increase in the mtDNA copy number together with a decrease in mitochondrial mass in MELAS fibroblasts. The MELAS fibroblasts also showed reduced respiratory chain enzyme activities. These data correlate with the reduced levels of mitochondrial proteins seen on immunoblots. Defects of complexes I and IV are common in patients with MELAS. However, because all four subunits of complex II are encoded by nuclear DNA, complex II activity is usually normal in fibroblasts, cybrids, and tissues harboring the MELAS mutation. Unexpectedly, complex II activity and protein levels of the 30-kDa subunit of complex II were also low in MELAS fibroblasts. These results are in agreement with recent investigations that also found a generalized reduction in mitochondrial enzyme activities in endothelial and astrocyte cells harboring the MELAS mutation (Davidson *et al.*, 2009). Low complex II activity observed in our study may be a consequence of the massive depletion of mitochondrial mass that we observed in MELAS fibroblasts by NAO staining and immunoblots of mitochondrial proteins. Furthermore, MELAS fibroblasts showed reduced levels of CoQ. Deficient respiratory chain enzyme activities, mitochondrial protein expression, and CoQ levels may impair normal mitochondrial electron flow and proton pumping, inducing a drop in $\Delta\Psi_m$. Our data showed that MELAS fibroblasts possess reduced $\Delta\Psi_m$, which may contribute to aggravation of mitochondrial dysfunction and perturbed cell bioenergetics. Reduced $\Delta\Psi_m$ will also affect protein import into mitochondria and amplify mitochondrial disorganization. Secondarily, critical components of the mitochondrial respiratory chain, such as CoQ, whose biosynthesis depends on mitochondrial proteins encoded by the nucleus, will also be affected. Furthermore, CoQ supplementation reverts many of the pathological alterations found in MELAS fibroblasts. Detection of secondary CoQ deficiency in mitochondrial diseases in general, and in MELAS patients in particular, is of great importance because CoQ supplementation could be particularly beneficial for the patients. Putative roles for CoQ supplementation include enhancement of electron transport and ATP production; antioxidant protection; a beneficial alteration in redox signaling; and stabilization of the MPT pore protecting against autophagy and apoptotic cell loss.

ROS production and oxidative stress is a common consequence of dysfunctional mitochondria and CoQ deficiency. Our results showed a significant increase in ROS generation in MELAS fibroblasts that was partially mitigated by CoQ supplementation. As mentioned previously, ROS damage can induce MPT by the opening of non-specific high conductance permeability transition pores in the mitochondrial inner membrane. This in turn leads to a simultaneous collapse of $\Delta\Psi_m$. Our results verify this hypothesis, showing the presence of MPT in MELAS fibroblasts. Therefore, oxidative stress in MELAS fibroblasts might cause mitochondrial damage, MPT, and autophagy activation. Elimination of these dysfunctional mitochondria would be critical to protect cells from the damage caused by altered mitochondrial function and the release of potentially pro-apoptotic molecules. Our data suggest that mitophagy could take place as a process that specifically targets dysfunctional mitochondria in MELAS fibroblasts. We postulated that the structural composition of mitochondria might be affected by increased ROS production, which in turn determines their self-elimination. We also demonstrated increased expression of autophagic genes and proteins in MELAS fibroblasts, suggesting the activation of autophagic machinery in these patients. Our results are in agreement with previous results which showed that mitochondria of fibroblasts from MELAS patients, but not from a normal control, undergo extensive autophagy in response to serum withdrawal (Gu et al., 2004).

Furthermore, lysosomal/autophagic markers (β-galactosidase, LC3, cathepsin D, and LysoTracker) were enhanced, indicating that autophagy was activated in MELAS fibroblasts. Increased autophagosomes and autophagolysosomes and selective degradation of dysfunctional mitochondria was also confirmed by electron microscopy and co-localization studies by immunofluorescence microscopy. Our results show too that secondary CoQ deficiency in MELAS fibroblasts plays a critical role in the activation of mitophagy because CoQ supplementation prevented mitophagy, and restored mitochondrial protein expression levels and respiratory enzymatic activities.

Besides autophagy activation, we found impairment in autophagosome degradation in MELAS fibroblasts. The fact that autophagic genes and protein were induced in MELAS fibroblasts suggests that accumulation of autophagosomes is due to both increased *de novo* autophagosome formation, and delayed or deficient fusion of autophagosomes with late endosomes/lysosomes. Our data suggest that impaired flux through the autophagic pathway and imbalance between induction and flux may contribute to the pathology of MELAS fibroblasts by causing the accumulation of incomplete degraded mitochondria. As a result of partial degradation of mitochondria, we can clearly observe co-localization of cytochrome c with autophagosome markers in small fragmented mitochondria (Figure 10.2). Therefore, we postulate that although there is some fusion of lysosomes with autophagosomes, it is not sufficient for complete mitochondrial degradation and autophagosomal maturation. This alteration leads to autophagosome accumulation. As the autophagic–lysosomal pathway is dependent on intracellular ATP levels, impaired autophagic flux in MELAS fibroblasts might be due to decreased ATP levels and bioenergetic collapse as a result of massive sequestration and partial degradation of mitochondria. Incomplete mitochondrial degradation can also explain the presence of PicoGreen foci in these small rounded depolarized LC3-positive mitochondria, which suggests that mtDNA is not degraded. Therefore, partial mitochondrial protein degradation and incomplete mtDNA degradation, along with compensatory replication of mtDNA induced by OXPHOS alteration, might explain the increased mtDNA copy number and reduced mitochondrial mass found in MELAS fibroblasts. Disproportionate

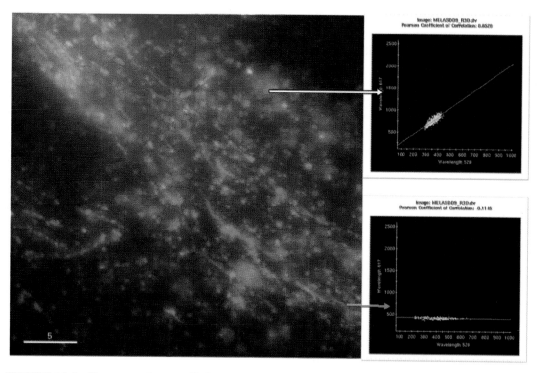

FIGURE 10.2 **Fluorescent images of LC3 protein (red) and cytochrome c (green) in MELAS fibroblasts.** Cell nuclei were stained with Hoechst (blue). Bar = 5 μm. White arrow, autophagosomes showing co-localization of LC3 and cytochrome c signal in autophagosomes (orange). Red arrow, normal tubular mitochondria without co-localization of LC3 and cytochrome c signal.

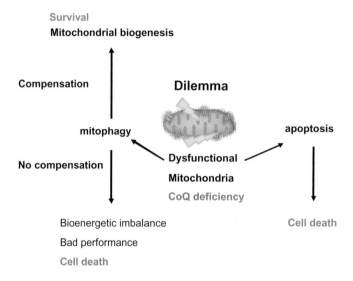

FIGURE 10.3   Scheme showing the relationships between CoQ deficiency, mitochondrial dysfunction, mitophagy, mitochondrial biogenesis, and cell death.

induction and impaired flux through the autophagic pathway (frustrated autophagy) has been demonstrated in other disease models, and can lead to cell stress and may trigger cell death (Gottlieb and Mentzer, 2010).

Secondary CoQ deficiency and autophagy activation were also demonstrated in transmitochondrial cybrids harboring the A3243G mutation, indicating that both processes are produced as a consequence of the mutation in mtDNA and are not the product of a concomitant nuclear gene defect.

Are ROS and MPT essential for autophagy in MELAS fibroblasts? To address this question, we tested the effects of N-acetyl-cysteine (NAC), and BHA, two general antioxidants, and the MTP inhibitor cyclosporine on the formation of autophagosomes in MELAS fibroblasts using Lysotracker as a marker. Results showed that both antioxidants and MPT inhibitors reduced Lysotracker staining. These data suggest that ROS generation and MPT are involved in MELAS-induced autophagy.

Protective Role of Mitophagy in Secondary Coenzyme Q_{10} Deficiency

If mitophagy removes damaged mitochondria in MELAS fibroblasts that would otherwise activate caspases and apoptosis, then mitophagy could be protective, as in primary CoQ deficiency. In agreement with this hypothesis, we demonstrated that disruption of autophagic processing in MELAS fibroblasts by 3-MA or wortmannin promoted apoptosis. To verify this hypothesis, we examined the effects of silencing the Atg5 gene by siRNA in MELAS fibroblasts. The absence of this essential autophagy gene in MELAS cells sensitized them to apoptosis. Together, these findings indicate that inhibition of autophagy in MELAS fibroblasts can promote cell death, suggesting a protective role of autophagy in this disease. However, massive mitophagy, mitochondrial loss, and autophagosome accumulation could impair autophagic flux and cell bioenergetics, and may also induce cell death.

CONCLUSIONS

In normal physiology, cells utilize autophagy to eliminate damaged, dysfunctional, and superfluous cytoplasmic components to maintain cellular homeostasis and adjust to changing physiological demands.

In this respect, mitochondrial degradation by autophagy (mitophagy) may play an essential role in maintaining cellular homeostasis in CoQ deficiency. We propose that mitophagy is triggered in our model as a "stress-induced" mechanism involved in the degradation of dysfunctional CoQ-deficient mitochondria, suggesting a protective role. However, massive mitophagy and autophagosome accumulation could impair cell bioenergetics and also induce cell death (Figure 10.3).

Acknowledgments

This work was supported by grants FIS PI10/00543 and FIS EC08/00076, Ministerio de Sanidad, Spain, and Fondo Europeo de Desarrollo Regional (FEDER-Unión Europea); grant SAS 111242t, Servicio Andaluz de Salud-Junta de Andalucía, Proyecto de Investigación de Excelencia de la Junta de Andalucía CTS-5725; and by AEPMI (Asociación de Enfermos de Patología Mitocondrial), FEEL (Fundación Española de Enfermedades Lisosomales) and Federación Andaluza de Fibromialgia y Fatiga Crónica (ALBA Andalucía).

References

Artuch, R., Brea-Calvo, G., Briones, P., et al., 2006. Cerebellar ataxia with coenzyme Q_{10} deficiency: diagnosis and follow-up after coenzyme Q_{10} supplementation. J. Neurol. Sci. 246, 153–158.

Boitier, E., Degoul, F., Desguerre, I., et al., 1998. A case of mitochondrial encephalomyopathy associated with a muscle coenzyme Q_{10} deficiency. J. Neurol. Sci. 156, 41–46.

Chen, Y.F., Kao, C.H., Chen, Y.T., et al., 2009. Cisd2 deficiency drives premature aging and causes mitochondria-mediated defects in mice. Genes Dev. 23, 1183–1194.

Cordero, M.D., De Miguel, M., Moreno Fernandez, A.M., et al., 2010. Mitochondrial dysfunction and mitophagy activation in blood mononuclear cells of fibromyalgia patients: implications in the pathogenesis of the disease. Arthritis Res. Ther. 12, R17.

Cotan, D., Cordero, M.D., Garrido-Maraver, J., et al., 2011. Secondary coenzyme Q_{10} deficiency triggers mitochondria degradation by mitophagy in MELAS fibroblasts. FASEB J. 25, 2669–2687.

Crane, F.L., Hatefi, Y., Lester, R.L., et al., 1957. Isolation of a quinone from beef heart mitochondria. Biochim. Biophys. Acta 25, 220–221.

Crouser, E.D., Julian, M.W., Huff, J.E., et al., 2006. Carbamoyl phosphate synthase-1: a marker of mitochondrial damage and depletion in the liver during sepsis. Crit. Care Med. 34, 2439–2446.

Davidson, M.M., Walker, W.F., Hernandez-Rosa, E., 2009. The m.3243A>G mtDNA mutation is pathogenic in an *in vitro* model of the human blood brain barrier. Mitochondrion 9, 463–470.

Di Giovanni, S., Mirabella, M., Spinazzola, A., et al., 2001. Coenzyme Q_{10} reverses pathological phenotype and reduces apoptosis in familial CoQ_{10} deficiency. Neurology 57, 515–518.

Gomes, L.C., Scorrano, L., 2008. High levels of Fis1, a pro-fission mitochondrial protein, trigger autophagy. Biochim. Biophys. Acta 1777, 860–866.

Gottlieb, R.A., Mentzer, R.M., 2010. Autophagy during cardiac stress: joys and frustrations of autophagy. Annu. Rev. Physiol. 72, 45–59.

Gu, Y., Wang, C., Cohen, A., 2004. Effect of IGF-1 on the balance between autophagy of dysfunctional mitochondria and apoptosis. FEBS Lett. 577, 357–360.

Kanki, T., Klionsky, D.J., 2008. Mitophagy in yeast occurs through a selective mechanism. J. Biol. Chem. 283, 32386–32393.

Kanki, T., Klionsky, D.J., 2009. Atg32 is a tag for mitochondria degradation in yeast. Autophagy 5, 1201–1202.

Kanki, T., Klionsky, D.J., 2010. The molecular mechanism of mitochondria autophagy in yeast. Mol. Microbiol. 75, 795–800.

Kanno, T., Sato, E.E., Muranaka, S., et al., 2004. Oxidative stress underlies the mechanism for Ca(2+)-induced permeability transition of mitochondria. Free Radic. Res. 38, 27–35.

Kubli, D.A., Quinsay, M.N., Huang, C., et al., 2008. Bnip3 functions as a mitochondrial sensor of oxidative stress during myocardial ischemia and reperfusion. Am. J. Physiol. Heart Circ. Physiol. 295, H2025–H2031.

Kundu, M., Lindsten, T., Yang, C.Y., et al., 2008. Ulk1 plays a critical role in the autophagic clearance of mitochondria and ribosomes during reticulocyte maturation. Blood 112, 1493–1502.

Narendra, D., Tanaka, A., Suen, D.F., et al., 2008. Parkin is recruited selectively to impaired mitochondria and promotes their autophagy. J. Cell Biol. 183, 795–803.

Okamoto, K., Kondo-Okamoto, N., Ohsumi, Y., 2009. A landmark protein essential for mitophagy: Atg32 recruits the autophagic machinery to mitochondria. Autophagy 5, 1203–1205.

Quinzii, C.M., Hirano, M., 2011. Primary and secondary $CoQ_{(10)}$ deficiencies in humans. Biofactors 37, 361–365.

Quinzii, C.M., Lopez, L.C., Von-Moltke, J., et al., 2008. Respiratory chain dysfunction and oxidative stress correlate with severity of primary CoQ_{10} deficiency. FASEB J. 22, 1874–1885.

Quinzii, C.M., Lopez, L.C., Gilkerson, R.W., et al., 2010. Reactive oxygen species, oxidative stress, and cell death correlate with level of CoQ_{10} deficiency. FASEB J. 24, 3733–3743.

Rodriguez-Enriquez, S., Kim, I., Currin, R.T., et al., 2006. Tracker dyes to probe mitochondrial autophagy (mitophagy) in rat hepatocytes. Autophagy 2, 39–46.

Rodriguez-Hernandez, A., Cordero, M.D., Salviati, L., et al., 2009. Coenzyme Q deficiency triggers mitochondria degradation by mitophagy. Autophagy 5, 19–32.

Rotig, A., Appelkvist, E.L., Geromel, V., et al., 2000. Quinone-responsive multiple respiratory-chain dysfunction due to widespread coenzyme Q_{10} deficiency. Lancet 356, 391–395.

Sandoval, H., Thiagarajan, P., Dasgupta, S.K., et al., 2008. Essential role for Nix in autophagic maturation of erythroid cells. Nature 454, 232–235.

Santos-Ocana, C., Do, T.Q., Padilla, S., et al., 2002. Uptake of exogenous coenzyme Q and transport to mitochondria is required for bc1 complex stability in yeast coq mutants. J. Biol. Chem. 277, 10973–10981.

Schagger, H., Pfeiffer, K., 2001. The ratio of oxidative phosphorylation complexes I–V in bovine heart mitochondria and the composition of respiratory chain supercomplexes. J. Biol. Chem. 276, 37861–37867.

Schatz, G., 2007. The magic garden. Annu. Rev. Biochem. 76, 673–678.

Scherz-Shouval, R., Shvets, E., Fass, E., et al., 2007. Reactive oxygen species are essential for autophagy and specifically regulate the activity of Atg4. EMBO J. 26, 1749–1760.

Shen, X., Zheng, S., Thongboonkerd, V., et al., 2004. Cardiac mitochondrial damage and biogenesis in a chronic model of type 1 diabetes. Am. J. Physiol. Endocrinol. Metab. 287, E896–E905.

Tran, U.C., Clarke, C.F., 2007. Endogenous synthesis of coenzyme Q in eukaryotes. Mitochondrion 7 (Suppl.), S62–71.

Yorimitsu, T., Klionsky, D.J., 2005. Autophagy: molecular machinery for self-eating. Cell Death Differ. 12 (Suppl. 2), 1542–1552.

Zorov, D.B., Juhaszova, M., Sollott, S.J., 2006. Mitochondrial ROS-induced ROS release: an update and review. Biochim. Biophys. Acta 1757, 509–517.

The Presence of Dioxin in Kidney Cells Induces Cell Death with Autophagy

Filomena Fiorito and Luisa De Martino

Abstract

Autophagy is a cellular process of "self-eating," which involves the digestion of cytoplasmic components via the lysosomal pathway as resources during starvation or other limiting conditions. However, many studies have indicated that autophagy may represent a cellular response to stress conditions. As a consequence, autophagy can directly induce cell death or act as a mechanism of cell survival.

It is well established that 2,3,7,8-tetrachlorodibenzo-p-dioxin (TCDD) may promote a multiplicity of toxic effects in mammalian cells. In particular, kidney anomalies are correlated with dioxin exposure by inducing augmented renal immune complex deposition, glomerulonephritis, and hydronephrosis. In Madin–Darby Bovine Kidney (MDBK), a kidney epithelial cell line, our group demonstrated that TCDD provokes cell proliferation and impairs cellular iron homeostasis, leading to changes in the extent of the labile iron pool. These processes could be associated with neoplastic transformation of the bovine kidney cell. Analysis of MDBK cell morphology revealed some death alterations in a large number of exposed cells where signs of

© 2014 Elsevier Inc. All rights reserved.

neither apoptosis nor necrosis were detected, but we found that dioxin activated cell death with autophagy. Our data establish the requirement for autophagy in the maintenance of MDBK cells exposed to dioxin, as well as providing evidence suggesting that autophagy protects against proliferative effects induced by non-genotoxic compounds such as TCDD. Indeed, multiple evidences indicate that autophagy plays a critical role in kidney maintenance, diseases, and aging. Generally, autophagy serves as a protective mechanism, but persistent activation of autophagy can result in cell death, mainly after exposure to toxic agents.

INTRODUCTION

Generally, autophagy is described as a homeostatic "self-eating" process, first recognized in yeast cells, that has been conserved among eukaryotic cells. The autophagic pathway begins with formation of the autophagosome, which consists of cytoplasmic material sequestered inside a double-membrane vesicle. The autophagosome then fuses with the lysosome and the cytoplasmic material is digested by hydrolases, as cellular resources during starvation or other limiting conditions. Starvation-induced autophagy is generally assumed to be non-selective, with the aim of generating building blocks essential for cell survival. Hence, in mammals autophagy is often a protective response activated by the cells as a response to stress, and its inhibition accelerates, rather than prevents, cell death. The role of autophagy extends beyond the general homeostatic removal, degradation, and recycling of damaged proteins and organelles, to many specific physiological and pathological processes such as development, immunity, energy homeostasis, cell death, or tumorigenesis (Rosenfeldt and Ryan, 2011). In the late 1960s, autophagy was found to be enhanced in various organs, including newborn kidney (Periyasamy-Thandavan *et al.*, 2009). Accumulating evidence indicates that ischemic, immunological, oxidative, and toxic stresses can cause induction of autophagy in renal epithelial cells, modifying not only the course of various kidney diseases but also kidney maintenance and aging. Most often, autophagy serves as a protective mechanism, but persistent activation of autophagy can result in cell death. This is true for many toxic agents, such as 2,3,7,8-tetrachlorodibenzo-p-dioxin (TCDD), commonly referred to as dioxin, which is a highly toxic and widely distributed environmental contaminant. In this chapter we will first discuss the general toxic effects of TCDD, and then consider how dioxin initiates divergent pathways of cell proliferation and cell death with autophagy in an epithelial kidney cell line.

Tetrachlorodibenzo-p-Dioxin (TCDD)

TCDD is a prototype of a group of compounds known as polyhalogenated aromatic hydrocarbons. Dioxin is a compound which is not intentionally generated. Certainly, it is a byproduct in some industrial processes, including chlorination of phenolic substances, but in fact uncontrolled waste combustion represents a large source of dioxin. TCDD is persistent in the environment and bioaccumulative in the body, where, being highly lipophilic, it accumulates in the adipose fraction of organs and tissues. Humans are generally exposed to TCDD, which is incorporated into food (products of animal origin rich in fat, such as meat, milk, cheese, and seafood) and is also present drinking water, soil, dust, smoke, and air. It causes a wide range of tissue- and species-specific toxic effects, such as chloracne, which is a persistent cystic and hyperkeratotic skin condition, thymic atrophy and immune dysfunction, hepatic damage and steatosis, gastric epithelial hyperplasia, embryonic teratogenesis, and several types of cancer (White and Birnbaum, 2009). As reviewed by these authors, there is a long history of anthropogenic dioxin production, which still persists today. The earliest evidence of man-made dioxin molecules was from a German chemical production plant in Lampertheim, South Hesse, that manufactured washing soda; there, chloracne, which represents a hallmark of dioxin exposure, was first identified and characterized in 1897 in German industrial workers. In general, most reported human exposures have been the result of unintentional production or spills, as was the case following its formation as a byproduct of Agent Orange. This herbicide, containing 2,4,5-trichlorophenoxyacetic acid (2,4,5-T) and contaminated with dioxin, was used as a defoliant in Vietnam between 1962 and 1970 to reduce enemy ground cover, as part of Operation Ranch Hand, and persistent chloracne was observed in exposed individuals. Recent studies of the Ranch Hand cohort revealed that American military exposures to Agent Orange are also associated with an increased risk of diabetes and of multiple cancers. The Institute of Medicine found sufficient evidence of association between Agent Orange exposure and soft-tissue sarcomas, non-Hodgkin's lymphoma, Hodgkin's disease, and chronic lymphocytic leukemia. In 1976, in Seveso, Italy, an explosion occurred at a chemical plant producing 2,4,5-trichlorophenol, an intermediate in 2,4,5-T synthesis. Within several weeks of the accident, some of the exposed community members were exhibiting skin lesions consistent with chloracne. In the years that followed, continuing studies of the exposed population supported the potential for TCDD to act as a carcinogen in humans and to increase risk for diabetes, adverse cardiovascular effects, and altered endocrine function. Just after the Seveso disaster, laboratory cancer studies in rats revealed that chronic 2-year exposure to TCDD at as low a dose as 0.01 µg/kg per day resulted in increased risk of hepatocellular carcinomas and various squamous cell carcinomas. Finally, one of the most recent incidents involved the Ukrainian Prime Minister Viktor Yushchenko, who may have been intentionally poisoned with TCCD as a measure to weaken his political influence and, potentially, remove him from the campaign. Two months prior to the presidential election, Yushchenko was hospitalized for pancreatitis; this was followed by profound facial acne and edema. The diagnosis of chloracne was confirmed when his dioxin blood levels were found to be three orders of magnitude above average.

Several studies, including our own research, demonstrate the involvement of dioxin in the genesis of tumors. Although the molecular mechanisms for carcinogenicity by dioxin have not been elucidated until very recently, in 1997 TCDD was classified as a cancer promoter by the International Agency for Research on Cancer (IARC, 1997). This classification is based on studies performed in laboratory animals showing that TCDD promotes the formation of neoplastic lesions in the liver, lung, oral mucosa, and skin. For instance, in the mouse, TCDD exposure induces continued proliferation of epithelial cells within the skin tissue in a tissue-dependent manner, as well as increasing proliferation of cultured cells, such as human keratinocytes (Ray and Swanson, 2009), late gestational ureteric cells (Bryant et al., 2001), and human breast cells (Ahn et al., 2005).

TCDD and the Kidney

Exposure of human and animals to acute and chronic toxic levels of TCDD causes a wide range of gene-, tissue- and species-specific adverse effects. These observations were made in studies carried out in mice and rats by examining a variety of different diseases. Furthermore, transgenerational transmission of adult onset diseases has implications of disease risk not only for current exposed human and animal populations, but also for future generations. For example, recent studies have supported temporal considerations and suggest that the Seveso accident may have resulted in consequences to a second generation – children, born to exposed parents, with increased risk for developmental neurologic, reproductive, or immune effects (White and Birnbaum, 2009). As reported above, toxic effects induced by TCDD include hepatotoxicity, carcinogenicity, teratogenicity, chloracne, and neurobehavioral disturbance, but also interference with lipid metabolism, endocrine disruption, wasting syndrome, thymic atrophy, developmental and reproductive toxicity, and immunosuppression. In general, chronic kidney disease in humans is correlated with high dioxin levels (Couture et al., 1990).

In 1971, Courtney and Moore described an example of dioxin-induced renal abnormalities where TCDD was identified as a teratogen (Courtney and Moore, 1971). They observed that the subcutaneous administration of TCDD to pregnant mice at a dose of 3 mg/kg on gestational days 6 through 15 induced cleft palate and kidney anomalies in offspring. The kidney anomaly, described as cystic kidney, consisted of renal papillae which were markedly reduced in size or non-existent with a large renal pelvis. The incidence of kidney abnormalities was 95%. Moreover, prenatal TCDD exposure has been shown to augment renal immune complex deposition, glomerulonephritis, and mesangial proliferation (Mustafa et al., 2011), while lactational exposure of mice to TCDD caused hydronephrotic kidney (Nishimura et al., 2008).

It is known that environmental compounds can promote epigenetic transgenerational inheritance of adult-onset disease in subsequent generations following ancestral exposure during fetal gonadal sex determination. A recent study examined the ability of TCDD to promote epigenetic transgenerational inheritance of disease and DNA methylation epimutations in sperm in rats. Gestating F0 generation females were exposed to dioxin during fetal days 8 to 14, and adult-onset disease was evaluated in F1 and F3 generation rats. The incidences of total disease and multiple disease increased in the F1 and F3 generations. In particular, kidney disease incidence was higher in the transgenerational F3 generation dioxin lineage males (Manikkam et al., 2012).

Recently, our group showed that TCDD induced significant ($P < 0.001$, $P < 0.01$, and $P < 0.05$) cell proliferation in Madin–Darby Bovine Kidney (MDBK) cells (Fiorito et al., 2008a, 2011), a kidney epithelial cell line. Here, TCDD induced concomitant Iron Regulatory Protein (IRP) 1 downregulation and IRP2 upregulation, thus determining a marked enhancement of transferrin receptor 1 expression and a response in ferritin content which impairs cellular iron homeostasis, leading to changes in the extent of the labile iron pool (Santamaria et al., 2011). Deregulation of cell proliferation/differentiation processes induced by TCDD in kidney cells coupled to an iron excess could be associated with neoplastic transformation of the bovine cell and with cancer development, as pro-oncogenic activity for IRP2 to induce the growth of tumor xenografts was described (Maffettone et al.,

2010). In general, the mechanism of action by which TCDD exerts biochemical effects on vertebrate species is through activation of the Aryl hydrocarbon Receptor (AhR), a ligand-activated basic helix–loop–helix transcription factor and a member of the PER-ARNT-SIM (PAS) superfamily of transcription factors. Binding of AhR/ARNT leads to changes including induction of the cytochrome P-450 1A1 (White and Birnbaum, 2009). In a recent paper, it was been reported that activation of the aryl hydrocarbon receptor pathway enhances cancer cell invasion and is associated with poor prognosis in upper urinary tract urothelial cancer (Ishida *et al.*, 2010).

Autophagy and the Kidney

As described previously, autophagy is a homeostatic "self-eating" process that has been conserved among eukaryotic cells, and involves digestion of cytoplasmic components via the lysosomal pathway. The autophagic pathway begins with formation of the autophagosome, which consists of cytoplasmic material sequestered inside a double-membrane vesicle; the autophagosome then fuses with the lysosome and the cytoplasmic material is digested by hydrolases, as cellular resources during starvation or other limiting conditions. However, many studies have indicated that autophagy may represent a cellular response to stress conditions. As a consequence, autophagy can either act directly as a mechanism of cell survival, or induce cell death. For many years, autophagy was considered to be primarily involved in cellular architectural changes that prevail during differentiation and development. However, in the late 1960s autophagy was found to be enhanced in various organs, including newborn kidney (De Duve and Wattiaux, 1966). It seems that autophagy is specifically linked to the pathogenesis of important renal diseases such as acute kidney injury, diabetic nephropathy, and polycystic kidney disease (see review by Huber *et al.*, 2012). Dysregulation of autophagy can result in the accumulation of autophagosomes, an event that has been noted in several kidney diseases. Depending upon the disorder involved, the accumulation of autophagosomes may be due to their increased formation or the result of their reduced degradation. Most of the studies performed to date relate to evidence of autophagy in kidney diseases, while very few works concern autophagy in kidney induced by toxic substances. For example, as reviewed by Orrenius *et al.* (2013), the toxic heavy metal cadmium accumulates within lysosomes of renal proximal convoluted tubule cells, where it triggers cell proliferation and autophagy. Such activation of autophagy is an adaptive mechanism, and it has been proposed as a biomarker for renal injury after cadmium exposure. Treatment of rats with the immunosuppressive drug cyclosporine has been found to increase the formation of autophagosomes in kidney tubular cells. In this study, autophagy was suggested to represent a cytoprotective mechanism, as inhibition of autophagy increased cyclosporine toxicity in human renal proximal tubular cells (Orrenius *et al.*, 2013). However, another study demonstrated that the Ca^{2+}-activated, calmodulin (CaM)-regulated serine/threonine kinase death-associated protein kinase (DAPk) triggered caspase activation and autophagic cell death in response to tunicamycin-mediated ER stress, and that $DAPk^{-/-}$ mice were protected from kidney damage caused by injection of this compound (Orrenius *et al.*, 2013). Thus, in kidney cells, activation of autophagy may have dual and opposing effects. Moreover, the highly toxic environmental pollutant TCDD activates cell death in bovine kidney cells (Fiorito *et al.*, 2011, see below).

TCDD AND AUTOPHAGY IN KIDNEY CELLS

In recent years, levels of TCDD exceeding the European Union tolerance have been detected in dairy products and milk from cows and water buffalo raised on some areas of the Campania Region (South Italy) (Esposito *et al.*, 2010). As a consequence, within a research project aimed to investigate the effects of dioxin on cattle, our group evaluated some morphological and biochemical effects due to TCDD using MDBK – a kidney epithelial cell line that represents a useful and standardized *in vitro* model for studying TCDD exposure in mammalian cells. Different doses of TCDD (0.01, 1 and 100 pg/mL) and different times of exposure (from 4 to 48 hours) were used (Fiorito *et al.*, 2008a,b, 2010, 2011; Santamaria *et al.*, 2011). As reported above, TCDD induces significant cell proliferation in bovine cells, where, by performing nuclear staining with propidium iodide, neither nuclear (apoptosis) nor membrane (necrosis) alterations were observed (Fiorito *et al.*, 2011). Moreover, our previous study demonstrated that TCDD induced no signs of apoptosis in bovine cells; in fact, neither chromatin condensation by acridine orange staining nor DNA laddering was observed (Fiorito *et al.*, 2008a). Furthermore, western blot analysis showed no activation of caspases 8, 9, or 3 (data not shown).

Morphological and Biochemical Changes Related to Autophagy

As reported in recommendations of the Nomenclature Committee on Cell Death 2012, autophagic cell death is defined not only by morphological definitions but also by a series of precise, measurable biochemical features (Galluzzi *et al.*, 2012). Thus, we described the morphological and biochemical results of experiments indicating that TCDD exposure increased autophagy in bovine kidney cells in a time- and dose-dependent manner (Fiorito *et al.*, 2011). Analysis of bovine cell morphology by Giemsa staining displayed significant signs of autophagic cell death in TCDD-exposed groups, where a large number of cells exhibited alterations such as expanded cytoplasm (magnified cells), increase in intercellular spaces, some pyknotic nuclei with central condensed chromatin, and an elevated degree of vacuolization, which often indicates increased autophagic flux, as previously described (Galluzzi *et al.*, 2012; Lamparska-Przybysz *et al.*, 2005). Moreover, the effects of different concentrations of TCDD on autophagic markers in MDBK cells at various times post-exposure were evaluated. Specifically, we performed western blot analysis and immunofluorescence for LC3, a recognized marker for mammalian autophagy, which is processed during autophagocytosis from an 18-kD protein (LC3-I) to a membrane-bound 16-kD protein (LC3-II) (Klionsky *et al.*, 2012). Our data reported that TCDD induced autophagic features in MDBK cells by increasing the amount of LC3-II in a dose-dependent manner when bovine cells were exposed to TCDD from 4–36 h; however, on examining treated cells at 0.01 and 100 pg/mL of TCDD compared to 1 pg/mL of TCDD, at 48 h we detected an inverted U-shaped dose responsiveness in LC3-II protein levels (Fiorito *et al.*, 2011). This modulation with an inverted U-shaped dose responsiveness induced by dioxin represents a typical cell response to dioxin (Ahn *et al.*, 2005; Fiorito *et al.*, 2008a,b, 2010, 2011). Furthermore, TCDD increased punctate staining for LC3 compared to controls, as detected by immunofluorescence for LC3, using epitope-specific antibody on methanol-fixed cells, in which there was a strong accumulation of LC3-II (Figure 11.1) (Fiorito *et al.*, 2011, and here). It is well known

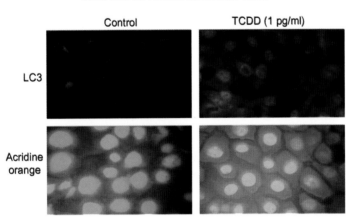

FIGURE 11.1   **TCDD induces autophagy in MDBK cells.** Immunofluorescence for LC3 in MDBK cells treated with TCDD (1 pg/mL) for 24 hours, or not treated (magnification ×400). Microphotographs of cells staining with acridine orange using a fluorescence microscope revealed the induction of acidic vesicular organelles. Detection of green and red fluorescence in acridine orange-stained cells was achieved using a fluorescence microscope in MDBK cells treated or with TCDD (1 pg/mL) for 24 hours, or not treated (magnification ×1000).

that the amount of LC3 is correlated with the extent of autophagosome formation. Indeed, when autophagosome–lysosome fusion is blocked, larger autophagosomes are detected, possibly due to autophagosome–autophagosome fusion (Klionsky *et al.*, 2012). As shown in Figure 11.1, LC3 was sometimes strongly detected in the nucleus and sometimes not. We also hypothesized that TCDD, like other toxins (Cummings *et al.*, 1998), could induce formation of toxic proteins and their import to the nucleus, which represents the primary site of action of proteotoxins. The data presented herein suggested that some nuclei were protected environments that provided a place for toxic protein aggregates to escape degradation by autophagy. Autophagy thus appeared to be relatively ineffective at clearing toxic protein aggregates which accumulated within some nuclei.

Autophagy is a process of sequestrating cytoplasmic proteins into the lytic component. To evaluate the formation of acidic vesicular organelles (AVOs), which further characterize autophagy, we performed vital staining with acridine orange in MDBK cells, where the cytoplasm and nucleolus fluoresced bright green and dim red (control group) whereas TCDD enhanced acidic compartments which fluoresced bright red (Figure 11.1). The intensity of the red fluorescence, proportional to the degree of acidity of the cellular acidic compartment, was increased by dioxin in a dose-dependent manner (Fiorito *et al.*, 2011, and here). Finally, treatment of MDBK cells with proteasome inhibitor MG-132, in the presence or absence of TCDD, was used to assess the autophagic flux by TCDD. As described in Fiorito *et al.* (2011), MG-132 increased LC3-II accumulation in the presence of all doses of TCDD at 12 h post-exposure, when significant TCDD-induced autophagy started. These results confirmed that TCDD activated autophagic flux in kidney cells, as autophagy can increase as a compensatory means of protein degradation when the proteasomal pathway is blocked (Pandey *et al.*, 2007). As reported above, autophagic cell death is not only accompanied by the accumulation of autophagic vacuoles, but also involves an increase in autophagy that contributes to cell death (Galluzzi *et al.*, 2012).

Downregulation of Telomerase Activity, bTERT, and c-Myc Protein Levels

Generally, the regulated lysosomal degradation pathway of autophagy prevents cellular damage and thus protects from malignant transformation. Deregulation of autophagy is known to affect many processes that can control the formation and existence of a cancer cell, but contradictions still exist regarding the relationship between autophagy and cancer (Rosenfeldt and Ryan, 2011). Anticancer compounds could induce antitumor activity through both inhibition of telomerase activity and autophagy modulation (Ko *et al.*, 2009). The enzyme responsible for telomere elongation, called telomerase, is a cellular reverse transcriptase that catalyzes the synthesis and extension of telomeric DNA repeats. Structurally, telomerase is a ribonucleoprotein enzyme complex that contains an essential RNA component and a catalytic protein subunit, the telomerase reverse transcriptase activity. In humans, the telomerase reverse transcriptase (hTERT) catalytic subunit is a protein which is actively upregulated by c-Myc (Wu *et al.*, 1999). Telomerase activity is specifically expressed in immortal cells, cancer and germ cells, where it compensates for telomere shortening during DNA replication and thus stabilizes telomere length. A variety of cell lines and malignant tumors have been found to express high levels of telomerase activity (Greider, 1996), suggesting that telomerase activation may be a critical step in cell immortalization and oncogenesis. Thus, we evaluated the effects of dioxin on telomerase activity by TRAP assay, and analyzed bovine TERT (bTERT) and c-Myc by western blot. TCDD significantly downregulated telomerase activity in kidney cells, with significant repression of both bTERT and c-Myc protein levels (Fiorito *et al.*, 2011). Until now there have been very few reports describing how TCDD impacts on telomerase activity. Specifically, TCDD did not affect telomerase activity in normal human epidermal cells, immortalized cells, or malignant keratinocytes (Rea *et al.*, 1998). Nevertheless, in human choriocarcinoma cells exposed to TCDD a dose-dependent increase in telomerase activity and an increase in hTERT copy number were detected (Sarkar *et al.*, 2006). Conversely, dioxin downregulated telomerase activity in kidney cells, with a decrease in bTERT protein levels (Fiorito *et al.*, 2011), in the presence of cell proliferation. Even though this may seem paradoxical, it has been shown that telomerase activity was reported in liver samples from patients with hepatitis and liver cirrhosis but no tumor pathology (Greider, 1996). Furthermore, as reported recently, approximately 10–15% of human cancers lack detectable telomerase activity (Heaphy *et al.*, 2011). Finally, the expression of c-Myc has been closely associated with cellular proliferation/cell death and hTERT activity; these were consistent with the inhibition of c-Myc by TCDD and the resulting decrease in telomerase activity in kidney cells (Fiorito *et al.*, 2011).

Changes in Protein Expression Levels

Since, in response to DNA damage or oncogene activation, the key tumor-suppressor p53 can be activated and subsequently orchestrate biological outputs such as modulation of autophagy (Botti *et al.*, 2006), we used western blot analysis to examine the protein levels of both p53 and the cell cycle inhibitor p21$^{Waf1/Cip1}$ in kidney cells and showed that TCDD significantly upregulated their expression levels (Fiorito *et al.*, 2011). Furthermore, we elected to study Ser315 phosphorylation. Ser315, located within the nuclear localization signal (aminoacids 305–322) of the C-terminal region of p53, is phosphorylated by kinases involved in cell cycle progression (Radhakrishnan and Gartel, 2006). In kidney cells, we detected p53 phosphorylation at serine 315 from 8 h to the end of treatment, suggesting that both activation by dioxin and phosphorylation levels increased with prolonged incubation (Fiorito *et al.*, 2011). These results, together with inhibition of telomerase activity, may represent some of the tumor suppressor mechanisms that protect MDBK cells from proliferation induced by dioxin, as reported by others (Shay and Wright, 2005). Moreover, by measuring the p-p53/p53 ratio we distinguished an increase in exposed groups only in the presence of 0.01 or 100 pg/mL of TCDD, at all times studied, whereas 1 pg/mL of TCDD induced, after an increase at 8 h, a decrease from 12 h until the end of exposure (Fiorito *et al.*, 2011). It is well known that p53 is phosphorylated at 23 sites, mostly found within the N- and C-terminal domains that form the molecule's regulatory regions, but generally, even though the total quantity of p-p53 might be significant for its transcription function, a decrease in the ratio might also lead to a dilution effect. In the presence of 1 pg/mL of TCDD, we detected an increase of p53 protein levels even if the ratio decreased, suggesting that this dose of TCDD was sufficient to induce maximal effects on the parameters studied (Fiorito *et al.*, 2011). A peculiar modulation of p53 phosphorylation induced by TCDD has already been found by Pääjärvi *et al.* (2005). Generally, ATM is considered as protein kinase that serves as a critical mediator of signaling pathways facilitating the response of mammalian cells to agents that induce DNA damage (Maya *et al.*, 2001). Mdm2 is the main regulator of p53, and ATM may target both p53 and Mdm2 (Maya *et al.*, 2001). Analysis of bovine kidney cells exposed to TCDD displayed a significant time-dependent augmentation of both ATM phosphorylation and the p-ATM/ATM ratio in the presence of a slow but significant time-dependent decline in Mdm2 protein levels (Fiorito *et al.*, 2011). A previous study showed that TCDD increased basal levels of Mdm2 protein and induced the rapid onset of p53 degradation in rat hepatocytes, where dioxin decreased apoptosis rates (Pääjärvi *et al.*, 2005). Conversely, our data indicated that TCDD induced cell death with autophagy in bovine cells, where decreased Mdm2 and intensified p53 protein levels were shown (Fiorito *et al.*, 2011). These results indicated that both p53 and p21[Waf1/Cip1] activations may be involved in stimulation of cell death in TCDD-treated bovine kidney cells. Furthermore, exposure of cells to dioxin activated the ATM checkpoint pathway, inducing both ATM and p53 phosphorylation, and inhibiting Mdm2 protein levels.

CONCLUSION

The kidney offers an opportunity to study autophagy in the context of highly specialized epithelia. However, the precise role of autophagy in the course of kidney diseases is still poorly understood. The influence of autophagy on cell survival in the kidney is likely to be an important component of any form of stress to which the kidney is subjected; however, in general, autophagy can act as a mechanism of cell survival or directly induce cell death. Exposure to dangerous environmental contaminants can trigger autophagy in the kidney, in which, until now, there have been few examples that describe autophagy after exposure to toxicants. Among the potential factors that affect autophagy in kidney cells are environmental contaminants like dioxin. This is accompanied by conversion of LC3 and formation of acidic vesicles, suggesting that autophagy contributes to TCDD-induced cell death in this experimental model.

Acknowledgments

Filomena Fiorito was supported by a fellowship from Polo delle Scienze e delle Tecnologie per la Vita dell'Universitá di Napoli "Federico II" (2012-4/STV-Progetto FORGIARE), co-funded by Compagnia San Paolo di Torino, Italy.

References

Ahn, N.S., Hu, H., Park, J.S., et al., 2005. Molecular mechanisms of the 2,3,7,8-tetrachlorodibenzo-p-dioxin-induced inverted U-shaped dose responsiveness in anchorage independent growth and cell proliferation of human breast epithelial cells with stem cell characteristics. Mutat. Res. 579, 189–199.

Botti, J., Djavaheri-Mergny, M., Pilatte, Y., et al., 2006. Autophagy signaling and the cogwheels of cancer. Autophagy 2, 67–73.

Bryant, P.L., Reid, L.M., Schmid, J.E., et al., 2001. Effects of 2,3,7,8-tetrachlorodibenzo-p-dioxin (TCDD) on fetal mouse urinary tract epithelium *in vitro*. Toxicology 162, 23–34.

Courtney, K.D., Moore, J.A., 1971. Teratology studies with 2,4,5-T and 2,3,7,8-tetrachlorodibenzo-p-dioxin. Toxicol. Appl. Pharmacol. 20, 396–403.

Couture, L.A., Abbott, B.D., Birnbaum, L.S., 1990. A critical review of the developmental toxicity and teratogenicity of 2,3,7,8-tetrachlorodibenzo-p-dioxin: recent advances toward understanding the mechanism. Teratology 42, 619–627.

Cummings, C.J., Mancini, M.A., Antalffy, B., et al., 1998. Chaperone suppression of aggregation and altered subcellular proteasome localization imply protein misfolding in SCA1. Nat. Genet. 19, 148–154.

De Duve, C., Wattiaux, R., 1966. Functions of lysosomes. Annu. Rev. Physiol. 28, 435–492.

Esposito, M., Serpe, F.P., Neugebauer, F., et al., 2010. Contamination levels and congener distribution of PCDDs, PCDFs and dioxin-like PCBs in buffalo's milk from Caserta province (Italy). Chemosphere 79, 341–348.

Fiorito, F., Pagnini, U., De Martino, L., et al., 2008a. 2,3,7,8-tetrachlorodibenzo-p-dioxin increases bovine herpesvirus type-1 (BHV-1) replication in madin-darby bovine kidney (MDBK) cells *in vitro*. J. Cell. Biochem. 103, 221–233.

Fiorito, F., Marfè, G., De Blasio, E., et al., 2008b. 2,3,7,8-tetrachlorodibenzo-p-dioxin regulates bovine herpesvirus type 1 induced apoptosis by modulating Bcl-2 family members. Apoptosis 13, 1243–1252.

Fiorito, F., Marfè, G., Granato, G.E., et al., 2010. 2,3,7,8-Tetrachlorodibenzo-p-dioxin modifies expression and nuclear/cytosolic localization of bovine herpesvirus 1 immediate-early protein (bICP0) during infection. J. Cell. Biochem. 111, 333–342.

Fiorito, F., Ciarcia, R., Granato, G.E., et al., 2011. 2,3,7,8-Tetrachlorodibenzo-p-dioxin induced autophagy in a bovine kidney cell line. Toxicology 290, 258–270.

Galluzzi, L., Vitale, I., Abrams, J.M., et al., 2012. Molecular definitions of cell death subroutines: recommendations of the Nomenclature Committee on Cell Death 2012. Cell Death Differ. 19, 107–120.

Greider, C.W., 1996. Telomere length regulation. Annu. Rev. Biochem. 65, 337–365.

Heaphy, C.M., Subhawong, A.P., Hong, S.M., et al., 2011. Prevalence of the alternative lengthening of telomeres: telomere maintenance mechanism in human cancer subtypes. Am. J. Pathol. 179, 1608–1615.

Huber, T.B., Edelstein, C.L., Hartleben, B., et al., 2012. Emerging role of autophagy in kidney function, diseases and aging. Autophagy 8, 1009–1031.

IARC, 1997. IARC monographs on the evaluation of carcinogenic risks to humans. In: Polycholorinated Dibenozo-Paradioxins and Polychlorinated Dibenzofurnas. IARC Monograph.

Ishida, M., Mikami, S., Kikuchi, E., et al., 2010. Activation of the aryl hydrocarbon receptor pathway enhances cancer cell invasion by upregulating the MMP expression and is associated with poor prognosis in upper urinary tract urothelial cancer. Carcinogenesis 31, 287–295.

Klionsky, D.J., Abdalla, F.C., Abeliovich, H., et al., 2012. Guidelines for the use and interpretation of assays for monitoring autophagy. Autophagy 8, 445–544.

Ko, H., Kim, Y.J., Park, J.S., et al., 2009. Autophagy inhibition enhances apoptosis induced by ginsenoside Rk1 in hepatocellular carcinoma cells. Biosci. Biotechnol. Biochem. 73, 2183–2189.

Lamparska-Przybysz, M., Gajkowska, B., Motyl, T., 2005. Cathepsins and BID are involved in the molecular switch between apoptosis and autophagy in breast cancer MCF-7 cells exposed to camptothecin. J. Physiol. Pharmacol. 56 (S3), 159–179.

Maffettone, C., Chen, G., Drozdov, I., et al., 2010. Tumorigenic properties of iron regulatory protein 2 (IRP2) mediated by its specific 73-amino acids insert. PLoS ONE 5, e10163.

Manikkam, M., Tracey, R., Guerrero-Bosagna, C., et al., 2012. Dioxin (TCDD) Induces epigenetic transgenerational inheritance of adult onset disease and sperm epimutations. PLoS ONE 7, e46249.

Maya, R., Balass, M., Kim, S.T., et al., 2001. ATM-dependent phosphorylation of Mdm2 on serine 395: role in p53 activation by DNA damage. Genes Dev. 15, 1067–1077.

Mustafa, A., Holladay, S., Witonsky, S., et al., 2011. Prenatal TCDD causes persistent modulation of the postnatal immune response, and exacerbates inflammatory disease, in 36-week-old lupus-like autoimmune SNF1 mice. Birth Defects Res. B Dev. Reprod. Toxicol. 92, 82–94.

Nishimura, N., Matsumura, F., Vogel, C.F., et al., 2008. Critical role of cyclooxygenase-2 activation in pathogenesis of hydronephrosis caused by lactational exposure of mice to dioxin. Toxicol. Appl. Pharmacol. 231, 374–383.

Orrenius, S., Kaminskyy, V.O., Zhivotovsky, B., 2013. Autophagy in toxicology: cause or consequence? Annu. Rev. Pharmacol. Toxicol. 53, 275–297.

Pääjärvi, G., Viluksela, M., Pohjanvirta, R., et al., 2005. TCDD activates Mdm2 and attenuates the p53 response to DNA damaging agents. Carcinogenesis 26, 201–208.

Pandey, U.B., Nie, Z., Batlevi, Y., et al., 2007. HDAC6 rescues neurodegeneration and provides an essential link between autophagy and the UPS. Nature 447, 859–863.

Periyasamy-Thandavan, S., Jiang, M., Schoenlein, P., et al., 2009. Autophagy: molecular machinery, regulation, and implications for renal pathophysiology. Am. J. Physiol. Renal Physiol. 297, F244–F256.

Radhakrishnan, S.K., Gartel, A.L., 2006. CDK9 phosphorylates p53 on serine residues 33, 315 and 392. Cell Cycle 5, 519–521.

Ray, S., Swanson, H.I., 2009. Activation of the aryl hydrocarbon receptor by TCDD inhibits senescence: a tumor promoting event? Biochem. Pharmacol. 77, 681–688.

Rea, M.A., Phillips, M.A., Degraffenried, L.A., et al., 1998. Modulation of human epidermal cell response to 2,3,7,8-tetrachlorodibenzo-p-dioxin by epidermal growth factor. Carcinogenesis 19, 479–483.

Rosenfeldt, M.T., Ryan, K.M., 2011. The multiple roles of autophagy in cancer. Carcinogenesis 32, 955–963.

Santamaria, R., Fiorito, F., Irace, C., et al., 2011. 2,3,7,8-Tetrachlorodibenzo-p-dioxin impairs iron homeostasis by modulating iron-related proteins expression and increasing the labile iron pool in mammalian cells. Biochim. Biophys. Acta 1813, 704–712.

Sarkar, P., Shiizaki, K., Yonemoto, J., et al., 2006. Activation of telomerase in BeWo cells by estrogen and 2,3,7,8-tetrachlorodibenzo-p-dioxin in co-operation with c-Myc. Int. J. Oncol. 28, 43–51.

Shay, J.W., Wright, W.E., 2005. Senescence and immortalization: role of telomeres and telomerase. Carcinogenesis 26, 867–874.

White, S.S., Birnbaum, L.S., 2009. An overview of the effects of dioxins and dioxin-like compounds on vertebrates, as documented in human and ecological epidemiology. J. Environ. Sci. Health C Environ. Carcinog. Ecotoxicol. Rev. 27, 197–211.

Wu, K.J., Grandori, C., Amacker, M., et al., 1999. Direct activation of TERT transcription by c-MYC. Nat. Genet. 21, 220–224.

Molecular Mechanisms Underlying the Activation of Autophagy Pathways by Reactive Oxygen Species and their Relevance in Cancer Progression and Therapy

Noemí Rubio Romero and Patrizia Agostinis

O U T L I N E

M.A. Hayat (ed): Autophagy, Volume 1
DOI: http://dx.doi.org/10.1016/B978-0-12-405530-8.00012-1

© 2014 Elsevier Inc. All rights reserved.

Abstract

Reactive oxygen species (ROS) have emerged as signaling molecules in pathways regulating cell growth and differentiation, inflammation, immune responses, survival, and death. ROS have been shown to promote autophagy, a lysosomal pathway for degradation of dysfunctional unnecessary cellular components. In fact, recent works have revealed a complex cross-talk between these intertwined signals. Whereas ROS can modulate autophagy activation in response to different types of stimuli, autophagy, in turn, may modulate ROS production by degrading, for example, dysfunctional mitochondria that generate aberrant amounts of ROS. Autophagy pathways can act both as tumor-promoter and tumor-suppressor mechanisms, with involvement of ROS in both cases. Paradoxically, whereas ROS and autophagy regulation may contribute to cancer initiation and progression, many antineoplastic treatments are precisely based on the massive production of ROS and activation of autophagy to induce cell death and eradication of diseased tissue. Nevertheless, autophagy activation has also shown a cytoprotective role against the efficiency of the therapy, and the mechanism that controls the switch between these two cellular functions in still unknown. In this chapter we will review the molecular mechanisms by which ROS modulate autophagy, and those modulated by autophagy to control ROS production, in the context both of cancer development and of cancer treatment.

INTRODUCTION

The term autophagy (from the Greek "self-eating") was coined by Christian de Duve in 1963 after the discovery of membrane-bound vesicles containing cytosolic material and lysosomal hydrolases using electron microscopy (De Duve and Wattiaux, 1966). Autophagy is an evolutionarily conserved intracellular process that involves the digestion of cytoplasmic components (from proteins, sugars, lipids, and nucleotides to organelles and invading pathogens) through the lysosomal pathway. At a basal level, this catabolic process acts as a quality control mechanism with housekeeping functions to maintain cellular homeostasis by removing aggregate-prone proteins and damaged organelles. However, multiple stress conditions such as aminoacids or glucose deprivation, hypoxia, endoplasmic reticulum (ER) stress, and oxidative stress can stimulate autophagy. Several factors and signaling pathways are involved in autophagy activation. Among these, reactive oxygen species (ROS) are principally involved in the modulation of autophagy responses. ROS is a term that describes oxygen-derived free radicals, such as superoxide ($O_2^{\bullet-}$), hydroxyl ($^{\bullet}OH$), hydroperoxyl ($HOO^{\bullet}$), alkoxyl ($RO^{\bullet}$), and peroxyl ($ROO^{\bullet}$) radicals, and non-radicals, such as hydrogen peroxide (H_2O_2) or singlet oxygen ($^1O_2$). Depending on their chemical reactivity, lifetime and lipid solubility, ROS may mediate in signaling mechanisms supporting cell growth and survival. Nevertheless, when excessively produced, ROS production results in a condition of oxidative stress that inflicts oxidative damage to vital molecules, like DNA, lipids and proteins impairing cellular integrity. Accumulating evidence indicates that loss of cellular redox homeostasis is associated to cancer initiation and progression (Kongara and Karantza, 2012), although it is also crucial in mediating the cellular response to various therapeutic agents, including chemo-, radio- and photodynamic therapy (PDT) (Agostinis *et al.* 2011; Ozben, 2007; Trachootham *et al.*, 2009). It is well established that excessive ROS can instigate apoptosis (Circu and Aw, 2010), but emerging data have also revealed a signaling role for ROS in the activation of autophagy pathways. In fact, activation of autophagy in response to ROS production during cancer progression and in response to anticancer therapy plays a role in the modulation of cellular redox homeostasis with consequences that depend on the genetic background of the cancerous cells, their ability to undergo apoptosis, progression stage and type of ROS insults (Dewaele *et al.*, 2010; Kongara and Karantza, 2012; Li *et al.*, 2012; Scherz-Shouval and Elazar, 2011). In cancer initiation and progression, autophagy can act both as a tumor promoter and tumor suppressor mechanism, whereas in ROS- based anticancer therapies, it plays a pivotal role in the regulation of survival functions and cell death processes. In this chapter, we will review the molecular mechanisms behind the modulation of autophagy by ROS and those modulated by autophagy to control ROS production. These mechanisms will be discussed both in the context of cancer development and cancer treatment.

OVERVIEW OF AUTOPHAGY CORE MACHINERY AND SIGNALING PATHWAYS

Three different autophagy mechanisms have been identified in mammalian cells: macroautophagy, microautophagy, and chaperone-mediated autophagy. (Macro)autophagy is a process of bulk degradation for cytoplasmic components characterized by the formation of double-membrane vesicles called autophagosomes responsible for cargo sequestration and delivery to lysosomes for hydrolytic degradation. Nevertheless, this process can be directed to degrade specific targets such as ubiquitinated protein aggregates (aggrephagy), or organelles like mitochondria (mitophagy), endoplasmic reticulum (reticulophagy), peroxisomes (pexophagy), or ribosomes (ribophagy). Microphagy is a non-selective process in which lysosomal membrane directly invaginates cytosolic components for degradation. The third type of autophagy, chaperone-mediated autophagy (CMA), is a selective process where soluble cytosolic proteins bearing a KFERQ-related sequence are recognized by the cytosolic heat shock cognate 70 (Hsc70), which is in a complex with several co-chaperones, to be delivered to the lysosomes. The lysosomal membrane receptor Lamp-2A (lysosome-associated membrane protein-2A) recognizes the substrate–chaperone complex, which is rapidly translocated into the lysosomes for degradation with the assistance of lysosomal Hsc70. Both macroautophagy and CMA are induced as acute adaptation responses to a variety of metabolic stressors, such as oxidative stress, nutrient starvation, growth factor withdrawal, high lipid content challenges, or hypoxia.

The molecular understanding of macroautophagy (hereafter referred to as autophagy) is linked to the discovery of the autophagy-related (Atg) genes. The autophagy "core" molecular machinery is composed of: (1) two kinase-systems, the Atg1/unc-51-like kinase (ULK) complex and the class III phosphatidylinositol 3-kinase/Vps34 (PI3KC3) complex; (2) two ubiquitin-like protein conjugation systems (Atg12 and Atg8/LC3); and (3) the transmembrane proteins Atg9/mAtg9 (Wirawan *et al.*, 2012).

In mammalian systems, autophagosome initiation is controlled by the ULK:Atg13:FIP200:Atg101 complex. The unc-51-like kinases 1 (ULK1) and 2 (ULK2) and the focal adhesion kinase family interacting protein of 200 kDa (FIP200) form a nutrient-independent stable complex with the mammalian (m)Atg13, which is stabilized by Atg101. The functional status of this complex is regulated by the mammalian target of rapamycin complex 1 (mTORC1), a central inhibitor of autophagy, a signaling hub on which different signaling pathways converge. The mTORC1 complex is composed by mTOR, regulatory associated protein of mTOR (raptor), proline-rich AKT substrate 40 kDa (PRAS40),

G-protein β-subunit-like protein (GβL/mLST8), and DEP domain containing mTOR-interacting protein (DEPTOR). Under nutrient-rich conditions and adequate presence of growth factors, Akt is activated by class I phosphatidylinositol 3-kinase (PI3KC1), leading to subsequent mTORC1 activation. By binding to the ULK complex the raptor subunit of mTORC1 binds to the PS domain of ULK1, inhibiting autophagy. Several phosphorylation steps occur under these conditions: ULK1 and ULK2 are phosphorylated by mTORC1, Atg13 is phosphorylated by ULK1, ULK2, and mTORC1, and FIP200 is phosphorylated by ULK1 and ULK2. On the other hand, in response to nutrient and growth factor deprivation or rapamycin treatment autophagy is induced due to mTORC1 inactivation. Under these conditions, mTORC1 dissociates from the ULK complex, which in turn translocates into the autophagosomal formation site, promoting dephosphorylation of ULK1, ULK2, and Atg13, and activation of ULK1 and ULK2, which phosphorylate Atg13 and FIP200. Reduced cellular energy (ATP) levels are detected by AMP-activated protein kinase (AMPK), which is activated by the upstream LKB1 kinase and binds to ULK1. Association between ULK1 and AMPK plays an important role in autophagy induction, since AMPK-mediated phosphorylation of raptor suppresses the inhibitory effect of mTOR on the ULK complex.

Nucleation and assembly of the initial phagophore membrane depends on the class III phosphatidylinositol 3-kinase (PI3KC3) complex, essential for autophagosome formation, which contains class III PI3K or Vps34, its regulatory protein kinase p150 or Vps15 and Beclin 1. This complex produces phosphatidyl-inositol-3-phosphate (PI3P), which recruits proteins like WIPI1 and WIPI2 (WD repeat domain phosphoinositide interacting 1 and 2), mAtg2, and double-FYVE containing protein-1 (DFCP1) to the site of autophagosome formation to initiate its nucleation. Beclin 1 can also bind to Atg14-like protein (Atg14L), also known as Barkor (Beclin 1-associated Atg key regulator), and Ambra 1 (activating molecule in Beclin 1-regulated autophagy 1) to increase the complex activity. There are other proteins that either can promote or inhibit autophagy by modulating this complex activity: the ultraviolet irradiation resistance-associated gene (UVRAG), when interacting with Bif-1 (Bax-interacting factor 1), binds to Beclin 1 to modulate autophagosome maturation. Binding of Rubicon to UVRAG, however, negatively regulates the activity of the PI3KC3 complex and, consequently, autophagosome maturation. Interestingly, UVRAG and Atg14L are mutually exclusive, since they compete for binding to Beclin 1. The role of Beclin 1 in autophagy is regulated by the anti-apoptotic Bcl-2 (B cell lymphoma/leukemia-2), which inhibits autophagy by binding to Beclin 1 under nutrient-rich conditions. Autophagy activation, in fact, is modulated by dissociation of Bcl-2 from Beclin 1. Interestingly, a recent study has shown the involvement of the ULK complex in the proper localization of the PI3KC3 complex (Di Bartolomeo et al., 2010). In nutrient-rich conditions, the PI3KC3 complex is connected to the cytoskeleton through Ambra 1, which links this complex to the microtubule-associated dynein motor complex. Under starvation conditions, however, ULK1 phosphorylates Ambra1. This phosphorylation event releases the PI3KC3 complex from the microtubules and enables its relocalization to the endoplasmic reticulum (ER), an organelle considered to be the major contributor to autophagosome formation. Moreover, in basal conditions, ULK1 has an important role in regulating the trafficking of the multispanning transmembrane protein mAtg9, the only transmembrane Atg protein that traffics between the trans-Golgi network and late endosomes. In response to starvation, mAtg9 is recruited to the growing autophagosome, where it supplies the lipids required for membrane elongation and acts as a platform for recruiting effectors to the phagophore.

Two ubiquitin-like conjugation systems are involved in the expansion, shaping, and sealing of the autophagosomal membrane. Atg5 is conjugated to Atg12, and Atg7 and Atg10 (E-1 and E-2 like enzymes, respectively) are required for this interaction. The Atg5–Atg12 conjugate interacts with Atg16L to form the large multimeric Atg16L complex. This complex is transiently associated to the autophagosomal membrane of the growing autophagosome, affecting its curvature. The second ubiquitin-like conjugation system involves LC3 (microtubules-associated light chain-3), which is cleaved at the C-terminus by the cysteine protease Atg4 to produce the cytosolic LC3-I. This cytosolic form contains a glycine residue that conjugates to phosphatidylethanolamine (PE) with the assistance of Atg7, the E2-like enzyme Atg3, and the Atg16L complex to produce the lipidated form LC3-II, which localizes to both leaflets of the autophagosomal membrane. The human LC3 family is composed of the three members LC3A–C, and the LC3 paralogues GABARAP1, 3, GATE-16, and Atg18L. After autophagosome formation, the Atg5–Atg12–Atg16L complex leaves the autophagosome, and LC3-II associated to the autophagosomal cytosolic surface is decoupled from PE by Atg4 for recycling. Prior to fusion with lysosomes, autophagosomes can also merge with endocytic vesicles. Fusion of the outer membrane of the autophagosomes with lysosomes results in release of the inner autophagosomal membrane and its cargo into the lysosomal lumen, and requires the lysosomal membrane protein Lamp-2 and the small GTPase Rab7. Degradation of the inner vesicle after fusion is performed by a series of lysosomal/vacuolar acid hydrolases, such as cathepsins B, D, and L. Small molecules, particularly amino acids, resulting from autolysosome degradation are released to the cytosol and recycled in different anabolic pathways, resulting in maintenance of energy metabolism and protein functions under starvation or stressful conditions.

As previously stated, in addition to the "in bulk" non-selective degradation of cytosolic components, autophagy can also be directed to sequestration of specific cargo substrates like ubiquitinated proteins and protein aggregates (aggrephagy), or organelles like mitochondria (mitophagy). Selective (macro)autophagy uses the same essential components of the autophagy machinery for "in bulk" degradation, with an additional step for cargo recognition mediated by the cargo recognition proteins. p62/SQSTM1 (sequestosome-1) and NBR1 (neighbor of BRCA1 gene 1) are adaptor proteins that connect ubiquitinated protein aggregates with the degradation machinery, whereas Nix and the pair PINK1 (PTEN-induced putative protein kinase 1)/E3 ubiquitin ligase Parkin recognize mitochondria. Recent studies suggest that PINK1/Parkin interacts directly with the Beclin 1/PI3KC3 complex. In fact, Parkin-dependent recruitment of Ambra 1 to the mitochondria, upon their depolarization, would lead to induction of the Beclin 1 complex and nucleation of pre-autophagosomal membranes surrounding damaged mitochondria (Ashrafi and Schwarz, 2013).

REACTIVE OXYGEN SPECIES: CELLULAR SOURCES AND SIGNALING ROLE

Reactive oxygen species, when produced at high concentrations that disturb the cellular pro-oxidant–antioxidant balance, lead to a condition known as oxidative stress. Excess ROS cause oxidative damage to essential biomolecules like lipids, proteins, and DNA, interfering with vital cellular functions. Nevertheless, when produced at low concentrations, ROS may act as secondary messengers in signal transduction pathways regulating cell growth, differentiation, inflammation, immune responses, survival, and cell death. The main source of ROS is mitochondria, where aerobic respiration through the mitochondrial electron transport chain (mETC) produces $O_2^{\bullet-}$. Enzymes such as membrane-localized NADPH oxidase, xanthine oxidase, or cytochrome P450 are also cellular sources of $O_2^{\bullet-}$, whereas the Ero1-DPI oxidative folding system in the ER produces H_2O_2. Organelles like peroxisomes are also cellular sources of cytosolic H_2O_2. The systematic characterization of ROS as molecular mediators in cellular signaling pathways is, however, somehow complex, because ROS can be rapidly neutralized or interconverted from one to another by the action of, for example, endogenous antioxidants. For example, $O_2^{\bullet-}$, a membrane-impermeable and thus more spatially confined ROS, can be converted by SOD into H_2O_2, a less reactive species with the ability to cross membranes and a lifespan long enough to diffuse out of the cells. In turn, H_2O_2 can be removed by catalase, glutathione peroxidases, and peroxiredoxins, or can be further converted into the most reactive ROS, $^{\bullet}OH$, by metal ions. The main ROS involved in cell signaling are $O_2^{\bullet-}$ and H_2O_2. The sulfur-containing residues in proteins are targets for H_2O_2 and have the ability to function as molecular switches in signal transduction. In fact, this ROS can oxidize the thiol groups in cysteine residues located at the catalytic center of cellular enzymes. Reactive oxygen species can regulate the activity of protein phosphatases, such as PTEN; tyrosine kinases, such as Scrl; and serine/threonine kinases, such as MAPKs (p38, ERK, and JNK) and PKB/Akt. These oxidants also regulate key transcription factors such as hypoxia-inducible factor -1 (HIF-1) in response to hypoxic conditions, nuclear factor kappaB (NF-κB) in immune responses, p53 in cell growth and proliferation, the activator protein 1 (AP-1) during cell growth and apoptosis, NF-E2-related factor 2 (Nrf2), and the activation of antioxidant responses or the forkhead box protein O (FOXO) to induce either cell death or a quiescent state characterized by a certain tolerance to oxidative stress.

ROS AND AUTOPHAGY

The interplay between ROS and autophagy is quite complex, because each of these elements can be involved in the regulation of the other. This cross-talk will be review in this section. First, we will discuss how ROS can modulate the autophagy pathway, and how different autophagy-activating stressors generate specific ROS that affect the autophagy pathways by regulating different elements of its molecular machinery. Secondly, we will discuss how autophagy in turn can control excessive ROS production by removing oxidized proteins and organelles such as mitochondria that, when dysfunctional, lead to aberrant generation of ROS.

Modulation of Autophagy by ROS

ROS and (Macro)autophagy

The existence of a complex interplay between ROS and autophagy pathways in the modulation of cellular responses to stress stimuli has emerged recently. Involvement of

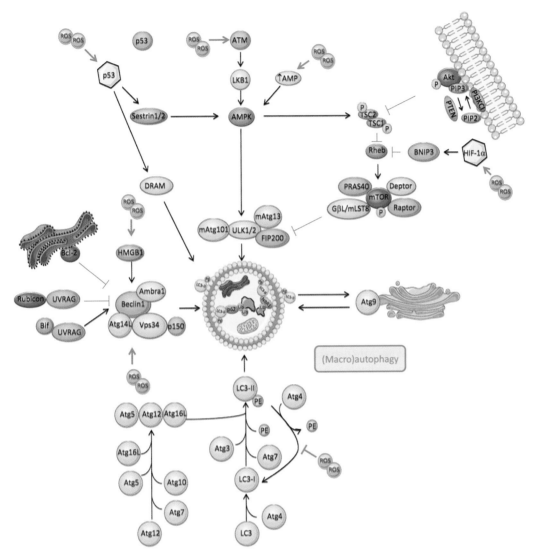

FIGURE 12.1   Molecular mechanisms underlying the activation of autophagy by ROS.

ROS in the activation of autophagy, however, is not only limited to situations of oxidative stress; low levels of ROS have also been shown to regulate cell signaling by reversibly oxidizing essential signaling components. Depending on the type of stress, cells will respond by producing specific types of ROS that in turn, depending on the cell type and its genetic background, will activate signaling pathways that induce autophagy (Figure 12.1). In the function of the overall cellular context, autophagy stimulation will have a prosurvival role or will act as a prodeath mechanism.

First evidences about the signaling role of ROS in autophagy were suggested by the study of the pathway leading to neuronal cell death in response to nerve growth factor (NGF) deprivation (Kirkland et al., 2002; Xue et al., 1999). Accumulation of mitochondrial ROS in sympathetic neurons by NGF deprivation led to cardiolipin peroxidation, which resulted in autophagic cell death (Kirkland et al., 2002).

In contrast, starvation-induced autophagy has largely been shown to be cytoprotective in certain situations. Scherz-Shouval et al. (2007) reported that mitochondrial H_2O_2 produced in a partially PI3K3C-dependent manner after amino acid deprivation was essential for activation of autophagy in response to starvation, with a clear cytoprotective role. H_2O_2 oxidizes the protease Atg4, specifically at its Cys81 residue near the catalytic site. Inactivation of Atg4 in turn promotes LC3 lipidation and formation of the autophagosome. When the autophagosome matures and fuses to the lysosome, it apparently localizes to an H_2O_2-poor environment, therefore promoting LC3 de-lipidation by Atg4, now active, in order to be recycled. Moreover, the PI3K3C inhibitors wortmannin and 3-methyladenine (3-MA) or partial silencing of Beclin 1 or Vps34 reduced starvation-induced ROS production. In contrast, another study on the activation of autophagy by starvation showed that $O_2^{\bullet-}$ was selectively induced by starvation of glucose, pyruvate, l-glutamine and serum, whereas amino acid and serum starvation induced $O_2^{\bullet-}$ and H_2O_2 formation (Chen et al., 2009). Both types of starvation clearly induced autophagy, which in turn was reduced when antioxidant enzymes such as SOD2 (manganese superoxide, located at the mitochondria) and catalase were overexpressed. The same study showed that blockage of the mETC, inhibition of SOD, and addition of exogenous H_2O_2 increased intracellular levels of $O_2^{\bullet-}$, leading to autophagy activation, thereby revealing a major role for this species in the activation of this pathway under these stress conditions. In this case, wortmannin or 3-MA treatment as well as Beclin 1 and Atg7 siRNA did not affect $O_2^{\bullet-}$ and H_2O_2 production after starvation-induced autophagy, revealing that increased levels of $O_2^{\bullet-}$ occur upstream of the activation of the Beclin 1–PI3K3C complex.

Interestingly, autophagy regulation by intracellular ROS produced under starvation or metabolic stress also appeared to involve the p53-inducible protein TP53-induced glycolysis and apoptosis regulator, TIGAR (Bensaad et al., 2009). This protein functions to hydrolyze fructose-2,6-biphosphate, so TIGAR expression, by decreasing the levels of this fructose, decreases the glycolytic rate, which results in an increased NADPH production that promotes ROS scavenging by reduced glutathione and increases cellular protection against oxidative stress. In fact, attenuation of TIGAR levels using siRNA techniques was sufficient to stimulate ROS production and autophagy in an mTOR- and p53-independent manner. Autophagy activation by loss of TIGAR is cytoprotective and decreases apoptosis by reducing the levels of ROS (probably by eliminating dysfunctional mitochondria), and this inhibitory role of TIGAR on autophagy is independent of the p53-inducible autophagy-promoter gene damage regulated autophagy modulator (DRAM). These results propose that nuclear p53 can control the level of starvation-induced autophagy by regulating the balance between DRAM, a protein that stimulates autophagy activation, and TIGAR, a protein that inhibits autophagy by decreasing the levels of ROS. In this case, ROS act as signaling molecules generated upstream of the autophagic response, although autophagy activation controls the oxidative stress levels by removing dysfunctional ROS-generating mitochondria. In fact, under conditions of oxidative stress, basal p53 expression induces the expression of different antioxidant targets such as MnSOD or SOD2, GPx1, ALDH4, and TPP53INP1. The family of stress-responsive and p53-regulated proteins, Sestrins, is also involved in the regulation of ROS. Sestrin1 and Sestrin2 are critical links between p53 activation and mTORC1 activity. In fact, these proteins are negative regulators of mTOR signaling through activation of AMPK and TSC2 (Budanov, 2011).

p53, however, can also increase the generation of ROS. Silibinin, an active constituent extracted from blessed milk thistle (*Sylibum marianium*) applied in liver disease has been shown to activate p53; this leads to an increase in ROS levels, which simultaneously appear to regulate p53 activity in a positive feedback loop, resulting in autophagy activation. Further works suggest that sibilinin stimulates p53-mediated autophagic cell death through activation of ROS-p38 and JNK MAPK pathways, and inhibition of PI3K/Akt and MERK/ERK pathways (Duan *et al.*, 2011). Therefore, the specific role and response of p53 to different stimuli and its relation with ROS generation is highly context- and cellular stress-specific.

As previously mentioned, reduced cellular energy levels (i.e., low ATP/AMP ratios) are detected by AMPK, which activates autophagy to restore those levels. Nevertheless, the AMPK signaling pathway is highly sensitive to oxidative stress. Interestingly, AMPK is also activated by exogenous addition of H_2O_2. This ROS evokes ATP depletion leading to subsequent accumulation of AMP and phosphorylation of AMPK. Interestingly, addition of dimethylsulfoxide (DMSO), a known $^{\bullet}OH$ scavenger, blocked both ATP depletion and AMPK activation caused by H_2O_2 (Choi *et al.*, 2001).

Ataxia-telangiectasia mutated (ATM) is a DNA damage sensor that preserves genomic integrity. In addition, it is involved in metabolic regulation and has a cytoplasmic function that participates in the cellular damage response to ROS. Under conditions of oxidative stress, ATM activates the TSC2 via the LKB1/AMPK metabolic pathway in the cytoplasm to inhibit mTORC1 and induce autophagy (Alexander *et al.*, 2010).

Although HIF-1 is the key transcription factor that regulates cellular responses to hypoxia, multiple works have reported that hypoxic conditions activate AMPK. In fact, activation of this protein kinase by low O_2 concentrations occurs through LKB1, and is not associated to an increase of the AMP levels. Moreover, hypoxic activation of AMPK depends on the production of mitochondrial ROS generated by the mETC and not by oxidative phosphorylation (Emerling *et al.*, 2009). AMPK activation by hypoxia inhibits mTOR (Liu *et al.*, 2006).

Hypoxia induces mitochondrial ROS production, which contributes to HIF-1α stabilization and, consequently, transcription of different target genes, such as BNIP3 (Bcl-2/E1B 19-kDa interacting protein 3) and BNIP3L or NIX, that lead to autophagy activation in response to low oxygen conditions. Under these conditions, autophagy activation is due to the direct binding between BNIP3 and the Ras-related small GTPase Rheb, an upstream activator of mTOR (Li *et al.*, 2007). Interestingly, apart from this induction under hypoxia, BNIP3 is also activated by the addition of H_2O_2 in C6 glioma cells leading to autophagy induction, which results in cell death. BNIP3-mediated autophagy activation after addition of H_2O_2 is due to dephosphorylation of mTOR at the Ser2481 and the p70 ribosomal protein S6 kinase (p70S6K) at the Thr389 residue, therefore inhibiting mTOR activity (Byun *et al.*, 2009). In agreement with this Bcl-2 family members/mTOR pathway interaction, another study performed on malignant human glioma U251 cells showed that autophagy induction by addition of H_2O_2 to these cells occurs by the Beclin 1 and Akt/mTOR pathways in a Bcl-2 dependent way (Zhang *et al.*, 2009).

High-mobility group box 1 (HMGB1) is a chromatin-binding nuclear protein that also works as an extracellular signaling molecule in cell migration, cell differentiation, inflammation, and tumor metastasis. Intriguingly, intracellular HMGB1 has been identified as a Beclin 1 binding protein that promotes autophagy in response to cellular stress. In fact, ROS produced by cellular stress promotes HMGB1 translocation from the nucleus to the cytosol, which activates autophagy by disrupting the Beclin 1–Bcl-2 interaction and enhancing ERK1/2 activity. Binding of HMGB1 to Beclin 1 and, consequently, activation of autophagy requires an intramolecular disulfide bridge between cysteins 23 and 45 (Tang *et al.*, 2010). Moreover, exposure of pancreatic tumor cells to H_2O_2 leads to an increase of the HMGB1 receptor RAGE (receptor for advanced glycation end-products), in a NF-κB-dependent manner, and activation of autophagy (Kang *et al.*, 2011).

Activation of autophagy by disruption of the Beclin 1–Bcl-2 interaction under conditions of oxidative stress has also been reported to occur via the DAPk–PKD pathway. The serine/threonine kinase protein kinase D1 (PKD) regulates the traffic from the trans-Golgi network and several signaling processes, such as motility, proliferation and cell death. Under conditions of oxidative stress (H_2O_2 addition), the tumor-suppressor death-associated protein kinase (DAPk) has been reported to activate autophagy in two ways: (1) by phosphorylation of Beclin 1, resulting in Bcl-2 release, and (2) by PKD phosphorylation that subsequently phosphorylates and activates Vps34 (Eisenberg-Lerner and Kimchi, 2011). All these studies together highlight that ROS modulation of the autophagy pathway is dependent on the type of ROS, and the cell type and its context.

ROS and CMA

Chaperone-mediated autophagy, and (macro)autophagy are induced in response to both metabolic stressors (e.g., nutrient starvation, growth factor withdrawal, hypoxia, or high lipid content challenges) and oxidative stress (Kaushik and Cuervo, 2006). Autophagy and CMA constitute different mechanisms with non-redundant functions. As described earlier, CMA is a selective process by which cytosolic proteins bearing a KFERQ-related sequence are recognized and removed for degradation through a system of chaperones. It has been estimated than approximately 30% of cytosolic proteins contain this motif. Nevertheless, while, under conditions of oxidative stress, oxidation of some aminoacids (e.g., oxidation of histidine to aspartic acid) may result in the generation of this motif in proteins previously lacking it, some proteins already bearing this sequence can lose it by the same oxidation process. Recent studies have shown that, under oxidative stress conditions, an important cross-talk between these autophagy mechanisms is established, and loss of either of these pathways tends to be compensated by the other. Cells with compromised (macro)autophagic activity show a constitutive upregulation of CMA, whereas cells displaying CMA deficiency activate autophagy as a compensatory mechanism. Therefore, both CMA and autophagy represent important mechanisms to cope with oxidative damage: CMA in the specific removal of soluble oxidized cytosolic proteins, and autophagy, via p62 recruitment or organelle-selective autophagy, in degradation of protein aggregates or dysfunctional organelles.

Modulation of ROS by Autophagy

Although ROS play an important role in the regulation of autophagy in response to several cellular stressors, this process also plays a key role in controlling excessive production

of ROS. While antioxidant enzymes such as SOD, catalase, glutathione peroxidases, peroxiredoxins, etc., play a key role in first-line defense against oxidative stress, autophagy acts at
a secondary level to remove oxidized proteins and organelles that otherwise would contribute to expand the oxidative damage throughout the cell.

Autophagy-Mediated Removal of Protein Aggregates

Oxidative conditions favor the unfolding of proteins that tend to form protein aggregates and initiate apoptosis if not removed properly. In fact, protein aggregates cannot be
removed by the proteasome system, and therefore other mechanisms, like autophagy,
need to be activated in order to remove them. Autophagy has been largely considered to
be a fairly unselective process. Nevertheless, recent works have identified that the protein
adaptors p62/SQSTM1 and NBR1 act both as cargo receptors for the degradation of ubiquitinated protein aggregates through autophagy and as autophagy substrates (Johansen
and Lamark, 2011). These protein adaptors have similar domain architecture with a LC3-
interacting region (LIR) allowing binding to the Atg8 family proteins, and a UBA (ubiquitin-
associated) domain to bind to mono- and polyubiquitin.

Oxidative stress can induce p62 by the transcriptional activation of Nrf2. In fact, the p62
promoter contains an antioxidant response element (ARE) region where Nrf2 binds to initiate transcription of this gene, leading to p62 mRNA expression. Interestingly, p62 itself
has also an important role in the regulation of the Nrf2/KEAP1 pathway. Specifically, p62
interacts with the Kelch-like ECH-associated protein 1 (KEAP1) at the Nrf2 binding site,
promoting Nrf2 release and subsequent activation of the antioxidant response. Binding
of p62 with Nrf2 in this non-canonical mechanism of Nrf2 activation occurs through the
KEAP1-interacting region (KIR) of p62. As a consequence, p62 creates a positive feedback
loop regulating its own transcription by controlling Nrf2 activation. Therefore, under conditions of oxidative stress where a major concentration of protein aggregates are accumulated,
increased expression of p62 helps in removing these aggregates by delivering them to the
autophagosome for degradation while at the same time modulating Nrf2 activity to induce
an antioxidant response that quenches ROS and restores homeostatic conditions.

Interestingly, Mathew *et al.* (2009) showed that metabolic stress produced in autophagy-
deficient tumor cells led to accumulation of p62, and elevated expression of both ER chaperones and protein disulfide isomerases, indicating protein quality-control malfunction. Defects
in the autophagy machinery led to accumulation of damaged mitochondria and, consequently, increased levels of ROS resulting in DNA damage. Interestingly, addition of the antioxidant N-acetylcysteine (NAC) in Beclin$^{+/-}$ and Atg5$^{-/-}$ IBMK cells increased cell survival
which was associated with decreased p62 accumulation during metabolic stress, suggesting
that ROS-mediated oxidative stress leads to protein damage and accumulation of p62.

Autophagy-Mediated Removal of Damaged ROS-Producing Organelles

Autophagy can also be directed to degrade damaged and dysfunctional organelles such as
mitochondria (in a process called mitophagy), ER (reticulophagy), ribosomes (ribophagy), or
peroxisomes (pexophagy). As described earlier in the chapter, mitochondria are the main cellular sources of ROS, especially in response to conditions of oxidative stress. Mitophagy is an
essential mechanism to ensure proper cellular homeostasis and viability, and mainly protects
in two essential ways: (1) by removing the damaged source of ROS that, when dysfunctional,

increases the production of the reactive species, and (2) by degrading damaged mitochondria that otherwise would release apoptotic factors (e.g., cytochrome c, apoptotic-induced factor (AIF), and other factors) to activate cell death. Mitophagy uses the components of the autophagy machinery with an additional step for cargo recognition mediated by the cargo recognition proteins Nix and the pair PINK1 (PTEN-induced putative protein kinase 1) and E3 ubiquitin ligase Parkin (Ashrafi and Schwarz, 2013). Supporting the role of mitophagy in controlling oxidative stress levels, increased levels of ROS produced in autophagy-defective Atg5$^{-/-}$ MEFs or Atg7$^{-/-}$ T cells have been associated with increased accumulation of dysfunctional mitochondria (Kongara and Karantza, 2012).

Autophagy-Mediated Removal of Antioxidants and Cell Death

Caspase-8 inhibition or depletion has been shown to promote selective degradation of the antioxidant enzyme catalase (which converts H_2O_2 into H_2O and O_2), leading to subsequent enhanced lipid peroxidation and autophagic cell death. Interestingly, only catalase was found to be selectively degraded, but not SOD (the enzyme that dismutates $O_2^{\bullet-}$ into H_2O_2), thereby suggesting a signaling role of H_2O_2 in this cell death modality (Yu et al., 2006). Therefore, it is possible that the selective removal of catalase by autophagy initiates a loop in which increased H_2O_2 accumulation further promotes the aberrant induction of autophagy that ultimately causes cell death. Although ROS are also produced in response to starvation-induced autophagy (see below), which has a cytoprotective function, nutrient deprivation did not induce selective catalase degradation. It has been suggested that increased accumulation of H_2O_2 produced by specific catalase degradation could be the signal that switches the outcome from cell survival to cell death and possibly decides which cell death modality takes place (Scherz-Shouval and Elazar, 2007).

AUTOPHAGY, ROS, AND CANCER

The increased metabolic activity observed in cancer cells, when compared to normal cells, mainly mediated by anaerobic metabolism to increase cellular proliferation, is known as the Warburg effect, and is a characteristic hallmark of cancer. Incomplete oxidative phosphorylation in addition to the accumulation of dysfunctional mitochondria leads to increased production of ROS in cancer cells. This basally high production of ROS is in turn amplified by constant exposure of cancer cells to metabolic and oxidative stress conditions (e.g., low nutrients and oxygen concentrations, or low pH of the microenvironment). As already mentioned, ROS can activate different signaling pathways, autophagy being one of them. In fact, autophagy and ROS are extensively involved in both cancer initiation and cancer progression, and modulation of these factors has been used in different therapeutic strategies to eradicate tumor-diseased tissue. The cross-talk between these factors both in cancer pathogenesis and treatment is discussed in this section.

Autophagy and ROS in Cancer Development

Basal levels of autophagy have a key function in maintaining cellular homeostasis and quality control by degrading damaged or misfolded proteins as well as malfunctioning or aged organelles. From this point of view, the process probably acts in promoting cell survival both in the early and late stages of cancer progression. From the perspective of tumor pathogenesis and development, however, autophagy plays a critical dual role both as a tumor promoter and as a tumor suppressor mechanism. In addition, ROS activate the transcription factors Nrf2, NF-κB, HIF-1, AP-1, STAT3, and others that are involved in the expression of genes involved in antioxidant responses, inflammation, cell transformation, tumor cell survival, proliferation, invasion, metastasis, and angiogenesis. Therefore, the cross-talk between ROS and autophagy in cancer pathogenesis and development is a complex interplay that will be affected by different factors, such as cancer cell type, its genetic background, and the microenvironment in which the tumor grows.

In the early stages of tumorigenesis, autophagy can act as a tumor suppressor mechanism. A driving cause in tumor initiation involves mutation of and damage to both genomic and mitochondrial DNA due to a lack of repair systems and histone protein protection, caused by oxidative stress and by exposure to chemicals, radiation (e.g., UV radiation), contaminants, and other factors. Whereas mitochondrial ROS are produced as a byproduct of mETC, dysfunctional mitochondria can increase ROS production, resulting in further oxidative DNA damage; this leads to chromosomal instability, which is associated with malignant transformation. Activation of mitophagy, for example, can remove damaged and dysfunctional mitochondria, alleviating the oxidative burden and consequently preventing tumorigenesis. Therefore, autophagic defects shown by some tumor cells can be associated with the accumulation of oncogenic mutations and malignant transformation. Interestingly, Mathew et al. (2009) reported that defects in the autophagy machinery produced an accumulation of damaged mitochondria and a subsequent increase in ROS production that leads to DNA damage. Increased cell survival observed after addition of the antioxidant NAC to Beclin$^{+/-}$ and Atg5$^{-/-}$ IBMK cells during metabolic stress suggested a key role of ROS in protein damage and p62 accumulation. These responses associated with p62 accumulation led to genome instability driving tumorigenesis (Mathew et al., 2007). Moreover, p62 accumulation due to the inability of autophagy-deficient cells to remove this protein was sufficient, for example, to modify NF-κβ regulation and gene expression to promote tumorigenesis. Monoallelic deletion of Beclin 1, for example, has been detected in prostate, ovarian, and breast cancer. Moreover, tumor suppressor proteins such as phosphatase and tensin homologue (PTEN), Bif-1, Atg4c, UVRAG, nuclear p53, DAPkinase, AMPK, TSC, and retinoblastoma proteins (RB) have been reported to positively regulate autophagy, whereas the products of common oncogenes, such as PI3KC1, PKB, TOR, and Bcl-2, have been shown to act as autophagy repressors. In fact, constitutive activation of the PI3K–Akt–mTOR axis (LoPiccolo et al., 2008), which inhibits autophagy while promoting tumor cell growth, proliferation, and survival, is a common feature in cancer.

On the other hand, autophagy can also act as a tumor promoter mechanism. Increased metabolic stress detected in cancer cells – especially in solid hypoxic regions as result of nutrient and oxygen deficiency – increases the energetic demands of rapidly dividing tumors, leading to autophagy activation. Hypoxia-inducible factor (HIF)-1, a key transcription factor stimulated in conditions of oxygen deprivation and/or mitochondrial generation of ROS, activates several target genes involved in the control of cellular metabolism, promotion of cellular survival, and angiogenesis. Deregulation of mTOR activates this transcription factor, leading to an increase in HIF-1α translation and its accumulation. Mitophagy-related

II. CANCER

genes such as BNIP3 (Bcl-2/E1B 19-kDa interacting protein 3) and BNIP3-related proteins have a key role in hypoxia-mediated mitophagy. In fact, BNIP3 and the related protein NIX localize to mitochondria, where they could directly stimulate mitophagy via the interaction with LC3 and GARABAP proteins. Additionally, these two proteins may have a more general role under hypoxia-induced autophagy by disrupting the Bcl-2/Beclin 1 interaction and subsquent activation of the PI3KC3 complex. Therefore, metabolic stress leads to ROS generation that contributes to autophagy activation sustaining cell survival.

Interestingly, autophagy has been shown to be upregulated in many cancer cell lines in which H-Ras or K-Ras oncogenes are expressed. Cancers with these oncogene mutations, which have poor prognosis, use autophagy as a means to survive starvation. In fact, recent works supporting a tumor-promoting role of autophagy have shown that ROS-mediated JNK activation leads to autophagy induction which is involved in the oncogenic K-Ras-induced malignant transformation of human normal breast epithelial cells, MCF10A (Kim et al., 2011).

The tumorigenic roles of ROS and autophagy are not only limited to the tumor itself, but can also involve the tumor environment, which in fact plays a key role in tumor progression and metastasis in different cancer types. Loss of stromal Caveolin-1 (Cav-1) in the tumor-associated fibroblast compartment has been associated with early tumor recurrence and metastasis. Indeed, Cav-1-deficiency has been reported to produce oxidative stress, mitochondria dysfunction, and autophagy that recycles proteins and dysfunctional mitochondria to provide nutrients and energy for the bystander cancer cells (Pavlides et al., 2010).

Interestingly, CMA has also be shown to have a relevant role in promoting tumor growth in a great variety of cancer cells and human tumors, such as lung cancer and melanoma, independently of the (macro)autophagy status. CMA blockage delays tumor growth and regression, thus revealing a key role of this pathway in tumor promotion (Kon et al., 2011).

Autophagy and ROS in Cancer Therapy

Understanding the specific roles that ROS production and autophagy play at the different stages of cancer progression, and how cell type and genetic context affect the cross-talk/interplay between both factors, is essential for the development and optimization of anticancer strategies. This is particularly relevant for those therapies based on ROS production, such as photodynamic therapy, some chemotherapeutics, or radiotherapy, since the ability to modulate prosurvival signaling pathways may lead to increased cancer cell death. Autophagy when activated with cell survival functions is an undesired side effect that should be inhibited to ensure a successful therapeutic outcome, whereas when it acts to promote cell death it is a pathway that should be potentiated. Moreover, activation of autophagy with prodeath functions can be a useful strategic alternative in apoptosis-resistant cells. Therefore, understanding of the role that autophagy plays in each case is a basic necessity in designing strategies that potentiate either induction or inhibition of this pathway.

On the other hand, since cancer cells show persistent high levels of ROS when compared to normal cells, many cancer cells have developed adaptive mechanisms that enhance the endogenous antioxidant capacity, thus making malignant cells more resistant to exogenous levels of oxidative stress. Paradoxically, ROS-based therapies can be cytotoxic to tumor cells, because they generate massive oxidative stress levels that push cancer cells to their limit and overwhelm their high antioxidant levels, thus causing cell death.

Photodynamic Therapy of Cancer (PDT)

Photodynamic therapy is an antineoplastic modality based on the combination of a light-absorbing molecule (i.e., a photosensitizer) that preferentially accumulates in cancer cells, molecular oxygen, and light to generate high concentrations of ROS that overwhelm the cellular antioxidant defense system, leading to tumor cell death and shutdown of the vascular supply (Agostinis et al., 2011). Specifically, excitation of the photosensitizer with visible light generates ROS, mainly in the form of singlet oxygen ($^1O_2$), although other ROS such as superoxide ($O_2^{\bullet-}$) or hydroxyl ($^\bullet OH$) can also be produced in this initial step. The excitation level of the light should ideally be in the therapeutic range of 600–800nm, to which biological tissues are most transparent and where the excited states are energetic enough to efficiently produce the cytotoxic ROS $^1O_2$. Depending on the chemical structure, photosensitizers accumulate preferentially in a specific subcellular location, the most common of which are the endoplasmic reticulum (ER), mitochondria, lysosomes, Golgi body, or plasma membrane. This subcellular location is crucial for initiation of the different cellular responses activated by photodynamic stress. As already mentioned, the photodynamic reaction mainly produces $^1O_2$, the only ROS that is an excited state and therefore has an inherent lifetime of few microseconds, which limits its area of reaction with proteins, phospholipids, etc. to the subcellular location of the photosensitizer. Nevertheless, the primary oxidation products can either break down and generate secondary ROS or activate enzymatic sources of ROS that can extend the oxidative damage throughout the cell, thereby activating either prosurvival responses or cell death mechanisms that eventually lead to eradication of the diseased tissue. In fact, PDT can induce autophagy and apoptotic cell death both in normal and in transformed cells (Reiners et al., 2010). Using hypericin (Hyp), a naturally occurring photosensitizer that accumulates preferentially at the ER of different cell lines, we showed that one of the primary photooxidation events produced by $^1O_2$ was sarco(endo)plasmic reticulum Ca^{2+}-ATPase (SERCA) pump photodamage, which initiated different subcellular responses leading to apoptotic cell death of different cancer cell lines. Hyp-mediated PDT (Hyp-PDT), however, also stimulated autophagy by a rapid downregulation of the Akt–mTOR–p70S6K pathway, resulting in a cytoprotective mechanism as revealed by the increased levels of apoptotic cell death detected after Hyp-PDT when Atg5 levels were attenuated (Buytaert et al., 2006; Dewaele et al., 2011). Moreover, we observed that whereas photodamage at the ER activated early reticulophagy, phospholipid hydroperoxides (produced in this organelle mainly by reaction of $^1O_2$ with ER phospholipids) and H_2O_2 propagated ROS damage to mitochondria, thereby amplifiying the oxidative damage. Mitochondrial ROS were involved both in the activation of cytoprotective mitophagy and in apoptotic cell death (Rubio et al., 2012) (Figure 12.2). In fact, our results supported a model in which cardiolipin hydroperoxides could act as molecular switches that initiate pre-apoptotic events when the oxidative pressure inside the mitochondria is too high and mitophagy fails to effectively remove the oxidatively damaged cellular components. Therefore, in this case we observed an ROS-induced ROS release process, which critically regulates both cytoprotective autophagy and apoptosis cell death.

Other photosensitizers that accumulate preferentially at the ER and/or the mitochondria, such as the porphycene CPO, benzoporphyrin derivative BPD, and silicon phthalocyanine

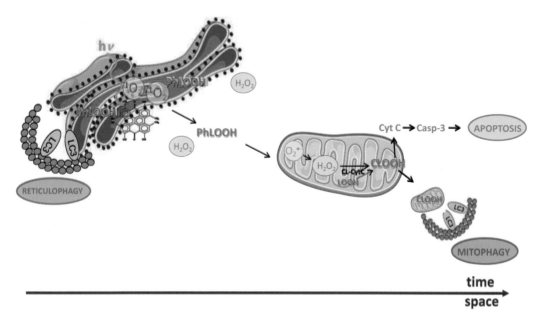

FIGURE 12.2   **Spatio-temporal autophagic degradation of oxidatively damaged organelles after Hyp-PDT.** Phospholipid hydroperoxides produced after photodamage at the ER are involved in the activation of reticulophagy, as well as in propagation of the oxidative damage to the mitochondria, which amplifies the oxidative damage. Mitochondrial ROS are involved both in the activation of cytoprotective mitophagy and in apoptotic cell death. Cardiolipin hydroperoxides could act as molecular switches between the two processes.

Pc4, have been shown to photodamage Bcl-2. This event disrupts Bcl-2 association with the pro-autophagic protein Beclin 1, thereby launching autophagy, which was shown to be cytoprotective. Regulation of the autophagic cascade by ROS-mediated redox-sensitive events induced by PDT is exemplified by the amphiphilic endolysosomal-localized aluminum sulfonated phthalocyanine (AlPcS$_{2a}$). Photoactivation of this photosensitizer directly targets the mTOR signaling network, causing a partial loss of both total mTOR and the Ser (2448) phosphorylated form in cultured adenocarcinoma cell lines and tumor xenograft (Reiners *et al.*, 2010).

Interestingly, we also reported for the first time that ROS-based PDT activates CMA, and this pathway appears to be the major autophagic mechanism for removal of damaged proteins after Hyp-mediated PDT, keeping and establishing a direct cross-talk with autophagy which is crucial to resist ROS-mediated photokilling (Dewaele *et al.*, 2011).

Although PDT stimulates autophagy activation in apoptosis-competent cells with a cytoprotective function, autophagy function in cells unable to activate an apoptotic response may differ. Hyp-PDT in Bax$^{-/-}$Bak$^{-/-}$ double knockdown cells activated a strong autophagy response which exhibited a prodeath role in response to photodynamic killing (Buytaert *et al.*, 2006). In agreement with this, apoptotic-resistant MCF7 human breast cancer cells treated with Pc4, an ER/mitochondria-localized photosensitizer, rely on autophagy for cell death after treatment (Reiners *et al.*, 2010). Therefore, activation of autophagy by PDT using photosensitizers that accumulate preferentially at the ER or mitochondria has a cytoprotective function. Accordingly, in order to optimize the therapeutic outcome of PDT, this treatment could be applied in combination with autophagy inhibitors to maximize cancer cell death mechanisms.

Another interesting way to prevent cytoprotective autophagy is to use lysosome-localized photosensitizers. In fact, photogeneration of ROS at the lysosomes/endosomes using the chlorine NPe6 and the palladium bacteriophephorbide WST11 results in either lysosomal permeabilization and subsequent alkylation or destruction of endosomes and lysosomes, therefore disrupting the autophagic flux process and inducing, or amplifying, apoptotic responses (Kessel *et al.*, 2012).

Chemotherapeutics

Many commonly used chemotherapeutic agents induce both ROS production and autophagy activation, which in some cases has a prosurvival role and should be inhibited to increase the therapy effectiveness, while in others it contributes to cell death and should therefore be potentiated, especially in apoptotic-deficient cancer cells.

Arsenium trioxide (AS_2O_3) is a chemotherapeutic agent with a cytotoxic action based on the generation of oxidative stress. This agent activates apoptosis, but also autophagy, which has been shown to contribute to cell death in various types of cancer cells, such as acute promyelocytic leukemia, gliomas, or ovarian carcinomas. Studies in leukemia cells treated with AS_2O_3 revealed that this agent increases $O_2^{\bullet-}$ generation by hindering mitochondrial respiration (Dewaele *et al.*, 2010). Consequently, AS_2O_3-induced ROS were associated with depletion of the antioxidant glutathione (GSH). AS_2O_3-treated human T lymphocytic leukemia and myelodysplastic syndrome (MDS) cell lines showed autophagy activation by upregulation of Beclin 1. Interestingly, studies performed on glioma cells revealed that AS_2O_3 damaged mitochondrial membrane integrity and upregulated BNIP3 and BNIP3-L, both events involved in the induction of autophagy, which in this case promotes cell death (Dewaele *et al.*, 2010). In fact, BNIP3 can displace Bcl-2 from its complex with Beclin 1 and therefore activate autophagy. Otherwise, studies in ovarian carcinoma cells have shown that SnoN/SkiL, a TGF-β signaling mediator, modulates autophagy induction after AS_2O_3-treatment in a Beclin 1-independent but Vps34-dependent way (Smith *et al.*, 2010). Moreover, human hepatocellular carcinoma and myeloid leukemia cells treated with AS_2O_3 have shown dephosphorylation of Akt, although other works on leukemia cells have reported activation of Akt and mTOR after treatment (Dewaele *et al.*, 2010).

2-Methoxyestradiol (2-ME) is an inhibitor of both the mETC complex I and the antioxidant enzyme SOD that is used as a chemotherapeutic agent able to activate apoptosis but also independent autophagy, with prodeath functions in several transformed (human embryonic kidney HEK293 cell line) and cancer cells (human glioma cancer cell line U87 and human cervical cancer cell line HeLa). 2-ME-induced autophagy is mediated by $O_2^{\bullet-}$ (Chen *et al.*, 2009). This agent is used in Phase II clinical trial studies for treatment of different types of cancer (Bruce *et al.*, 2012; Harrison *et al.*, 2011).

Valproic acid is an anti-epileptic and chemotherapeutic agent that activates autophagy with prodeath functions by the ROS-induced extracellular signal-regulated kinase 1/2 (ERK 1/2) pathway in glioma cells (Fu *et al.*, 2010).

In some cases, inhibition of autophagy can accelerate the kinetics of chemotherapeutic-induced cell death. Chloroquine (CQ) is a lysosomotropic antimalarial drug that neutralizes lysosomal acidification, thus blocking autophagosomal degradation. Currently, CQ is used in Phase II clinical trials to treat solid tumors in combination with standard chemotherapeutics such as tamoxifen, an oxidative stress-producing agent (Chen and Karantza, 2011).

Radiotherapy

Ionizing radiation (IR) is an antineoplastic modality whose cytotoxic effect is also based on the production of oxidative stress. As in the previous ROS-based anticancer modalities, radiotherapy can activate autophagy with either a prosurvival role or a prodeath function, depending on the cancer type, genetic background of the cancer cell, and microenvironment, as well as the therapeutic strategy. For example, blockage of Beclin 1 decreased cell survival in radio-resistant carcinoma cell lines after 1 Gy irradiation, whereas cell survival in radiosensitive carcinoma cancer cells was increased (Apel *et al.*, 2008).

CONCLUSIONS AND PERSPECTIVES

Current studies on the interplay between ROS and autophagy have revealed a complex cross-talk between these intertwined processes. While ROS are molecules involved in the activation and modulation of autophagy pathways, these processes can in turn control excessive ROS production, thus inducing a feedback loop. In addition, modulation of autophagy pathways by ROS may occur at the different mediators of the signaling pathway, which adds an additional level of complexity.

Dysfunctions in autophagy regulation contribute to cancer initiation, while cancer cells show increased levels of ROS when compared to normal cells. Autophagy pathways can act as tumor suppressor mechanisms by removing damaged proteins or dysfunctional mitochondria that otherwise would generate aberrant concentrations of ROS leading to DNA damage, genomic instability, and, eventually, cancer pathogenesis. However, autophagy pathways can also act as tumor promoter processes, supporting tumor growth. In solid tumors, for example, nutrient and oxygen scarcity can activate autophagy for nutrients provision and energy metabolism, and this process is also associated with ROS generation. Whereas ROS and autophagy regulation contribute to cancer initiation and progression, many anticancer treatments are based on the production of cytotoxic ROS, often, if not always, accompanied by activation of autophagy. Autophagy induction by ROS-based therapeutics has, in most instances, a prosurvival role, suggesting that its inhibition may improve therapy outcomes. On the other hand, in some circumstances autophagy may be recruited to favor cancer cell death. The mechanism by which autophagy switches between these two cellular functions is still unknown, although it appears to be influenced by the nature and duration of the ROS-based treatment as well as tumor characteristics, such as type of cancer, genetic background, and expression of proteins regulating autophagy and apoptosis. In conclusion, although prediction of the outcome of ROS and autophagy interplay is quite complex and depends on several parameters, ROS-induced anticancer therapies where autophagy activity can be modulated, either by promoting or inhibiting it, have been shown to be quite powerful therapeutic strategies, and research should be focused on this direction, especially in those cases where tumors show apoptosis-resistance and alternative mechanisms are required to mediate cell death.

Acknowledgments

This work was supported by grants from the Fund for Scientific Research Flanders (FWO-Vlaannderen, G0661.09, G0728.10, and G.0584.12N) to PA. Figures were designed using Servier Medical Art (www.servier.com).

References

Agostinis, P., Berg, K., Cengel, K.A., et al., 2011. Photodynamic therapy of cancer: an update. CA Cancer J.Clin. 61, 250–281.

Alexander, A., Cai, S.L., Kim, J., et al., 2010. ATM signals to TSC2 in the cytoplasm to regulate mTORC1 in response to ROS. Proc. Natl. Acad. Sci. USA 107, 4153–4158.

Apel, A., Herr, I., Schwarz, H., et al., 2008. Blocked autophagy sensitizes resistant carcinoma cells to radiation therapy. Cancer Res. 68, 1485–1494.

Ashrafi, G., Schwarz, T.L., 2013. The pathways of mitophagy for quality control and clearance of mitochondria. Cell Death Differ. 20, 31–42.

Bensaad, K., Cheung, E.C., Vousden, K.H., 2009. Modulation of intracellular ROS levels by TIGAR controls autophagy. EMBO J. 28, 3015–3026.

Bruce, J.Y., Eickhoff, J., Pili, R., et al., 2012. A phase II study of 2-methoxyestradiol nanocrystal colloidal dispersion alone and in combination with sunitinib malate in patients with metastatic renal cell carcinoma progressing on sunitinib malate. Invest. New Drug 30, 794–802.

Budanov, A.V., 2011. Stress-Responsive sestrins link p53 with redox regulation and mammalian target of rapamycin signaling. Antiox. Redox Sign. 15, 1679–1690.

Buytaert, E., Callewaert, G., Hendrickx, N., et al., 2006. Role of endoplasmic reticulum depletion and multidomain proapoptotic BAX and BAK proteins in shaping cell death after hypericin-mediated photodynamic therapy. FASEB J. 20, 756–758.

Byun, Y.J., Kim, S.K., Kim, Y.M., et al., 2009. Hydrogen peroxide induces autophagic cell death in C6 glioma cells via BNIP3-mediated suppression of the mTOR pathway. Neurosci. Lett. 461, 131–135.

Chen, N., Karantza, V., 2011. Autophagy as a therapeutic target in cancer. Cancer Biol. Ther. 11, 157–168.

Chen, Y., Azad, M.B., Gibson, S.B., 2009. Superoxide is the major reactive oxygen species regulating autophagy. Cell Death Differ. 16, 1040–1052.

Choi, S.L., Kim, S.J., Lee, K.T., et al., 2001. The regulation of AMP-activated protein kinase by H_2O_2. Biochem. Biophys. Res. Commun. 287, 92–97.

Circu, M.L., Aw, T.Y., 2010. Reactive oxygen species, cellular redox systems, and apoptosis. Free Radic. Biol. Med. 48, 749–762.

De Duve, C., Wattiaux, R., 1966. Functions of lysosomes. Annu. Rev. Physiol. 28, 435–492.

Dewaele, M., Maes, H., Agostinis, P., 2010. ROS-mediated mechanisms of autophagy stimulation and their relevance in cancer therapy. Autophagy 6, 838–854.

Dewaele, M., Martinet, W., Rubio, N., et al., 2011. Autophagy pathways activated in response to PDT contribute to cell resistance against ROS damage. J. Cell. Mol. Med. 15, 1402–1414.

Di Bartolomeo, S., Corazzari, M., Nazio, F., et al., 2010. The dynamic interaction of AMBRA1 with the dynein motor complex regulates mammalian autophagy. J. Cell Biol. 191, 155–168.

Duan, W.J., Li, Q.S., Xia, M.Y., et al., 2011. Silibinin Activated p53 and induced autophagic death in human fibrosarcoma HT1080 cells via reactive oxygen species-p38 and c-Jun N-Terminal kinase pathways. Biol. Pharm. Bull. 34, 47–53.

Eisenberg-Lerner, A., Kimchi, A., 2011. PKD is a kinase of Vps34 that mediates ROS-induced autophagy downstream of DAPk. Cell Death Differ. 19, 788–797.

Emerling, B.M., Weinberg, F., Snyder, C., et al., 2009. Hypoxic activation of AMPK is dependent on mitochondrial ROS but independent of an increase in AMP/ATP ratio. Free Radic. Biol. Med. 46, 1386–1391.

Fu, J., Shao, C.J., Chen, F.R., et al., 2010. Autophagy induced by valproic acid is associated with oxidative stress in glioma cell lines. Neuro-Oncology 12, 328–340.

Harrison, M.R., Hahn, N.M., Pili, R., et al., 2011. A phase II study of 2-methoxyestradiol (2ME2) NanoCrystalA (R) dispersion (NCD) in patients with taxane-refractory, metastatic castrate-resistant prostate cancer (CRPC). Invest. New Drug 29, 1465–1474.

Johansen, T., Lamark, T., 2011. Selective autophagy mediated by autophagic adapter proteins. Autophagy 7, 279–296.

Kang, R., Tang, D., Livesey, K.M., et al., 2011. The receptor for advanced glycation end-products (RAGE) protects pancreatic tumor cells against oxidative injury. Antiox. Redox Sign. 15, 2175–2184.

Kaushik, S., Cuervo, A., 2006. Autophagy as a cell-repair mechanism: activation of chaperone-mediated autophagy during oxidative stress. Mol. Aspects Med. 27, 444–454.

Kessel, D.H., Price, M., Reiners, J.J., 2012. Atg7 deficiency suppresses apoptosis and cell death induced by lysosomal photodamage. Autophagy 8, 1333–1341.

Kim, M.J., Woo, S.J., Yoon, C.H., et al., 2011. Involvement of autophagy in oncogenic K-Ras-induced malignant cell transformation. J. Biol. Chem. 286, 12924–12932.

Kirkland, R.A., Adibhatla, R.M., Hatcher, J.F., et al., 2002. Loss of cardiolipin and mitochondria during programmed neuronal death: evidence of a role for lipid peroxidation and autophagy. Neuroscience 115, 587–602.

Kon, M., Kiffin, R., Koga, H., et al., 2011. Chaperone-mediated autophagy is required for tumor growth. Sci. Transl. Med. 3, 109–117.

Kongara, S., Karantza, V., 2012. The interplay between autophagy and ROS in tumorigenesis. Front. Oncol. 2, 171.

Li, L., Ishdorj, G., Gibson, S.B., 2012. Reactive oxygen species regulation of autophagy in cancer: implications for cancer treatment. Free Radic. Biol. Med. 53, 1399–1410.

Li, Y., Wang, Y., Kim, E., et al., 2007. Bnip3 mediates the hypoxia-induced inhibition on mammalian target of rapamycin by interacting with rheb. J Biol Chem. 282, 35803–35813.

Liu, L.P., Cash, T.P., Jones, R.G., et al., 2006. Hypoxia-induced energy stress regulates mRNA translation and cell growth. Mol. Cell 21, 521–531.

LoPiccolo, J., Blumenthal, G.M., Bernstein, W.B., et al., 2008. Targeting the PI3K/Akt/mTOR pathway: effective combinations and clinical considerations. Drug Resist. Updat. 11, 32–50.

Mathew, R., Kongara, S., Beaudoin, B., et al., 2007. Autophagy suppresses tumor progression by limiting chromosomal instability. Genes Dev. 21, 1367–1381.

Mathew, R., Karp, C.M., Beaudoin, B., et al., 2009. Autophagy suppresses tumorigenesis through elimination of p62. Cell 137, 1062–1075.

Ozben, T., 2007. Oxidative stress and apoptosis: impact on cancer therapy. J. Pharm. Sci. 96, 2181–2196.

Pavlides, S., Tsirigos, A., Migneco, G., et al., 2010. The autophagic tumor stroma model of cancer. Role of oxidative stress and ketone production in fueling tumor cell metabolism. Cell Cycle 9, 3485–3505.

Reiners, J.J., Agostinis, P., Berg, K., 2010. Assessing autophagy in the context of photodynamic therapy. Autophagy 6, 7–18.

Rubio, N., Coupienne, I., Di Valentin, E., et al., 2012. Spatiotemporal autophagic degradation of oxidatively damaged organelles after photodynamic stress is amplified by mitochondrial reactive oxygen species. Autophagy 8, 1312–1324.

Scherz-Shouval, R., Elazar, Z., 2007. ROS, mitochondria and the regulation of autophagy. Trends Cell Biol. 17, 422–427.

Scherz-Shouval, R., Elazar, Z., 2011. Regulation of autophagy by ROS: physiology and pathology. Trends Biochem. Sci. 36, 30–38.

Scherz-Shouval, R., Shvets, E., Fass, E., et al., 2007. Reactive oxygen species are essential for autophagy and specifically regulate the activity of Atg4. EMBO J. 26, 1749–1760.

Smith, D.M., Patel, S., Raffoul, F., et al., 2010. Arsenic trioxide induces a beclin 1-independent autophagic pathway via modulation of SnoN/SkiL expression in ovarian carcinoma cells. Cell Death Differ. 17, 1867–1881.

Tang, D., Kang, R., Livesey, K.M., et al., 2010. Endogenous HMGB1 regulates autophagy. J. Cell Biol. 190, 881–892.

Trachootham, D., Alexandre, J., Huang, P., 2009. Targeting cancer cells by ROS-mediated mechanisms: a radical therapeutic approach? Nat. Rev. Drug Discov. 8, 579–591.

Wirawan, E., Vanden Berghe, T., Lippens, S., et al., 2012. Autophagy: for better or for worse. Cell Res. 22, 43–61.

Xue, L.Z., Fletcher, G.C., Tolkovsky, A.M., 1999. Autophagy is activated by apoptotic signalling in sympathetic neurons: an alternative mechanism of death execution. Mol. Cell Neurosci. 14, 180–198.

Yu, L., Wan, F.Y., Dutta, S., et al., 2006. Autophagic programmed cell death by selective catalase degradation. Proc. Natl Acad. Sci. USA 103, 4952–4957.

Zhang, H., Kong, X., Kang, J., et al., 2009. Oxidative stress induces parallel autophagy and mitochondria dysfunction in human glioma U251 Cells. Toxicol. Sci. 110, 376–388.

CHAPTER

13

Induction of Autophagic Cell Death by Anticancer Agents

Karin Eberhart, Ozlem Oral, and Devrim Gozuacik

OUTLINE

Abstract

Autophagy is a cellular degradation and recycling pathway contributing to cell survival under stressful conditions (e.g., starvation and growth factor deprivation). Depending on the cellular context, excessive autophagy might sometimes lead to a non-apoptotic programmed death, namely autophagic cell death. Studies using various pharmacological agents and substances with anticancer properties revealed a role for autophagy in cancer cell elimination. In this chapter, we will document and analyze the contribution of autophagy to cell death activated by various anticancer agents. The chapter will be limited to cases where blockage of autophagy using chemical inhibitors or genetic approaches resulted in the survival of cancer

M.A. Hayat (ed): Autophagy, Volume 1
DOI: http://dx.doi.org/10.1016/B978-0-12-405530-8.00013-3

© 2014 Elsevier Inc. All rights reserved.

cells during drug treatment – hence, to examples of autophagy-related or autophagic cell death (ACD). In other words, in studies that will be discussed here, autophagy seemed to play a rate-limiting role in cellular demise, irrespective of the downstream executionary event. Paradoxically, autophagy was reported to play a prosurvival role (i.e., inhibition of autophagy potentiated cell death) in other cancer cell types treated with similar drugs, underlining the cellular context dependence of ACD. Usage of drugs downregulating anti-autophagic pathways (e.g., mTORC1 and AKT pathways) or stimulating dissociation of the key autophagy protein BECN1 (Beclin 1 protein) from an inhibitory complex with BCL-2 proteins as monotherapy or combination treatment seemed to strongly activate ACD and to overcome the death resistance of cancer cells in several cases. Yet death execution mechanisms downstream of autophagy have been revealed to be multiple. In addition to lysosomal degradation-mediated mechanisms, apoptosis, necroptosis, or lysosomal membrane permeabilization were involved in autophagy-related cell death. Nevertheless, the study and exploitation of autophagy and ACD certainly has the potential to give rise to novel and effective treatment strategies, especially in cancer types that are refractory to conventional chemotherapy and associated with poor prognosis.

INTRODUCTION

The ultimate goal of cancer treatment is the eradication of the maximum number of malignant cells from tissues and from the circulation. In many cases, genetic and epigenetic events leading to malignant transformation result in the resistance of cancer cells to apoptosis, the classical form of programmed cell death. Therefore, recent studies have focused on alternative, non-apoptotic cell death pathways with the hope that they might be manipulated or exploited for cancer treatment. In fact, several commonly used chemotherapy agents kill cells by non-apoptotic means. In this chapter, we will mainly focus on macroautophagy (autophagy herein) and cell death connection in the context of drug responses of cancer cells.

In fact, autophagy is a highly conserved and tightly regulated mechanism of protein degradation that is critical for the maintenance of homeostasis in all living organisms, from yeast to man (Mizushima *et al.*, 2011). It involves the degradation of cellular components and invaders, either because they are harmful (e.g., damaged organelles, mutant proteins or intracellular parasites) or because their recycling is required to support cellular metabolism. Autophagy is triggered by cellular stress pathways, and results in the segregation of cytosolic proteins, protein aggregates, membranes, and organelles in multi- or double-membrane vesicles (autophagosomes or autophagic vesicles) that eventually fuse with the vacuole in yeast, and with lysosomes in higher organisms. In the vacuole/lysosomes, the luminal contents of the vesicles are degraded by the digestive machinery of these compartments.

Autophagy is the major mechanism for the degradation of large cellular structures such as organelles and protein aggregates. In the absence of stress, basal autophagy has an important housekeeping function of waste disposal in the cells and supplies cellular metabolism with building blocks. Cellular turnover is important for all types of cells, but it is especially important in quiescent and terminally differentiated cells, where damaged components are not diluted by cell replication. During stressful conditions, including starvation, autophagy feeds cellular metabolism through nutrient recycling and helps the cell to adapt to unfavorable conditions, promoting cell survival.

MOLECULAR MECHANISMS OF AUTOPHAGY

Autophagy is a tightly regulated process requiring the concerted action of more than 30 known autophagy-related (Atg) proteins (Mizushima *et al.*, 2011, and references therein). The pathway proceeds in several distinct stages, namely the autophagic vesicle nucleation, membrane elongation, docking and fusion, and, finally, lysosomal degradation stages (Figure 13.1).

Activation of autophagy is negatively regulated by the mammalian target of rapamycin (mTOR) protein, a highly conserved serine/threonine kinase serving as the key component of the mTORC1 protein complex (Laplante and Sabatini, 2012; Mizushima *et al.*, 2011). In fact, there are two different mTOR complexes in mammalian cells: the mTORC1 and the mTORC2 complexes. Only mTORC1, consisting of mTOR, RAPTOR, mLST8/GβL, and the recently identified partners PRAS40 and DEPTOR, was shown to be a direct regulator of autophagy. mTORC1 complex integrates signals from nutrient sensing and growth factor pathways to regulate cell growth, protein synthesis, and autophagy according to the availability of cellular resources. Inactivation of mTORC1 during nutrient starvation or growth factor deprivation, or by mTOR inhibitors such as rapamycin, leads to the activation of autophagy through the Atg1/ULK1 complex, consisting of ULK1/2, mAtg13, FIP200, and Atg101 proteins. In

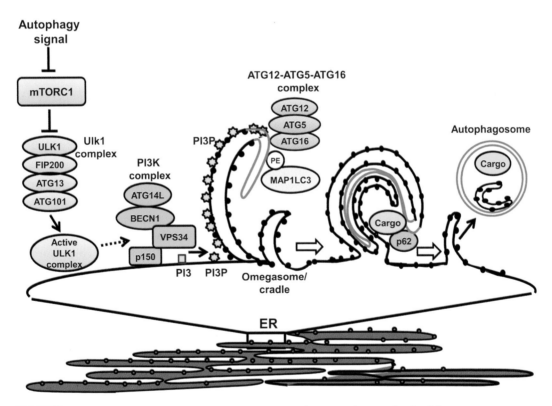

FIGURE 13.1   Molecular events leading to autophagosome formation (see text for details).

mammals, ULK1 interacts with mTORC1 under nutrient-rich conditions, and mTORC1 phosphorylates and inactivates ULK1 and its partner mAtg13. Stimuli such as starvation result in the dissociation of ULK1 from mTORC1, leading to its activation through dephosphorylation. Following activation, the ULK1 complex relays signals for the recruitment of other Atg proteins to autophagosome formation sites on cellular membranes, including the endoplasmic reticulum (Figure 13.1). These autophagosome sites are marked with phosphatidylinositol 3-phosphate (PI3P) molecules produced by a hVPS34 Class III phosphatidylinositol 3-kinase (PI3K) complex (Mizushima *et al.*, 2011, and references therein). Atg6/BECN1 (the Beclin 1 protein) is a subunit of the PI3K complex and has a central role in its regulation, hence in the regulation of the canonical autophagy pathway. After activation of autophagy, a cup-shaped structure (omegasome or cradle) is formed on the ER membrane, giving rise to the formation of autophagosome precursors called "isolation membranes." Elongation, which is a critical step in autophagosome formation, is controlled by two ubiquitin-like conjugation systems, namely Atg12–Atg5–Atg16L1 and Atg8/MAP1LC3 (or LC3) systems. Ubiquitination-like reactions result in the covalent conjugation of a lipid molecule, phosphatidylethanolamine (PE), to the LC3 protein. The Atg12–Atg5–Atg16L1 complex is suggested to play an E3-like activity in these reactions. LC3 lipidation is critical for proper autophagic vesicle formation and expansion. During selective autophagy, LC3 recruits autophagy-related adaptor/receptor proteins such as sequestosome 1 (SQSTM1/p62) that are able to recognize and tag substrate proteins, protein aggregates, and damaged organelles, and that allow cargo recruitment to autophagosomes. In higher eukaryotes, degradation and recycling of the engulfed cargo occur in lysosomes. Autophagosome/lysosome fusion is induced by dynein motor proteins which mediate vacuole movement along the microtubules. After fusion, the lytic vesicles are called "autolysosomes." Finally, cargo molecules in autolysosomes are degraded into their building blocks (e.g., proteins degraded into amino acids) that are eventually actively transported back to the cytosol for reuse.

Signals leading to autophagy activation are diverse, and they mainly converge with mTORC1 at the level of its upstream regulator TSC2/TSC1 complex (Laplante and Sabatini, 2012; Mizushima *et al.*, 2011). TSC2/TSC1 is a GTPase activating complex for the RHEB protein, an mTORC1 activator in its GTP-bound state. Favoring the hydrolysis of GTP to GDP on RHEB, TSC2/TSC1 acts as a negative regulator of mTORC1. Signals integrated by TSC2/TSC1 include those coming from the growth factor-activated PI3K/AKT pathway, the RAS/MEK/ERK pathway, Wnt ligand-activated GSK3β, and the energy (especially ATP) depletion and/or hypoxia-activated LKB1/AMPK pathway. Downstream effectors of mTORC1 include 4E-binding protein 1 (4EBP1) and p70S6K. Phosphorylation of 4E-BP1 by mTORC1 leads to its dissociation from eukaryotic translation initiation factor 4E (eIF4E) and upregulates translation. Phosphorylation of p70S6K by mTORC1 enhances p70S6K activity and allows it to phosphorylate downstream targets such as eEF2K (eukaryotic elongation factor 2 kinase). Therefore, dephosphorylation of 4EBP1 and p70S6K correlates with mTORC1 inactivation.

Another key event in autophagy regulation is the balance between anti-apoptotic BCL2 proteins (i.e., BCL2, BCL2L1/BCLXL, MCL1) and BECN1. BCL2 proteins inhibit autophagy through direct interaction with the BECN1 protein (Eisenberg-Lerner *et al.*, 2009, and references therein). BECN1 sequestered by BCL2 binding can no longer activate the VPS34–PI3K complex, resulting in autophagy downregulation. Direct phosphorylation of either BCL2 proteins or BECN1 by activated c-JUN N-terminal kinase (JNK) or the death-associated protein kinase-1 (DAPK1), respectively, was shown to promote dissociation of the complex and to stimulate the autophagy pathway. Conversely, an increase in BCL2 protein expression or a decrease in BECN1 levels, events that are observed in various malignancies, may tip the balance towards inhibition of autophagy.

PROGRAMMED CELL DEATH AND AUTOPHAGY

In addition to its homeostatic and cytoprotective roles in promoting cell survival under basal and stressful conditions, in certain biological scenarios autophagy might also induce a caspase-independent type of programmed cell death, namely autophagic cell death, or type 2 programmed cell death (type 1 cell death being classical apoptosis) (Galluzzi *et al.*, 2012; Gozuacik and Kimchi, 2007). In this chapter we will mainly focus on the cytotoxic role of autophagy, especially on the induction of autophagy-related or autophagic cell death (ACD) by anticancer agents.

Morphological and molecular manifestations of ACD are different from those of apoptosis or necrosis (Galluzzi *et al.*, 2012). Classical apoptotic or type 1 cell death manifests itself with morphological features including cell shrinkage, chromatin condensation (pyknosis), nuclear fragmentation (karyorrhexis), plasma membrane blebbing, formation of apoptotic bodies, and early phagocytosis. Phosphatidyl serine exposure (PS) on the outer leaflet of the plasma membrane serves as the major "eat-me" signal for apoptosis. Activation of caspases (CASPs), a family of cysteine-dependent aspartate-directed proteases, is mainly responsible for the characteristic morphological changes associated with the apoptotic cell death. Two distinct pathways might lead to caspase activation and cellular demise during apoptosis: the death receptor-dependent extrinsic pathway involving CASP8 activation, or the mitochondrial intrinsic pathway involving the release of mitochondrial factors such as cytochrome c, AIF, and Endo G into the cytosol, and activation of CASP9. Both pathways converge in the activation of downstream effector caspases such as CASP3 and CASP7.

Until recently, necrosis was characterized as an accidental, non-programmed cell death type. Recent studies revealed that there might be several forms of necrosis, and that necrosis can be programmed after all. A type of necrosis, called necroptosis, was studied in detail. Necroptosis was characterized as a caspase-independent but RIP- and/or RIP3-dependent necrotic programmed cell death type, activated by death receptors and blocked by RIP-inhibitor chemicals called necrostatins (Galluzzi *et al.*, 2012). Downstream executionary mechanisms of necroptosis are not well established to date, but have been reported to involve cellular bioenergetic problems, ROS overproduction, and lysosomal membrane permeabilization (Vandenabeele *et al.*, 2010).

Autophagic cell death (ACD) is achieved through a series of specific morphological and molecular changes (Gozuacik and Kimchi, 2007). The most prominent characteristic of autophagic cell death is the accumulation of autophagic vesicles in the cytosol of dying cells. These vesicles may be formed of double or multiple membranes, and engulf bulk cytoplasm and/or cytoplasmic organelles such as mitochondria. At least ultrastructurally, autophagosomes produced during ACD resemble those activated under moderate, physiological stress conditions. Nuclear changes such as chromatin condensation are less prominent and partial during ACD. Cells shrink but do not dissolve into fragments, yet blebbing and PS exposure may sometimes be observed. Nevertheless, phagocytosis of dying cells is less frequent, and delayed, compared to apoptosis. The extent of autophagic activity in ACD might sometimes reach such a level that the total area of autophagosomes and auto-lysosomes can be equal to or greater than that of the rest of cytosol and organelles, leading to cellular atrophy (Gozuacik and Kimchi, 2007, and references therein).

Since the original definition of ACD was based on morphology and did not include functional or molecular criteria, the term "autophagic cell death" was long used to refer to caspase-independent cell death progressing with autophagosome accumulation. Considering the role of autophagy as a cellular recycling and stress response mechanism, a debate evolved in the scientific community regarding whether accelerated autophagy observed in dying cells played a causal role in cellular demise, or whether it was part of an ultimate (but failing) rescue attempt of the cell to survive stress. Since the cytoprotective and cata-bolic role of autophagy was dominant in many studies, a direct role of autophagy in cell death execution began to be doubted. The question arose of whether ACD is cell death with or despite of autophagy, or cell death by autophagy. In a recent review, Shen and Codogno (2011) coined the definition of autophagic cell death as "a modality of non-apoptotic and non-necrotic programmed cell death in which autophagy serves as a death mechanism." According to this definition, ACD should define programmed cell death meeting the fol-lowing criteria: (1) cell death should occur without the involvement of apoptosis; (2) there should be an increase of the autophagic flux (degradation), and not just an increase of the autophagic markers, in dying cells; and (3) suppression of autophagy via pharmacologi-cal inhibitors (e.g., 3-MA, wortmannin or other PI3K inhibitors) and/or genetic approaches (e.g., gene knockout or RNAi mediated knockdown of essential autophagy related genes such as Atg3, Atg5, Atg7, BECN1) should rescue or prevent cell death. Therefore, the authors suggested that the term ACD should be used based on biochemical and functional considerations, and not only on morphological observations. This definition seems to be accepted by the majority of the scientific community. However, studies that conform to all the above-mentioned criteria are few, and attempts to analyze the role of ACD in cell death systematically have been limited to only a few specific cell lines (Shen *et al.*, 2011).

INDUCTION OF AUTOPHAGIC CELL DEATH BY ANTICANCER AGENTS

Although the role of autophagy in cancer is very complex, various pharmacologi-cal agents with different antineoplastic properties have been shown to induce autophagic activity resulting in massive death of cells in some cancer types. Apoptosis resistance is one of the major causes of chemoresistance, and an important challenge in the treatment of cancer is the development of therapies that overcome chemoresistance. Thus, activation of autophagy in apoptosis-resistant cancers could potentially provide a way to induce cell death and impede malignant growth.

This section describes some interesting examples of drugs and drug-like molecules induc-ing ACD in cancer cells. In this chapter, in line with the ACD criteria mentioned above, only cases in which cell death could be blocked by chemical or genetic inhibition of autophagy will be defined as ACD and discussed further (see Table 13.1 for a summary of drugs).

TABLE 13.1 Anticancer Agents Inducing Cell Death and Autophagy in Cancer Cell Lines

Drug Class	Anticancer Agent	Pathways Involved/ Targets	Autophagy Inhibition	Cancer Cell Type	Reference
Antimetabolites	Pemetrexed	AMPK, mTOR	3-MA, siRNA Beclin 1	Breast cancer cells (BT474), metastatic breast cancer cells (4T1), and hepatocellular carcinoma cells (HuH7), lung cancer cells (H460)	Bareford et al. (2011)
	3-Bromopyruvate + glutamine starvation	ATP↓, ROS	3-MA, siRNA Atg5	Cervical cancer cells (HeLa)	Cardaci et al. (2012)
Tyrosine kinase inhibitors	Lapatinib + obatoclax	Akt/mTOR, BCLXL/MCL1, AIF	siRNA Atg5, siRNA Beclin 1	Colon cancer cells (HCT116), breast cancer cells (MCF-7, SKBR3, BT474, MMTV-HER2, 4TI-luc-I2B, HCC1954)	Martin et al. (2009)
	Cetuximab + rapamycin	PI3K, mTOR	Chloroquine, siRNA Atg5	Vulvar squamous carcinoma cells (A431), head and neck cancer cells (HN5, FaDu)	Li et al. (2010)
	Imatinib	Akt/mTOR, ERK1/2 pathway	3-MA, siRNA Atg5, siRNA Atg10, siRNA Atg12	Glioblastoma cells (U87-MG, LN229, U373-MG, LNZ308)	Shingu et al. (2009)
	Sorafenib + pemetrexed	mTOR, Mcl-1 and Bcl-XL	3-MA, siRNA Beclin 1	Breast cancer cells (BT474), metastatic breast cancer cells (4T1), hepatocellular carcinoma cells (HuH7), lung cancer cells (H460)	Bareford et al. (2011)
Histone deacetylase inhibitors	SAHA	n.s.	3-MA	Chondrosarcoma cells (SW1353, RCS, OUMS-27)	Yamamoto et al. (2008)
	SAHA	Akt/mTOR	siRNA Beclin 1, siRNA Atg7, siRNA TSC2	Cervical carcinoma cells (HeLaS3)	Cao et al. (2008)
	OSU-HDAC42, SAHA	Akt/mTOR, ER stress	3-MA, siRNA Atg5	Hepatocellular carcinoma cells (Huh7, HepG2, Hep3B)	Liu et al. (2010)

(*Continued*)

TABLE 13.1   (Continued)

Drug Class	Anticancer Agent	Pathways Involved/ Targets	Autophagy Inhibition	Cancer Cell Type	Reference
Alkalyting agent	Temozolomide	n.s.	3-MA	Glioblastoma cell lines (U373-MG, T98G, U251-MG, GB-1,U87-MG, A172)	Kanzawa et al. (2004)
mTOR inhibitors	RAD001 + doxorubicin or radiation	Met dephos-phorylation	siRNA Atg5	Papillary thyroid cancer cells (TPC-1, 8505-C)	Lin et al. (2010)
	RAD001 + Z-DEVD + radiation	n.s.	siRNA Atg5, siRNA Beclin 1	Lung cancer cells (H460)	Kim et al. (2008)
Proteasome inhibitors	Bortezomib	Caspase-8 activation	3-MA, siRNA Atg5	Cervical carcinoma cells (HeLa Bcl-2 overexpressing), NSCLC cells (H460 Bcl-2 overexpressing)	Laussmann et al. (2011)
	Bortezomib	Lysosomal degradation of TRAF6	3-MA	Acute myeloid leukemia cells (TF-1, THP1, HL60), primary myelodysplastic syndrome cells (MDS-01, MDS-02)	Fang et al. (2012)
BH3 mimetics	(−)-Gossypol + temozolomide	mTOR	siRNA Atg5, siRNA Beclin 1	Glioblastoma cells (U87, U343, MZ-54)	Voss et al. (2010)
	Obatoclax + dexamethasone	mTOR, dissociation of Beclin 1/MCL-1 interaction	3-MA, bafilomycin A, siRNA Atg7, siRNA Beclin 1	GC-resistant acute lymphoblastic leukemia cells (CEM-C1, Jurkat)	Bonapace et al. (2010)
	Obatoclax + lapatinib	Akt/mTOR, AIF	siRNA Atg5, siRNA Beclin 1	Colon cancer cells (HCT116)	Martin et al. (2009)
Glucocorticoids	Dexamethasone	PML↑, Akt inhibition	3-MA, LY294002, siRNA Beclin 1	Acute lymphoblastic leukemia cells (RS4;11, SUP-B15)	Laane et al. (2009)
	Dexamethasone + obatoclax or rapamycin	mTOR, dissociation of Beclin 1/MCL-1 interaction	3-MA, bafilomycin A, siRNA Atg7, siRNA Beclin 1	GC-resistant acute lymphoblastic leukemia cells (CEM-C1, Jurkat)	Bonapace et al. (2010)
Others	STF-62247	Golgi trafficking and PI3K	3-MA, siRNA Atg5, siRNA Atg7, siRNA Atg9	Renal cell carcinoma cells (VHL deficient; RCC4, RCC10)	Turcotte et al. (2008)

(*Continued*)

TABLE 13.1 (Continued)

Drug Class	Anticancer Agent	Pathways Involved/ Targets	Autophagy Inhibition	Cancer Cell Type	Reference
Sphingolipids	CERS1 and C18-ceramide	Lethal mitophagy	siRNA Atg3, siRNA Atg5, siRNA Atg7	Head and neck squamous cell carcinoma cells (UM-SCC-22A)	Sentelle et al. (2012)
Others	Fenretinide	n.s.	3-MA	Breast cancer cells (MCF-7)	Fazi et al. (2008)
Vitamin D analogue	EB1089	n.s.	3-MA	Breast cancer cells (MCF-7)	Hoyer-Hansen et al. (2005)
Plant-based chemo-therapeutics	Resveratrol	Akt/mTOR	si RNA Atg7	Breast cancer (MCF-7)	Scarletti et al. (2008)
	Resveratrol	mTOR, JNK and AMPK	Bafilomycin A, siRNA Atg5, siRNA LC3, siRNA p62	Chronic myeloid leukemia cells (K562)	Puissant et al. (2010)
	Cannabinoids	ER stress, mTOR	siRNA Atg1/Ulk1, siRNA Atg5, siRNA Ambra1	Glioblastoma cells (U87MG)	Salazar et al. (2009)
	Cannabinoids	ER stress, Akt/mTOR	3-MA, E64d + pepstatin A, siRNA Atg5	Hepatocellular carcinoma cells (Huh7, HepG2)	Vara et al. (2011)
	β-Lapachone	ROS induction	3-MA, siRNA Atg6, siRNA Atg7, Bafilomycin A	Glioblastoma cells (U87MG)	Park et al. (2011)
	Avicin D	ATP↓, AMPK, mTOR siRNA	Atg5, siRNA Atg7, siRNA TSC2, chloroquine	Osteosarcoma cells (U2OS)	Xu et al. (2007)
	B10 betulinic acid derivative	Caspase-3, LMP	siRNA Atg5, siRNA Atg7, siRNA Beclin 1	Glioblastoma cells (U87MG)	Gonzalez et al. (2012)
	Polygonatum cyrtonema lectin	ROS, p38–p53 activation	3-MA	Melanoma cells (A375)	Liu et al. (2009)

n.s., not studied.

Antimetabolites

The antifolate and antimetabolite pemetrexed is already in clinical use for the treatment of non-small cell lung carcinoma (NSCLC). Pemetrexed interferes with cellular metabolism and leads to elevated 5-aminoimidazole-4-carboxamide-1-b-D-ribofuranosyl monophosphate (ZMP) levels, leading to the activation of AMPK, which in turn inactivates mTORC1. The end result is increased autophagy. Pemetrexed treatment of breast cancer cells was shown to cause a reduction in cell viability, an effect that was blocked by 3-MA or by knockdown of BECN1 (Bareford *et al.*, 2011). Combination of pemetrexed with another inducer of autophagy, rapamycin, further enhanced pemetrexed toxicity in multiple tumor cell types.

Another modulator of metabolism is 3-bromopyruvate (3-BP). Upon uptake into cells via solute carrier family 16 (SLC16), 3-BP inhibits complex II of the mitochondrial respiratory system (succinate dehydrogenase) through substitution of its normal substrate pyruvate. 3-BP treatment results in reduction in ATP levels, formation of reactive oxygen species (ROS), and metabolic oxidative stress leading to cell death. This effect could even be potentiated by prior glutamine starvation of cancer cells, thereby facilitating the cellular uptake of 3-BP. Upon glutamine withdrawal, 3-BP-induced carcinoma cell death was not executed through apoptosis, but showed features of ACD, as evidenced by the autophagic flux increase and significant reduction of cell death through either chemical (3-MA) or genetic (siRNA-mediated Atg5 knockdown) inhibition of the autophagic machinery (Cardaci *et al.*, 2012). Putative candidates in mediating ACD stimulated by 3-BP and ROS were proposed to be mitogen-activated protein kinase 8 (MAPK8/JNK), AMPK, and the death-associated protein kinase (DAPK1).

Tyrosine Kinase Inhibitors

Dysregulation or constitutive activation of tyrosine kinases plays a key role in tumor development and progression, making them attractive cancer therapy targets. For example, the tyrosine kinase inhibitor lapatinib was shown to target both ERBB1 and ERBB2 receptor kinases stimulating cancer growth – yet clinical studies showed that single agent therapy with ERBB1/ERBB2 inhibitors was frequently not effective. Resistance to lapatinib in colon cancer cells HCT116 was associated with an increased expression of cell death protective MCL1 and BCLXL proteins and a decrease in pro-apoptotic BAX levels (Martin *et al.*, 2009). Combination of the BH3 domain antagonist obatoclax, capable of inhibiting BCL2/BCLXL/MCL1 function, enhanced lapatinib-induced cytotoxicity in resistant HCT116 cells. This combinatory cytotoxic effect could also be observed in several breast cancer cell lines (MCF-7, SKBR3, BT474, MMTV-HER2, 4TI-luc-I2B, and HCC1954 mammary carcinoma cells). Potentiation of lapatinib-induced cytotoxicity correlated with caspase activation, increased cytosolic levels of AIF, expression of LC3, and the formation of large vesicles. Knockdown of Atg5 or BECN1 significantly reduced cell killing, providing evidence that ACD was in play. In this scenario, reduced AKT, mTOR, and S6K1 activation was observed and this contributed to autophagy induction by the agents. Since knockdown of MCL1 and BCLXL significantly enhanced cell death, obatoclax possibly contributed to the stimulation of a toxic form of autophagy by promoting BECN1 release from the BCL2 proteins.

Epidermal growth factor receptor (EGFR), a member of the ERBB family of tyrosine kinase receptors, was found to be overexpressed in many epithelial cancers. Dysregulation of EGFR contributes to cancer formation and growth through its effects on autonomous cell growth, cell death inhibition, angiogenesis, and tumor spread. Cetuximab was among the first EGFR monoclonal antibodies approved by the FDA for the treatment of solid tumors.

It effectively inhibits EGFR by blocking its ligand-induced activation; however, resistance to EGFR blocking drugs, including cetuximab, could develop in some tumors. In A431 human vulvar squamous carcinoma cells where cetuximab single therapy induces only weak apoptosis, combination of cetuximab with rapamycin was shown to result in the activation of ACD (Li et al., 2010). Similarly, ACD could be activated by the combination treatment in HN5 and FaDu head and neck cancer cells that normally respond to cetuximab by growth inhibition, and which are resistant to cetuximab-induced apoptosis. Cetuximab/rapamycin combination-induced autophagy and cell death was blocked by silencing Atg5, or by the treatment of cells with the lysosomal inhibitor chloroquine. Therefore, ACD induction achieved through a combination of cetuximab and rapamycin might increase the potency of cetuximab in resistant solid tumor types.

Imatinib was developed as a specific inhibitor for the BCR-ABL oncoprotein, but was later found to have some inhibitory effects on c-ABL, c-KIT, and PDGFR as well. Imatinib was shown to induce ACD in human malignant glioma cells (U87-MG, LN229, U373-MG, LNZ308) through inhibition of the AKT/mTOR pathway and activation of the ERK1/2 pathway (Shingu et al., 2009). Imatinib-induced cytotoxicity was attenuated by the inhibition of autophagy at an early stage, by 3-MA treatment, or Atg5, Atg10, or Atg12 silencing. Interestingly, cell death was augmented following the inhibition of autophagy at a later stage by the use of the autolysosome inhibitors, bafilomycin A or RTA203. Acceleration of imatinib-induced cytotoxicity by autolysosome inhibitors was associated with mitochondrial membrane depolarization and apoptosis. Therefore, although ACD might be activated by imatinib, agents disturbing lysosomal activity and/or lysosomal homeostasis could convert cell death into apoptosis, possibly through induction of lysosomal membrane permeabilization.

As explained in more detail above, under the subheading Antimetabolites, the AMPK-activating molecule pemetrexed was shown to induce ACD in cancer cells. Synergistic activation of autophagy and cell death was observed when the kinase inhibitor drug sorafenib was used in combination with pemetrexed in breast, liver, and lung cancer cells (Bareford et al., 2011). Sorafenib is a multikinase inhibitor drug originally designed as a RAF-1 inhibitor, but it was later shown to affect receptor tyrosine kinases such as VEGFR and PDGFR. Synergistic antitumor action of pemetrexed and sorafenib was shown in vitro in breast and liver cancer cells, and in vivo in a mice breast cancer model. Molecular mechanisms of the observed effects were studied. Pemetrexed/sorafenib drug combination led to the downregulation of MCL1 and BCLXL levels in MCF-7 cells, but caused an increase in BECN1 protein levels. Following treatment, Atg12–Atg5 expression levels were higher and AKT, mTOR, and p70 S6K protein kinases were inactivated. ACD activation was confirmed through knockdown of BECN1, resulting in the blockage of both autophagy and cell death observed under these conditions.

Histone Deacetylase Inhibitors

Aberrant epigenetic control is commonly observed as an early event in tumor progression, and abnormal acetylation has been implicated in tumorigenesis. Histone acetylation is controlled by histone acetyl transferases, which transfer acetyl groups to lysine residues, and histone deacetylases (HDACs), which deacetylate them. HDAC-mediated histone acetylation occurs in nucleosomes, and regulates changes in chromatin conformation and gene expression. HDACs also regulate the acetylation of a variety of non-histone substrates which include proteins involved in tumor progression, cell cycle control, apoptosis, and angiogenesis. Expression deregulation and mutations of HDAC genes are associated with tumor development through modification of gene transcription, as well as effects on non-histone HDAC substrates.

Inhibitors of HDACs were introduced as potent anticancer drugs. At least two histone deacetylase inhibitors, the hydroxamic acid-based vorinostat (also known as suberoylanilide hydroxamic acid, SAHA) and romidepsin (FK228), have been approved by the FDA. A number of studies showed that SAHA-induced cancer cell death could not be blocked by caspase inhibitors, suggesting that a non-apoptotic cell death pathway was in play. For example, SAHA treatment successfully inhibited growth of chondrosarcoma cell lines (Yamamoto *et al.*, 2008). Chondrosarcomas exhibit high resistance to conventional chemotherapy, yet SAHA administration was shown to successfully inhibit tumor growth in mice xenograft models. This inhibition was the result of a non-apoptotic cell death induced by the agent. In SAHA-treated chondrosarcoma cells, autophagic vesicle accumulation was observed and inhibition of autophagy by 3-MA restored cell viability, strongly indicating that cell death was autophagic. In line with this, Cao *et al.* (2008) reported a SAHA-induced caspase-independent cell death with autophagic features in HeLa S3 cells. SAHA-induced cell death occurred independently of caspase activity, but with a high degree of autophagy induction. Cell death was dependent on BECN1 and Atg7 protein expression, as shown by a decrease in death after siRNA-mediated knockdown of these autophagy genes. Following the treatment, activities of the autophagy- and cell survival-related kinases mTOR and AKT were reduced, and downregulation of the mTOR regulator TSC2 protein inhibited SAHA-induced autophagy. These data suggest that SAHA induced ACD through blockage of upstream autophagy inhibitory pathways.

In addition to SAHA, the HDAC inhibitor OSU-HDAC42 activated autophagy in hepatocellular carcinoma cells (Liu *et al.*, 2010). SAHA and OSU-HDAC42 inhibited mTOR phosphorylation, as well as phosphorylation of its downstream substrates p70/p85S6 kinases. SAHA led to a decrease in the AKT activity in a dose-dependent manner, and PERK activation followed by eIF2α phosphorylation was observed. Hence, SAHA and OSU-HDAC42 induced autophagy through downregulation of AKT/mTOR signaling and induction of the endoplasmic reticulum stress response. Inhibition of autophagy by 3-MA or Atg5 knockout reduced cytotoxicity, indicating that autophagy-induced by SAHA (and possibly by OSU-HDAC42) was responsible for the death of cells.

Temozolomide

Temozolomide (TMZ) is a small lipophilic alkylating agent in use as an anticancer agent for high-grade, aggressive brain tumors and melanoma. The action of TMZ depends on its ability to alkylate DNA, leading to DNA damage and tumor cell death. Malignant glioma cells mainly respond to TMZ by undergoing G2/M cell cycle arrest, or, rarely, by apoptosis. Kanzawa *et al.* (2004) showed that TMZ activated autophagy in a malignant glioma cell line, U373-MG. Inhibition of autophagy by 3-MA completely blocked the cytotoxic effects of TMZ, indicating that the drug activated ACD in U373-MG glioma cells. Yet blockage of autophagosome–autolysosome fusion by bafilomycin A (due to the lysosomal acidification defect) further increased the toxic effects of TMZ. Observation of cell death following bafilomycin A treatment, but not with 3-MA, was most probably due to an increase in the lysosomal membrane permeability (LMP) caused by this agent. Therefore, usage of lysosome destabilizer drugs might convert TMZ-induced ACD into a LMP- and apoptosis-dependent cell death in a glioma model.

mTOR Inhibitors

Rapamycin, binds to the FK506-binding protein FKBP12 and inhibits the mTOR pathway, the central negative regulator of autophagy. Rapamycin treatment exhibited anticancer properties, and is currently in clinical trials for the treatment of various malignancies. Several rapamycin analogues with improved solubility and stability have been developed, including CCI-779 (temsirolimus) and RAD001 (everolimus), which are already approved for the treatment of renal cell carcinoma and pancreatic neuroendocrine tumors. There is growing evidence suggesting the involvement of ACD in rapamycin-induced cell death. For example, in papillary thyroid cancer cells, RAD001 sensitized cells to treatment with the DNA damaging agent doxorubicin and radiation therapy (Lin *et al.*, 2010). The cytotoxic effect of RAD001 was attenuated by RNAi knockdown of Atg5, suggesting that cells died by ACD. Atg5 knockdown increased MET phosphorylation and everolimus treatment resulted in decreased MET activity, involving MET in autophagy-mediated sensitization to doxorubicin and radiation therapy. In line with these results, SU11274, a small molecule inhibitor of c-MET, led to ACD in A549 lung cancer cells. ERK and p53 activation and AKT inhibition were involved in the observed effect (Liu *et al.*, 2012).

Combined treatment of RAD001 with the caspase-3 inhibitor DEVD radiosensitized apoptosis-deficient lung cancer cells *in vitro* and *in vivo* in a mouse lung cancer xenograft model, and resulted in enhanced cytotoxicity and delayed tumor growth (Kim *et al.*, 2008). Increased cytotoxicity was linked to the induction of autophagy. Autophagy was required for susceptibility to cell death, as knockdown of Atg5 and BECN1 resulted in radiation resistance of lung cancer cells. mTOR inhibition also affected tumor vasculature, contributing to the antitumor activity of this rapamycin analogue.

Proteasome Inhibitors

The ubiquitin proteasome system (UPS) is the main mechanism for the degradation of short-lived proteins in cells. Due to their ability to specifically induce cell death in transformed cells, proteasome inhibitors were evaluated for their potential in cancer therapy as single agents or in combination with other treatment regimens. The reversible proteasome inhibitor bortezomib was approved by the FDA and is in clinical use for the treatment of multiple myelomas and mantle cell lymphomas. Treatment with proteasome inhibitors mainly induces apoptosis in cells. Interestingly, even in apoptosis-deficient cells, mouse embryonic fibroblasts (BAX/BAK knockout fibroblasts), BCL2 overexpressing HeLa cervical carcinoma cells, and H460 NSCLC cells, treatment with proteasome inhibitors (bortezomib, MG-132, or epoxomicin) led to significant cell death induction (Laussmann *et al.*, 2011). Cell death was independent of CASP3 and CASP7 activation, but was dependent on activation of CASP8. CASP8 activation in response to proteasome inhibition was not related to death receptors, but depended on autophagy activation; inhibition of autophagy with either 3-MA or by knocking down Atg5 reduced CASP8 processing and cell death. This study reveals a new autophagy-dependent cell death pathway involving, CASP8 activation in cells in which the canonical apoptotic pathway was blocked.

Bortezomib also induced autophagy and subsequent apoptosis in acute myeloid leukemia (AML) and myelodysplastic syndrome (MDS) cell lines (Fang *et al.*, 2012). TRAF6 was found to be the target of bortezomib-induced cytotoxicity in these cells. Reduction in TRAF6 protein levels was correlated with bortezomib-triggered autophagy, and subsequent apoptosis. In line with this, RNAi-mediated depletion of TRAF6 resulted in rapid apoptosis induction. Inhibition of autophagy by 3-MA not only restored cellular TRAF6 protein levels but also enhanced cell viability. These findings suggest that the mechanism of bortezomib-induced cell death in myeloid malignancies might involve the degradation of survival-related TRAF6 protein by autophagy.

BH3 Mimetics

Anti-apoptotic members of the BCL2 protein family function in the suppression of both apoptosis and autophagy, and they are of major importance in the therapy resistance of several cancer types, including malignant gliomas. In an attempt to specifically target BCL2 proteins, BH3 mimetics were developed as drugs. For example, a BH3 mimetic, pan-BCL2 inhibitor (−)-gossypol, efficiently activated death in malignant glioma cells exhibiting only limited sensitivity to monotherapies (Voss *et al.*, 2010). Furthermore, (−)-gossypol addition potentiated cell death induced by temozolomide (TMZ) in glioma cell lines U343 and U87. (−)-Gossypol induced autophagy and cytochrome c release, but cell death occurred in the absence of lysosomal damage and effector caspase activation. Knockdown of BECN1 or Atg5 strongly diminished the extent of cell death induced by (−)-gossypol/TMZ combination, indicating that autophagy contributed to this type of cell death. Stable knockdown of mTOR or combination of (−)-gossypol with rapamycin further increased ACD. These data suggest that pan-BCL2 inhibitors are promising drugs that induce caspase-independent ACD in apoptosis-resistant tumors, including gliomas, and these drugs may be effectively used alone or in combination with other chemotherapy agents.

Glucocorticoids

Glucocorticoids (GC) have been exploited in the treatment of lymphoid malignancies because of their ability to induce cell cycle arrest and apoptosis. Although they have been in clinical use for a long time, their mode of action and the mechanisms of resistance development during therapy remain unknown. In the treatment of childhood acute lymphoblastic leukemia, resistance to GC in the initial phases of therapy reflects a poor outcome. Therefore, elucidating the mechanism of GC-induced cell death and resistance development is important in order to establish new treatment regimens. There is evidence that, besides apoptosis, autophagy might be involved in GC-activated cell death, and this fact might be exploited in the treatment of resistant cells. In a recent study, it was suggested that GC-induced cell death in acute lymphoblastic leukemia cells was mediated through an autophagy-dependent mechanism (Laane et al., 2009). In this study, treatment with the GC dexamethasone stimulated autophagy followed by the activation of the intrinsic apoptotic pathway. Blockage of autophagy, by either chemical or genetic means, attenuated cell death rates. Moreover, a comparison between GC-sensitive and GC-resistant cells of CLL patients was performed, and autophagy induction after ex vivo dexamethasone treatment occurred only in GC-sensitive cells. Dexamethasone treatment resulted in the upregulation of the PML protein (the promyelocytic leukemia protein), which was found to form a complex with AKT. Initiation of autophagy and the onset of apoptosis were both dependent on PML-related AKT dephosphorylation. These data suggest that autophagy is indispensable for dexamethasone-induced cell death that is finally executed by apoptosis.

Bonapace and colleagues demonstrated that autophagy was activated by a combination of the BH3 mimetic obatoclax and dexamethasone (Bonapace et al., 2010). Combined treatment was sufficient to restore dexamethasone response in GC-resistant acute lymphocytic leukemia cells. The resensitization of GC-resistant cells to dexamethasone could be completely abrogated by inhibitors that interfere with the early (3-MA) or late (bafilomycin A) stages of the autophagic process, as well as the knockdown of essential Atg genes (BECN1 and Atg7) in ALL cells and GC-resistant BAX/BAK knockout fibroblasts. At a molecular level, as expected, obatoclax led to the dissociation of BECN1 from its inhibitory association with MCL1, and dexamethasone/obatoclax combination resulted in mTOR inhibition. Similarly, inhibition of mTOR by rapamycin also potentiated GC-related ACD. Cell death was dependent on the necroptosis mediators RIP-1 kinase and CYLD. Hence, autophagy was an early and limiting step to steroid sensitization by obatoclax, and it was triggered upstream to the CYLD and RIP-1 kinase-dependent necroptosis pathway. Data support a model in which the apoptotic blockade in GC-resistant ALL cells can be overcome by activating an autophagy-dependent necroptotic cell death pathway.

Small Molecule Drug STF-62247

In a screen of small molecule drugs using renal cell carcinoma (RCC) cell lines, Turcotte and colleagues identified a compound, STF-62247, that selectively killed von Hippel-Lindau (VHL) deficient cancer cells both in vitro in culture and in vivo in tumor implantation tests (Turcotte et al., 2008). The VHL tumor suppressor gene is inactivated in 75% of RCC patients. STF-62247 caused autophagy induction and massive vacuolization in VHL-deficient RCC cells, but it did not lead to apparent DNA damage or apoptosis. Blockage of autophagy using 3-MA, or Atg5, Atg7, or Atg9 knockdown counteracted STF-62247 toxicity in VHL deficient cancer cells, supporting the idea that STF-62247 induced ACD. In the yeast model, loss of proteins involved in Golgi trafficking was found to increase cell death-induced by STF-62247. It is possible that Golgi-related pathways were involved in the cell death induction mechanisms of this drug, but confirmation in the mammalian system is required. Therefore, STF-62247 activated ACD to kill VHL-deficient RCC cells, perhaps through a Golgi-related pathway.

Sphingolipids

Ceramides are bioactive sphingolipids that can mediate cell death and exhibit antitumor effects. The mammalian ceramide synthases 1–6 (CERS1 to CERS6) regulate de novo generation of ceramides, preferentially C_{18}- and C_{16}-ceramides, respectively. CERS1 and its product C_{18}-ceramide was shown to demonstrate tumor suppressor activity in head and neck squamous cell carcinomas (Sentelle *et al.*, 2012). C_{18}-ceramide was shown to localize to the mitochondria, reduce mitochondrial respiration, and induce mitophagy. Cell death activated by ceramide was dependent on Atg proteins (Atg3, Atg5, and Atg7), as shown by their siRNA mediated knockdown. Moreover, C_{18}-ceramide-triggered death was independent of BAX and BAK pro-apoptotic BCL2 family proteins and CASP3 and CASP7 in MEFs. C_{18}-ceramide stimulated LC3B lipidation and interacted with the LC3B protein on the outer membrane of mitochondria, targeting the organelle into autophagosomes following fission. These results implicate mitophagy (autophagy of mitochondria) and mitochondrial degradation in the mechanisms of ceramide-induced ACD. On the other hand, C_{16}-ceramide, not localizing to the mitochondrial outer membrane, showed no effect on autophagy or cell death.

Fenretinide

Fenretinide is a derivative of retinoic acid, the active metabolite of vitamin A. Whereas natural retinoids show only moderate efficacies on cancer cells and induce cell differentiation rather than death, the synthetic derivative fenretinide stimulated apoptosis and showed synergistic effects in combination with the anticancer agent cisplatin in several cancer cell lines (small cell lung carcinoma, breast cancer cells). In fact, fenretinide is in clinical trials for relapse reduction in breast cancer patients. Fazi and colleagues analyzed the effect of fenretinide in apoptosis-competent or -deficient MCF-7 breast cancer cells (Fazi *et al.*, 2008). Reconstitution of CASP3 in originally deficient MCF-7 cells led to the activation of apoptosis following fenretinide treatment; however, in apoptosis-resistant, non-reconstituted MCF-7 cells, fenretinide induced autophagy-dependent cell death that could be blocked by 3-MA addition. In line with this, BECN1 protein expression was induced by fenretinide. Induction of ACD in the CASP3-negative MCF-7 cell line indicates that this synthetic retinoid might be tested in the treatment of apoptosis-resistant breast tumors.

Vitamin D3 Analogue EB1089

The vitamin D3 analogue EB1089 was shown to be toxic for various malignant cells, including ovarian cancer and prostate cancer cells. In MCF-7 breast cancer cells, administration of EB1089 resulted in cell death associated with the hallmarks of autophagy, including accumulation of autophagic vesicles and increased lysosomal activity (Hoyer-Hansen *et al.*, 2005). More importantly, EB1089-induced cell death could be inhibited by 3-MA. In line with the involvement of PI3K activity in this type of cell death, restoration of BECN1 expression in low expressor MCF-7 cells sensitized the cells to EB1089-induced ACD.

Resveratrol

Resveratrol is a natural phenol with potent antioxidant and antitumorigenic activities, and is found in red grape skin and other fruits. Resveratrol inhibited proliferation and induced autophagy and cell death in breast cancer cells (Scarlatti *et al.*, 2008). Similar to fenretinide, resveratrol induced apoptosis only in MCF-7 breast cancer cells stably expressing

CASP3 but not in CASP3-deficient MCF-7 cells, whereas autophagy was induced in both cell lines. Activation of autophagy by resveratrol was associated with the inhibition of AKT phosphorylation and blockage of the mTOR pathway. In this context, autophagy induction and cell death were dependent on the Atg7 protein, since knockdown of Atg7 by siRNA blocked resveratrol-induced autophagy and cell death. Interestingly, downregulation of BECN1 and hVPS34 proteins or treatment with the autophagy inhibitor 3-MA blocked neither autophagy nor cell death in resveratrol-treated cells, revealing that a non-canonical, BECN1- and hVPS34-independent autophagy pathway was activated here.

In another study, resveratrol was shown to stimulate autophagy and cell death in imatinib-sensitive and -resistant CML cells (Puissant et al., 2010). In imatinib-resistant cells, cell death could be blocked by caspase inhibitors and bafilomycin A, suggesting a role for both cell death pathways – apoptosis and autophagy – in resveratrol-induced cytotoxicity. Resveratrol-induced death could be inhibited by Atg5 or LC3 knockdown, underlining the critical role of autophagy in cellular demise. Surprisingly, knockdown of the autophagy receptor p62 could also lead to cell death attenuation in this system. It is possible that degradation of a survival-related and p62-recruited target by autophagy could be involved in this ACD scenario. In this study, in addition to mTOR inhibition, autophagy induction by resveratrol was shown to depend on JNK and AMPK activation.

Cannabinoids

Cannabinoids, the active components of *Cannabis sativa* and *Cannabis indica*, exert a wide spectrum of pharmacological activities in the brain as well as in the periphery, and therefore the therapeutic potential of cannabinoids has gained much attention during the past few years. THC (delta-9-tetrahydrocannabinol) is the primary biologically active substance in cannabinoids, and is mainly known for its psychoactivity. Additionally, drugs containing THC as the active agent were approved by the FDA for the treatment of chemotherapy-related side effects. In a study exploring the anticancer properties of THC on glioblastomas, the substance was shown to induce cell death with autophagic features (Salazar et al., 2009). Indeed, knockdown of autophagy-related proteins Atg1/ULK1, AMBRA1, or Atg5 in U87MG astrocytoma cells, or knockout of Atg5 in fibroblasts, prevented the cytotoxic effects of THC. In this scenario, autophagy-dependent apoptosis was activated, and it contributed to cellular demise. Additionally, blockage of autophagy in cells resulted in the preservation of mitochondrial membrane potential and attenuation of ROS production. Requirement of autophagy for anticancer effects of THC was also shown *in vivo* in mice, in a MEF tumor xenograft model. As a molecular mechanism, THC stimulated *de novo* ceramide synthesis and led to endoplasmic reticulum stress with the upregulation of stress-related p8, ATF4, CHOP, and TRB3 proteins. THC treatment led to a decrease in the phosphorylation of AKT, TSC2, and PRAS40 (AKT targets in the mTORC1 pathway), as well as mTORC1 inhibition. AKT inhibition was TRB3 dependent, and TRB3/AKT inhibitory interaction was a key event leading to the observed effects on the downstream targets. Therefore, THC could activate an ER stress and AKT inhibition-related and autophagy-dependent cell death program to kill cancerous cells. Strikingly, normal, non-transformed primary astrocytes were not sensitive to the toxic effects of THC, making the substance a promising chemotherapy agent candidate. Moreover, in hepatocellular carcinoma cells (HCC), treatment with THC led to autophagy-dependent cell death induction and reduced the growth of HCC subcutaneous xenografts (Vara *et al.*, 2011).

β-Lapachone

β-Lapachone is a quinone-containing compound that was originally isolated from the lapacho tree in South America. Previous studies introduced β-lapachone as a potential chemotherapeutic and radiosensitizing agent inducing death in a number of human breast and prostate cancer cell lines. Park and colleagues studied the anticancer effects of β-lapachone in U87MG malignant glioma cells (Park *et al.*, 2011). They discovered that cell death induced by this agent showed autophagic properties. Indeed, β-lapachone-induced cell death was not affected by apoptosis (zVAD-fmk) or necroptosis (necrostatin-1) inhibitors. Autophagic activity in cells was upregulated and ROS induction was prominent. In line with this, treatment of cells with antioxidants as well as inhibition of autophagy through BECN1 or Atg7 knockdown, or usage of 3-MA or bafilomycin A, blocked β-lapachone-induced death. ROS was activating autophagy in U87MG cells and inhibition of ROS accumulation blocked β-lapachone-induced autophagy and cell death, suggesting that ROS-induced ACD is responsible for the anticancer effects of this substance.

Avicins

Avicin D is a natural triterpenoid saponin originally isolated from the Australian desert tree *Acacia victoriae*. It inhibits cell growth and induces apoptosis in transformed tumor cell lines in *in vitro* and in *in vivo* mouse models, yet avicin D could activate cell death even in apoptosis-deficient cells (in zVAD-fmk treated cells or BAX/BAK knockout cells) (Xu *et al.*, 2007). Cell death was mediated by autophagy, since attenuation of autophagy using the inhibitor chloroquine and specific knockdown of Atg5 or Atg7 blocked cellular demise in U2OS and MEF cells. The mechanism of avicin D-activated autophagy was explored. The substance was shown to decrease cellular ATP levels, thereby activating AMPK. This led to the inhibition of the mTORC1 pathway and its downstream substrate S6 kinase. Suppression of AMPK by other means was effective in decreasing ACD by the substance; avicin D-induced ACD could be blocked by the AMPK inhibitor compound C, dominant-negative AMPK, and the knockdown of TSC2 (a key mediator linking AMPK to mTOR inhibition). These results suggest that the AMPK/TSC2/mTORC1 pathway is the primary pathway targeted by avicin D, and underline the therapeutic potential of ACD triggered by avicins.

Betulinic Acid Derivative B10

Betulinic acid is a triterpenoid initially derived from the white birch tree, and has received attention because of its multiple biological activities in mammalian cells. Gonzalez *et al.* (2012) reported a novel mechanism of action for B10, a semi-synthetic glycosylated derivative of betulinic acid. In glioblastoma cell lines, cell death activated by B10 was not consistent with the apoptotic morphology. Molecular analyses in U87MG glioblastoma cells supported this observation; in these cells, proCASP-3 downregulation could not completely prevent B10-induced toxicity and DNA fragmentation rates did not reflect cell death rates.

Therefore, a non-apoptotic cell death type could be induced upon B10 treatment. Indeed, B10 caused autophagy activation as well as lysosome destabilization resulting in cathepsin Z and B release into the cytoplasm. Consistently, a cathepsin inhibitor, Ca074Me, significantly decreased B10-induced cell death, indicating the contribution of cathepsins to the observed death phenotype. Knockdown of Atg5, Atg7, or BECN1 significantly decreased lysosomal permeabilization and cell death. All these results provided evidence that B10 induced ACD, and downstream lysosomal destabilization contributed to the anticancer effects of the substance on glioblastoma cells.

Plant Lectins

Plant lectins are proteins that can reversibly bind to carbohydrates, precipitate polysaccharides and glycoconjugates, and agglutinate cells. A high degree of glycosylation was found to be frequently associated with malignant and metastatic cells, and plant lectins were found to be able to discriminate between malignant and benign tissue, and to recover circulating tumor cells from blood. Moreover, plant lectins were reported to induce death of cancer cells. A plant lectin, *Polygonatum cyrtonema* lectin (PCL), was shown to induce both apoptosis and autophagy in the A375 melanoma cell line, but not in normal melanocytes (Liu *et al.*, 2009). PCL-induced cytotoxicity was inhibited by 3-MA, suggesting that, in this context, autophagy had a death-promoting role. PCL treatment led to classical signs of intrinsic apoptosis as well, including BAX upregulation, BCLXL and BCL2 downregulation, mitochondrial membrane potential reduction, cytochrome c release, and CASP9 activation. Moreover, PCL treatment resulted in mitochondrial ROS accumulation as well as p38 and p53 activation in cells, suggesting that a ROS-mediated p38–p53 pathway might be involved in apoptosis. In the case of PCL, apoptosis and autophagy seem to be connected and dependent on each other, but the exact molecular mechanism of this interaction needs to be further elucidated.

DISCUSSION

Chemotherapy is still the essential treatment modality for the majority of cancers. Many classical agents used in chemotherapy kill cells through apoptosis induction, yet apoptosis defects resulting from mutations of apoptosis genes, overexpression, or activation of anti-apoptotic proteins and pathways may reduce the efficacy of cancer treatment. Therefore, targeted induction of alternative cell death mechanisms in cancers might open new avenues for the treatment of apoptosis-resistant or -insensitive cancer types. In light of the studies presented above, autophagy activation and/or ACD induction remains one of the possible approaches for the elimination of these resistant cells.

Although the mechanism of action of some drugs on the autophagy pathway is not clear, many drugs or drug-like molecules have been observed to target similar upstream pathways in order to induce autophagy activation (see Table 13.1 and Figure 13.2). AKT pathway inhibition and mTORC1 pathway inactivation seem to be common denominators in the action of the majority of ACD-inducing agents (Table 13.1). Another important molecular outcome of drug treatments is a change in the balance between BECN1 and anti-apoptotic

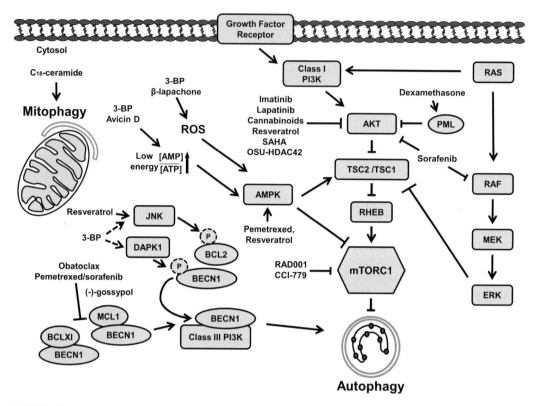

FIGURE 13.2 **Molecular targets of anticancer agents in the autophagy-activating upstream pathways.** AKT pathway inhibition and mTORC1 pathway inactivation seem to be common mechanisms in the action of several anticancer agents inducing ACD.

BCL2 proteins, either through stimulation of the dissociation of BECN1/BCL2 protein complexes (possibly involving the activation of JNK and/or DAPK proteins that stimulate dissociation), or by upregulating BECN1 protein levels. As a result, an increase in free BECN1 levels in cells seems to favor the stimulation of autophagy. ATP level changes and AMPK activation, stimulation of ceramide, ROS production, and ERK or p53 pathway activation were also important for the stimulation of autophagy by some drugs.

Several mechanisms were proposed to explain the toxic effects of autophagy during ACD. Proposed mechanisms include non-targeted consumption of cellular vital components or targeted destruction of prosurvival proteins (e.g., TRAF6 or p62-binding other targets), antioxidant proteins (e.g., catalase; see Gozuacik and Kimchi, 2007, and references therein), and important organelles such as mitochondria. Since these molecular events were not systematically studied in reports on ACD-inducing drugs, there is no substantial evidence about a common autophagy-related executionary mechanism shared by all drug types, and cell death induction mechanisms operating downstream to hyperactivated autophagy seem to be diverse. Moreover, in some cases autophagy was documented to be placed upstream (bortezomib, dexamethasone, and cannabinoid substance THC) of or possibly parallel (resveratrol and plant lectin PCL) to caspase activation and apoptosis. In other cases (dexamethasone/obatoclax), autophagy-related cell death manifested itself in a RIP-kinase-dependent necrotic fashion. Lysosomal permeability increase and cathepsin release was also reported to occur as an autophagy-dependent or -related downstream pathway and contributed to cell death (e.g., betulinic acid derivative B10).

In cases where autophagy inhibition rescued or delayed cell death phenotype following drug treatment, a clear implication of autophagic digestion reaching to its final stages in cancer cell demise was reported. Outcome of the blockage of autolysosomal degradation was studied at least in the case of resveratrol, cannabinoids, β-lapachone, avicin D and combination treatments with cetuximab/rapamycin, dexamethasone/obatoclax, and dexamethasone/rapamycin. Co-treatment of cancer cells with agents disturbing lysosomal degradation, such as cathepsin inhibitors, bafilomycin A, or chloroquine, was shown to result in the attenuation of cell death induced by these drugs or drug combinations (Table 13.1). In the case of the drugs imatinib and temozolomide, while inhibition of upstream autophagy pathways using inhibitors or knockout/knockdown strategies blocked cell death, prevention of lysosomal acidification by drugs such as bafilomycin A changed the character of the cell death routine. Thus, autophagy involving lysosomal degradation of cellular proteins/components might indeed be a contributor to the toxicity of ACD that is activated by some anticancer agents.

In biological scenarios involving a rate-limiting and crucial contribution of autophagy to cell death, a broader definition of ACD can be considered irrespective of the prominent downstream executionary mechanisms or simultaneously activated death routines. In fact, hierarchical relations between autophagy and apoptosis were reported for stress inducers or drugs other than anticancer drugs (Gozuacik and Kimchi, 2007). Moreover, mixed cell death types involving parallel activation of autophagy and apoptosis were observed, and independent contribution of these events to cellular demise was documented. Dynamic interactions between cell death pathways may also exist, and complicate the study of an isolated cell death routine. Involvement of the lysosomal activity in cell death remains an important criterion for the definition of ACD. Again, though, as stated above, it should be considered that inhibitors of the lysosomal activity that are commonly used to prove autophagic flux (i.e., modifiers of lysosomal pH and/or enzymatic activity) might also modify lysosomal membrane permeability. Lysosome destabilization may lead to the leakage of cathepsins and trigger cell death-related changes activated by these enzymes, resulting in modification of the initially studied cell death pathway.

Although there are now several reliable tools of autophagic activity detection, ACD-specific molecular markers are still missing. Discovery of these markers or ACD-specific events (e.g., specific and universal degradation of cell death/survival-related target protein(s)) would make both dissection of these complicated cell death programs and a more precise and clear molecular definition of ACD possible.

Another important issue is the dual role of autophagy in cell death and survival. In fact, autophagy plays a well-documented prosurvival role under conditions leading to cellular stress, including starvation and growth factor deprivation. Indeed, several anticancer agents, including some of those described in this chapter, were shown to activate prosurvival autophagy in other independent studies. When studies reporting ACD activation by a specific drug and those claiming a prosurvival role for autophagy in response to the same drug were compared, it became clear that cell lines and tumor types studied in those reports were different in the majority of cases (Oral, Eberhart and Gozuacik, unpublished data). Thus, the biological context resulting from the accumulation of various genetic and epigenetic hits and clonal evolution indeed seems to be the key factor determining the response of cancer cells to autophagy-inducing drugs.

In drug-resistant cancers, or in malignancies where autophagy was reported to play a role in cellular destruction, stimulation of autophagy using drug combinations including mTOR inhibitor rapamycin or its analogues temsirolimus (CCI-779) or everolimus (RAD001) enhanced the toxicity of primary anticancer agents. Similarly, drug combinations including BH3 mimetics such as obatoclax or (−)-gossypol, which stimulate the dissociation of BECN1/BCL2 protein complexes, increased anticancer drug potency through ACD activation. Thus, exploitation of ACD induction has the potential to be effective in single therapy regimens as well as in drug combination protocols, especially against therapy-resistant, apoptosis-refractory cancers.

A detailed and systematic analysis of the molecular pathways involved in ACD induction and execution, and characterization of the molecular, genetic, and/or epigenetic components of the cellular context rendering cells susceptible to ACD, would allow a more rational design of autophagy-activating treatment protocols. Impartial and unbiased studies in the autophagy field, and especially on ACD, will surely contribute to a better understanding of the molecular pathways and networks shaping cell death responses, and contribute to the rational design of more potent anticancer drugs.

Acknowledgments

This work was supported by Scientific and Technological Research Council of Turkey (TUBITAK) Grants, the European Molecular Biology Organization (EMBO), and Sabanci University. DG is a recipient of an EMBO Strategical Development and Installation Grant (EMBO-SDIG) and a Turkish Academy of Sciences (TUBA) GEBIP Award. KE and OO are recipients of TUBITAK-BIDEB Postdoctoral Scholarships.

References

Bareford, M.D., Park, M.A., Yacoub, A., et al., 2011. Sorafenib enhances pemetrexed cytotoxicity through an autophagy-dependent mechanism in cancer cells. Cancer Res. 71, 4955–4967.

Bonapace, L., Bornhauser, B.C., Schmitz, M., et al., 2010. Induction of autophagy-dependent necroptosis is required for childhood acute lymphoblastic leukemia cells to overcome glucocorticoid resistance. J. Clin. Invest. 120, 1310–1323.

Cao, Q., Yu, C., Xue, R., et al., 2008. Autophagy induced by suberoylanilide hydroxamic acid in Hela S3 cells involves inhibition of protein kinase B and up-regulation of Beclin 1. Int. J. Biochem. Cell. Biol. 40, 272–283.

Cardaci, S., Rizza, S., Filomeni, G., et al., 2012. Glutamine deprivation enhances antitumor activity of 3-bromopyruvate through the stabilization of monocarboxylate transporter-1. Cancer Res. 72, 4526–4536.

Eisenberg-Lerner, A., Bialik, S., Simon, H.U., et al., 2009. Life and death partners: apoptosis, autophagy and the cross-talk between them. Cell Death Differ. 16, 966–975.

Fang, J., Rhyasen, G., Bolanos, L., et al., 2012. Cytotoxic effects of bortezomib in myelodysplastic syndrome/acute myeloid leukemia depend on autophagy-mediated lysosomal degradation of TRAF6 and repression of PSMA1. Blood 120, 858–867.

Fazi, B., Bursch, W., Fimia, G.M., et al., 2008. Fenretinide induces autophagic cell death in caspase-defective breast cancer cells. Autophagy 4, 435–441.

Galluzzi, L., Vitale, I., Abrams, J.M., et al., 2012. Molecular definitions of cell death subroutines: recommendations of the Nomenclature Committee on Cell Death 2012. Cell Death Differ. 19, 107–120.

Gonzalez, P., Mader, I., Tchoghandjian, A., et al., 2012. Impairment of lysosomal integrity by B10, a glycosylated derivative of betulinic acid, leads to lysosomal cell death and converts autophagy into a detrimental process. Cell Death Differ. 19, 1337–1346.

Gozuacik, D., Kimchi, A., 2007. Autophagy and cell death. Curr. Top. Dev. Biol. 78, 217–245.

Hoyer-Hansen, M., Bastholm, L., Mathiasen, I.S., et al., 2005. Vitamin D analog EB1089 triggers dramatic lysosomal changes and Beclin 1-mediated autophagic cell death. Cell Death Differ. 12, 1297–1309.

Kanzawa, T., Germano, I.M., Komata, T., et al., 2004. Role of autophagy in temozolomide-induced cytotoxicity for malignant glioma cells. Cell Death Differ. 11, 448–457.

Kim, K.W., Hwang, M., Moretti, L., et al., 2008. Autophagy upregulation by inhibitors of caspase-3 and mTOR enhances radiotherapy in a mouse model of lung cancer. Autophagy 4, 659–668.

Laane, E., Tamm, K.P., Buentke, E., et al., 2009. Cell death induced by dexamethasone in lymphoid leukemia is mediated through initiation of autophagy. Cell Death Differ. 16, 1018–1029.

Laplante, M., Sabatini, D.M., 2012. mTOR signaling in growth control and disease. Cell 149, 274–293.

Laussmann, M.A., Passante, E., Dussmann, H., et al., 2011. Proteasome inhibition can induce an autophagy-dependent apical activation of caspase-8. Cell Death Differ. 18, 1584–1597.

Li, X., Lu, Y., Pan, T., et al., 2010. Roles of autophagy in cetuximab-mediated cancer therapy against EGFR. Autophagy 6, 1066–1077.

Lin, C.I., Whang, E.E., Donner, D.B., et al., 2010. Autophagy induction with RAD001 enhances chemosensitivity and radiosensitivity through Met inhibition in papillary thyroid cancer. Mol. Cancer Res. 8, 1217–1226.

Liu, B., Cheng, Y., Zhang, B., et al., 2009. *Polygonatum cyrtonema* lectin induces apoptosis and autophagy in human melanoma A375 cells through a mitochondria-mediated ROS–p38–p53 pathway. Cancer Lett. 275, 54–60.

Liu, Y.L., Yang, P.M., Shun, C.T., et al., 2010. Autophagy potentiates the anti-cancer effects of the histone deacetylase inhibitors in hepatocellular carcinoma. Autophagy 6, 1057–1065.

Liu, Y., Yang, Y., Ye, Y.C., et al., 2012. Activation of ERK-p53 and ERK-mediated phosphorylation of Bcl-2 are involved in autophagic cell death induced by the c-Met inhibitor SU11274 in human lung cancer A549 cells. J. Pharmacol. Sci. 118, 423–432.

Martin, A.P., Mitchell, C., Rahmani, M., et al., 2009. Inhibition of MCL-1 enhances lapatinib toxicity and overcomes lapatinib resistance via BAK-dependent autophagy. Cancer Biol. Ther. 8, 2084–2096.

Mizushima, N., Yoshimori, T., Ohsumi, Y., 2011. The role of Atg proteins in autophagosome formation. Annu. Rev. Cell. Dev. Biol. 27, 107–132.

Park, E.J., Choi, K.S., Kwon, T.K., 2011. beta-Lapachone-induced reactive oxygen species (ROS) generation mediates autophagic cell death in glioma U87 MG cells. Chem. Biol. Interact. 189, 37–44.

Puissant, A., Robert, G., Fenouille, N., et al., 2010. Resveratrol promotes autophagic cell death in chronic myelogenous leukemia cells via JNK-mediated p62/SQSTM1 expression and AMPK activation. Cancer Res. 70, 1042–1052.

Salazar, M., Carracedo, A., Salanueva, I.J., et al., 2009. Cannabinoid action induces autophagy-mediated cell death through stimulation of ER stress in human glioma cells. J. Clin. Invest. 119, 1359–1372.

Scarlatti, F., Maffei, R., Beau, I., et al., 2008. Role of non-canonical Beclin 1-independent autophagy in cell death induced by resveratrol in human breast cancer cells. Cell Death Differ. 15, 1318–1329.

Sentelle, R.D., Senkal, C.E., Jiang, W., et al., 2012. Ceramide targets autophagosomes to mitochondria and induces lethal mitophagy. Nat. Chem. Biol. 8, 831–838.

Shen, H.M., Codogno, P., 2011. Autophagic cell death: Loch Ness monster or endangered species? Autophagy 7, 457–465.

Shen, S., Kepp, O., Michaud, M., et al., 2011. Association and dissociation of autophagy, apoptosis and necrosis by systematic chemical study. Oncogene 30, 4544–4556.

Shingu, T., Fujiwara, K., Bogler, O., et al., 2009. Inhibition of autophagy at a late stage enhances imatinib-induced cytotoxicity in human malignant glioma cells. Int. J. Cancer 124, 1060–1071.

Turcotte, S., Chan, D.A., Sutphin, P.D., et al., 2008. A molecule targeting VHL-deficient renal cell carcinoma that induces autophagy. Cancer Cell 14, 90–102.

Vandenabeele, P., Galluzzi, L., Vanden Berghe, T., et al., 2010. Molecular mechanisms of necroptosis: an ordered cellular explosion. Nat. Rev. Mol. Cell. Biol. 11, 700–714.

II. CANCER

Vara, D., Salazar, M., Olea-Herrero, N., et al., 2011. Anti-tumoral action of cannabinoids on hepatocellular carci-
    noma: role of AMPK-dependent activation of autophagy. Cell Death Differ. 18, 1099–1111.
Voss, V., Senft, C., Lang, V., et al., 2010. The pan-Bcl-2 inhibitor (−)-gossypol triggers autophagic cell death in malig-
    nant glioma. Mol. Cancer Res. 8, 1002–1016.
Xu, Z.X., Liang, J., Haridas, V., et al., 2007. A plant triterpenoid, avicin D, induces autophagy by activation of
    AMP-activated protein kinase. Cell Death Differ. 14, 1948–1957.
Yamamoto, S., Tanaka, K., Sakimura, R., et al., 2008. Suberoylanilide hydroxamic acid (SAHA) induces apoptosis or
    autophagy-associated cell death in chondrosarcoma cell lines. Anticancer Res. 28, 1585–1591.

Immunogenicity of Dying Cancer Cells–The Inflammasome Connection: Autophagic Death Arrives on the Scene

Gizem Ayna*, Goran Petrovski*, and László Fésüs

O U T L I N E

*These authors contributed equally to the work.

© 2014 Elsevier Inc. All rights reserved.

Abstract

One of the natural functions of the immune system is to find and eradicate neoplastic and dysplastic cells in tissues. This immune surveillance can be impaired due to the unpredictable immune escape strategies of cancer cells. Induction of apoptotic cell death by chemotherapy is applied to kill malignant cells in patients with cancer even though it has many weak points, such as the fact that apoptotic cells are usually ignored by the immune system since they are immunologically silent and even suppress inflammation. Inducing immunogenic cell death can promote efficient clearance of cancerous cells before they become aggressive and lethal. Unlike the generally anti-inflammatory apoptotic cells, clearance of immunogenic apoptotic, necrotic, and autophagic dying cells often triggers an innate immune response through inflammasome activation with subsequent release of IL-1β and IL-18 from immune-competent cells. These immunogenic dying cells can expose or release danger-associated molecular pattern molecules (DAMPs), which are the inducers of inflammasome components' expression and/or assembly of the inflammasome to activate caspase-1 for the formation of active cytokines. In this chapter, we discuss which inflammasome-stimulant DAMPs have been recognized so far, and how immunogenic apoptotic, necrotic, and particularly autophagic dying cells may provoke inflammasome induction and/or activation.

INTRODUCTION

Under normal conditions, the immune system can recognize and discriminate foreign materials, pathogens (non-self) from healthy viable cells (self), and dying cells (altered-self) in order not to stimulate an inflammatory response to self and prevent possible damage to various tissues (Kersse *et al.*, 2011). It is also well known that not all non-self foreign elements (such as chimeric cells, fetus, commensal bacteria) trigger an immune response. The immune system does not ignore but instead interacts with and tolerates these harmless elements. The immunogenic response is induced due to antigenic difference, and not only because of the difference between self and non-self; proinflammatory and immunogenic cellular elements can be also recognized as harmful for the body via danger signals and specific antigenic properties (Kersse *et al.*, 2011). Macrophages and dendritic cells have the capacity to be activated by danger-associated molecular pattern molecules (DAMPs), and to trigger a proinflammatory response also mediating the development of a specific immune reaction depending on the appearance of antigens derived from pathogens, or endogenous sources such as tumor cells. These signals are recognized by membrane-bound or cytoplasmic pattern recognition receptors (PRRs), which include Toll-like receptors (TLRs), NOD-like receptors (NLRs), RIG-I-like receptors (RLRs), C-type lectin receptors (CLRs), and purinergic receptors (Kersse *et al.*, 2011). In this chapter, following a discussion on the apoptotic, necrotic, and autophagic cell death forms, and the mechanism as well as the influence of their clearance, we discuss further the NLRs and inflammasome activation by dying malignant cells in macrophages and dendritic cells.

DYING CELLS AND THEIR CLEARANCE BY IMMUNE-COMPETENT CELLS

In our body, billions of aged and damaged cells die daily and are replaced by new ones to maintain tissue homeostasis and immune regulation (Ravichandran, 2010). About 100 years ago, Ilya Mechnikov was awarded a Nobel Prize for his discovery of macrophage functions, which, as it turned out in later studies, are mainly responsible also for the removal of different types of dying cells and cellular debris generated during tissue remodeling and diseases such as cancers (Ravichandran, 2010). Under normal conditions basal clearance capacity is high and effective in tissues, but it can be defective, leading to autoimmune reactions due to imbalance between the number and types of dying cells, number of phagocytes, and low efficiency of the phagocytes' uptake mechanism. Upon clearance of dying cells and the cellular debris, macrophages release various immune mediators depending on how they are stimulated through phagocytosis receptors inducing production of either proinflammatory cytokines or anti-inflammatory molecules. The response of the macrophages strongly depends upon the type of cell death, which can be either immunogenic or non-immunogenic, according to their capacity to induce or inhibit the inflammatory pathways (Ravichandran, 2010). Here, we focus on the immunogenicity of necrotic, apoptotic, and autophagic dying cells mediated by inflammasome induction and activation in phagocytes as a result of danger molecules exposed on or released from these cells.

Necrosis has been considered to be an uncontrolled form of cell death without showing the features of apoptosis, leading to plasma membrane rupture and release of intracellular components (Galluzzi *et al.*, 2012). It can happen accidentally as a result of severe damage (such as hypoxia, hyperthermia, or detergent-induced cytolysis). Recently, it was observed that certain conditions can initiate *programmed necrosis (necroptosis)* with strictly regulated signaling events – for example, through TNF activation of its death receptor, PRR activation and excessive DNA damage via serine/threonine kinases receptor interacting proteins (RIP1–RIP3), and pronecrotic complex formation inducing the activity of these enzymes. Necrosis is generally observed with apoptosis as its back-up cell death mechanism; for instance, when caspases are inactive for some reasons (Galluzzi *et al.*, 2012).

Apoptosis is a programmed and controlled breakdown of the cell into apoptotic bodies during development and tissue homeostasis (Galluzzi *et al.*, 2012). There are two main evolutionarily conserved protein families that play crucial roles in apoptosis: caspases, and Bcl-2 family members. Caspases are cysteine proteases with a central role in the executive phase of apoptosis. Bcl-2 family members can be classified into two groups: pro-apoptotic proteins (apoptogens) and anti-apoptotic proteins. Bcl-2 proteins are the decision-makers on whether or not cell death occurs mainly through death receptors and via the mitochondrial pathway with a pivotal role in regulating caspase activation. Apoptosis may be initiated through distinct inducers and different biochemical routes, such as the extrinsic pathway (induced directly by the activation of death receptors and occurring through the mitochondrial-dependent or -independent pathway) and the intrinsic pathway (induced by loss of survival/trophic factors, toxins, radiation, hypoxia, oxidative stress, ischemia–reperfusion, and DNA damage) (Galluzzi *et al.*, 2012). Upon stimulation of the intrinsic apoptotic pathway, mitochondrial outer membrane permeabilization (MOMP) is promoted via the Bax/Bak complex and cytochrome c is released from the mitochondrial intermembrane space. Upon cytochrome c release to the cytosol, the apoptosome complex is formed by dATP (deoxyadenosine triphosphate) or adenosine triphosphate (ATP), apoptotic protease activation factor-1 (Apaf-1), and pro-caspase-9 oligomerization followed by effector caspase activation leading to death upon cleavage of cellular proteins (Galluzzi *et al.*, 2012).

Eukaryotic cells can adapt by autophagy to many external stress conditions, such as nutrient deprivation, ER stress, pathogens, and exposure to danger molecules. *Autophagy*, or self-eating, is a tightly regulated and conserved pathway in all eukaryotes, being a stress-induced catabolic and cell survival process (Galluzzi *et al.*, 2012). In macroautophagy (referred as autophagy throughout this chapter), double-membraned vesicles (autophagosomes) sequester targets such as organelles, proteins destined for degradation, or portions of the cytoplasm, and deliver them to the lysosome to be digested. Cells primarily use the basal level of autophagy to utilize cellular components through a catabolic pathway and recycle them to maintain nutrient and energy for survival. Excessive bulk self-destruction and selectively targeting key cell survival elements by autophagy can result in cell death. Autophagy-related cell death is difficult to define due to the mixed phenotypes of dying cells in a given cell population. Autophagy can trigger the upstream pathways of apoptosis, can occur parallel to apoptosis, can assist in eliminating the apoptotic corpses in the final stage of apoptosis, or can replace apoptosis when the apoptotic machinery is defective or caspases are inhibited (Galluzzi *et al.*, 2012). Some signaling pathways and central components of apoptosis and autophagy can regulate both pathways, which shows that there is cross-talk between these two processes. Autophagy can also trigger cell death independently of apoptosis in cases of excessive starvation-induced cell death in the involution of *Drosophila melanogaster* salivary glands – providing unique *in vivo* evidence that cell death can be induced by autophagy.

Cells start also to die also as a result of detachment from extracellular matrix (ECM) proteins. The fate of these cells is to die via **anoikis** (AN) (homelessness), which is generally an apoptotic process. Anoikis is a physiologically relevant cell death process, since correct adhesion of cells is essential to prevent reattachment of cells into improper locations, and dysplastic growth. When anchorage-dependent tumor cells which are apoptosis defective are detached, autophagy can lead first to survival and the cells can then eventually die by anoikis with an excess amount of autophagy (Petrovski *et al.*, 2007).

Circulating peripheral blood monocytes (PBMCs) develop from myeloid progenitor cells in bone marrow, and migrate into tissues in the steady state or in response to inflammation. They replenish the long-lived tissue **macrophages** of bone (osteoclasts), alveoli, the central nervous system (microglial cells), connective tissue (histiocytes), and the gastrointestinal tract, liver (Kupffer cells), spleen, and peritoneum, and are mainly responsible for the removal of dying cells. Additionally, macrophages that can be found in the tumor milieu are known as components of the stromal cells around tumor cells, or as tumor-associated macrophages. Upon their activation by living or dying cancer cells, they release soluble factors such as growth factors and inflammatory mediators promoting tumor cell growth and metastasis (Mantovani *et al.*, 2006). **Dendritic cells** (DCs) are professional phagocytes whose uptake of antigens is achieved by phagocytosis, macropinocytosis, and receptor-mediated endocytosis. Pathogens and inflammatory stimuli help mature the DCs and change their chemokine receptor expression pattern. Upon these changes, they can migrate from peripheral tissues to lymphoid organs to induce adaptive immune responses (Aymeric *et al.*, 2010).

The complex and dynamic interface between dying and engulfing cells shows that the efficient clearance of apoptotic dying cells is tightly regulated and connected to distinct signaling pathways (Ravichandran, 2010). **The engulfment process** comprises four major steps: (1) "find-me" signals, released from apoptotic cells to attract phagocytes to the target site in tissues; (2) "eat-me" signals, exposed on the apoptotic cells to promote recognition of the dying cells by the phagocytes; (3) ingestion of the engulfed cell corpses, which go through the phagosome formation and degradation processes; and (4) release of anti-inflammatory cytokines from phagocytes that have already recognized and engulfed the apoptotic cells (Ravichandran, 2010). "**Find-me**" signals include ATP/UTP, lysophosphatidylcholine (lysoPC), adhesion molecules, and chemokines which can affect the immunogenic or non-immunogenic immune response of the phagocytes to apoptotic cells. Apoptotic cells' exposure of phosphotidylserine (PS) is the most known "**eat-me**" signal molecule on the outer cellular leaflet. It has been also shown that changes in glycosylation pattern and sugar composition of the plasma membrane may occur in apoptotic cell death. Additionally, exposure of molecules such as calreticulin (CLR), annexin-1, pentraxin 3 (PTX3), DNA, or lysophosphatidylcholine (lyso-PC) has been observed during formation of the apoptotic cell death-associated molecular patterns (ACAMPs). Bridging molecules, such as thrombospondin 1 (TSP-1), C1q, collectins, (MFG-E8), mannose binding lectins (MBLs), and certain complements are essential for recognition of the apoptotic cells by the phagocytes. There are appropriate receptors on the phagocytes (such as scavenger receptors, PS receptors, thrombospondin (TSP) receptors, integrins, and complement receptors) that bind to molecules exposed on dying cells or the bridging molecules (Ravichandran, 2010).

It is not yet fully understood how necrotic and autophagic cells are cleared by macrophages. Recent studies have indicated that the internalization of necrotic cells is initiated via macrophage–necrotic cell interaction, and this internalization can be preceded by macropinocytic mechanisms. It was suggested that some macrophage receptors involved in the uptake mechanism of apoptotic cells can be also involved in clearance of necrotic cells (Marques-da-Silva et al., 2010). Besides, it has been shown that blocking the exposure of PS on autophagic dying MCF-7 can inhibit their phagocytosis by non-professional phagocytes (living MCF-7) but not professional phagocytes (macrophages) (Petrovski et al., 2007).

DYING CELLS AND THE INFLAMMATORY RESPONSE

The engulfment mechanism and the immune response differ according to the presented surface molecules on the outer leaflet of dying cells, and cytosolic or organelle-specific pathways in dying cells. For instance, necrotic cells are believed to be proinflammatory when they are recognized, internalized (macropinocytosis), and release DAMPs (Galluzzi et al., 2012). Due to the breakdown of the plasma membrane in necrotic cells, the cytoplasmic contents, including lysosomal enzymes, are released into the extracellular fluid, and therefore this type of cell death initiates an extensive inflammatory response (Gregory and Devitt, 2004). One of the reasons why necrotic cells lead to proinflammatory response is the extracellular appearance of DNA binding protein high-mobility group protein B1 (HMGB1), which leaks out of the ruptured necrotic cells; in its absence, late and leaky apoptotic cells are no longer proinflammatory. HMGB1 activates the Toll-like receptors (TLRs) 2 and 4 on macrophages similarly to lipopolysaccharide (LPS). Necrotic cells can release cellular contents other than HMGB1, such as proteases, inflammatory eicosanoids, granulocyte macrophage colony stimulating factor (GM-CSF), macrophage inflammatory protein 2 (MIP-2), interleukin (IL)-8, and tumor necrosis factor alpha (TNF-α), which may also initiate proinflammatory response as well as high levels of nucleotide release (Green et al., 2009). On the other hand, observations suggest that necrotic cell death is not always proinflammatory. It has been shown that when cell lysates or necrotic cells die by freeze-thawing or hypotonic shock and are then injected into mice subcutaneously, they do not evoke an immunogenic response (Chekeni *et al.*, 2010).

Apoptotic cells engulfed by either professional or non-professional phagocytes before the loss of their membrane integrity are thought to be immunologically silent and even suppress inflammation. Anti-inflammatory features of apoptotic cells can result from the exposure of cell surface apoptotic cell-associated molecular patterns (ACAMPs); phosphatidylserine (PS) was the first such molecule recognized. It was shown that, independent of phagocytosis, direct interaction of particular receptors with PS on apoptotic cells was enough to suppress the proinflammatory response (Ravichandran, 2010). In addition, LPS induced formation and secretion of proinflammatory cytokines, such as IL-1β, TNF-α, IL-6, IL-8, and IL-12, have been shown to be suppressed by apoptotic cells in phagocytes via inhibition of the NF-κB pathway and activation of some suppressor genes (Tassiulas *et al.*, 2007). There are also soluble factors (such as IL-10 and adenosine) released from human DCs after phagocytosis of apoptotic cells that act as an immune suppressor against proinflammatory cytokines, chemokines, and lipid mediators, depending on the cell death pathway and cell type (Majai *et al.*, 2010).

It would be an oversimplification to state that apoptotic cells are always anti-inflammatory, non-immunogenic, tolerogenic, and even immune-suppressive. During the past couple of years it has become clear that, under certain conditions, apoptotic cells can also be immunogenic due to their cell surface exposure or release of DAMPs; for instance, doxorubicin treatment of cancer cells can initiate immunogenic cell death *in vivo*, *ex vivo*, and *in vitro* (Krysko *et al.*, 2011). In contrast to other cytotoxic agents, including etoposide and mitomycin C, it was shown that anthracyclin-type antibiotics (DNA damaging agents, such as doxorubicin) can cause immunogenic apoptotic cell death in tumor cells most probably due to their high binding affinity to DNA (Casares *et al.*, 2005).

Upon uptake of apoptotic neutrophils by DCs, the cytokines at the site of inflammation, such as in vasculitis patients, may mature the DCs, leading to an autoimmune phenotype. Apoptotic cells can provide antigens which can be presented on DCs via MHC class I molecules to CD8+ T cells (cross-presentation) (Clayton *et al.*, 2003). Nuclear and cytoplasmic antigens obtained by an autophagic process can be presented to CD4+ T cells via MHC class II molecules on DCs (Crotzer and Blum, 2009). Additionally, it has been recently observed that specific subtypes of DCs respond to allogeneic apoptotic neutrophils during long-term interaction with proinflammatory cytokines and lead to T cell activation, which is also modulated by anti-inflammatory peroxisome proliferator-activated receptor gamma (PPARγ) (Majai *et al.*, 2010).

THE INFLAMMASOME AND ITS ACTIVATORS

NOD-like receptors (NLRs) are located in the cytoplasm of immune-competent cells, comprising 23 members in humans and almost 34 in mice (Kersse *et al.*, 2011). NLRs have three domains: the C-terminal domain contains a leucine-rich repeat (LRR), which is a sensing module; the N-terminal part has the caspase activation and recruitment (CARD) or pyrin (PYD) domain; and the intermediate region exhibits the nucleotide-binding and oligomerization (NACHT) domain, which mediates NLR oligomerization. NLRs are grouped into NLRA, NLRB, NLRC, NLRP, and NLRX (a subtype of NLRC) subfamilies, according to their N-terminal effector module (Kersse *et al.*, 2011).

NLRs such as NLRP1 (responds to anthrax lethal toxin), IPAF (responds to bacterial flagellin), NLRP3/NALP3 (responds to endogenous danger signals and pathogen-associated molecular patterns (PAMPs)), NLRP6 (responds to gut microbial ecology), RLRs (RIG-I-like receptors; respond to antiviral components), and the cytosolic hematopoietic interferon (IFN)-inducible nuclear protein 200aa (HIN200) and family member absent in melanoma 2 (AIM2) (responds to dsDNA) are capable of forming protein complexes called inflammasomes (Kersse *et al.*, 2011). Components of the NLRP1 and NLRC4 inflammasomes are constitutively expressed in cells, whereas NLRP3 transcription is usually triggered by bacterial components through the TLR4 pathway, a process that is also called "priming." Since inflammasome components are not fully expressed, priming of the phagocytes by ultra-pure LPS is often needed in cell culture experiments to respond to activators (Ayna *et al.*, 2012; Kersse *et al.*, 2011). Inflammasome activators such as ATP, amyloid-β (Aβ), asbestos, and nigericin trigger IL-1β and IL-18 secretion through initiating an assembly of a multiprotein inflammasome complex which promotes the proteolytic activation of an inactive form of caspase-1 (pro-caspase-1), which further cleaves a zymogen form of these cytokines. In addition, inflammasome activation may lead to caspase-1-dependent cell death (pyroptosis), transcription of certain cytokines and chemokines via the mitogen-activated protein kinase (MAPK) and NF-κB pathways, autophagy, and type 1 INF signaling. NALP-3 inflammasome complexes can be formed in the cytosol of granulocytes, monocytes, macrophages, DCs, astrocytes, T and B cells, epithelial cells, and osteoblasts (Kersse *et al.*, 2011).

It is widely accepted that NALP-3 activation requires generation/activation of signaling pathways and secondary messengers. ***P$_2$X$_7$ receptor activation by extracellular ATP*** is one of the most known danger signals among the DAMPs, and leads to NALP3 inflammasome activation. ATP released from immunogenic dying tumor cells acts on P$_2$X$_7$ purinergic receptors of dendritic cells, which can lead to inflammasome activation, K$^+$ efflux from the cytosol, and IL-1β secretion, which can prime INF-γ-producing T cells (Aymeric *et al.*, 2010). Recently, it has been observed that overexpression of an ATP degrading enzyme on the cell surface prevents the immunogenicity of cell death, thus making cancers resistant against chemotherapeutic agents such as anthracyclines or oxaliplatin. On the other hand, it has been observed that higher amounts of extracellular ATP (1 mM) can enhance the immune-suppressive effect of regulatory T cells (Tregs), can stimulate the proliferation and migration of tumor cells via activation of their purinergic receptors, and may lead to CD4+ T cell apoptosis (Michaud *et al.*, 2012). It was also indicated that certain types of necrotic cells can release ATP and activate the NALP3 inflammasome in engulfing macrophages that can further generate an inflammatory microenvironment for recruiting blood neutrophils to the site of sterile inflammation (Trabanelli *et al.*, 2012). ATP is also regarded as a critical "find-me" signal released from apoptotic cells to promote P$_2$Y purinoreceptor 2 (P2RY2)-dependent phagocyte recruitment and efficient phagocytosis of dying cells (McDonald, 2010). However, apoptotic cells, which are generally silent and even immune-suppressive, are not inducers of the inflammasome. This may be explained by the presence of ecto-ATPases expressed on the plasma membrane with externally oriented active sites for ATP (Ravichandran, 2010).

Pannexin-1 channels show homology to gap junction-forming invertebrate innexins. Recently, it has been shown that pannexin-1 channels in the brain may conduct small molecules (up to ~1 kDa) such as ions, ATP, inositol triphosphate, and amino acids, and can mediate ATP release from astrocytes as well as arachidonic acid and its metabolites from red blood cells (Qu *et al.*, 2011). Furthermore, pannexin-1 was identified as a plasma membrane channel mediating the regulated release of ATP and uridine triphosphate (UTP) (both are "find-me" signals for phagocytes) from apoptotic cells as a consequence of its caspase-3-dependent activation (Qu *et al.*, 2011). Using short hairpin (sh)RNA to silence pannexin-1 channels in neurons and astrocytes, it was demonstrated that these channels are needed for inflammasome activation (Chekeni *et al.*, 2010).

Reactive oxygen species such as singlet oxygen, hydroxyl radicals, superoxide, and hydrogen peroxide are highly reactive molecules containing unpaired electrons. They are continuously produced as byproducts of the mitochondrial respiratory chain in healthy cells at a tolerable level. ROS can damage cell structures due to their capability to oxidize lipids, proteins, and DNA. It was observed that NALP3 activators such as ATP, asbestos, and silica can trigger excess ROS production with K^+ efflux. ATP treatment of primed macrophages can lead to ROS production, which stimulates the phosphatidylinositide 3-kinases (PI3K) pathway, subsequently activating Akt and extracellular signal regulated kinase 1/2 (ERK1/2) (Tschopp and Schroder, 2010). These *endo-lysosomal proteases* such as *cathepsins* play a key role in immune responses upon exposure to foreign antigens. It has been shown that amyloid-beta (Aβ) can trigger the formation and activation of NALP3 inflammasome in macrophages, in a lysosomal damage-dependent manner (Halle *et al.*, 2008). In this model, these crystalline molecules can lead to lysosomal rupture due to their size, and upon being phagocytosed and released, the *cathepsin B* enzyme can lead to NALP3 inflammasome activation through a yet unknown mechanism. Aβ could not induce the NALP3 inflammasomes in cathepsin B-deficient macrophages (Halle *et al.*, 2008).

INFLAMMASOME-ACTIVATING DAMPS RELEASED FROM NECROTIC AND APOPTOTIC CELLS

How inflammasomes sense a particular inducer and initiate the secretion of IL-1β from macrophages and DCs has not been clarified in detail. Direct interaction between NALP3 and its activators has been shown only in a limited number of cases. Bacterial muramyl dipeptide (MDP) and the bacterial cell wall component peptidoglycans interact directly with the LRR part of NALP1 and NALP3, respectively (Kersse *et al.*, 2011). It is believed that pore-forming toxins such as maitotoxin and nigericin directly decrease cellular K^+ by perforating the plasma membrane and mediating an exchange of other cations (H^+, Na^+, and Ca^{2+}), which can induce inflammasome activation (Mariathasan *et al.*, 2006). However, NALP3 inflammasome activation pathways have not been defined for most of the PAMPs and DAMPs, and it seems improbable that the different activators are specifically sensed by the inflammasome.

A **"danger theory"** proposed by Matzinger and colleagues states that the immune system can discriminate not only self from non-self, but also DAMPs from innocuous cellular and molecular disturbances in the body (Matzinger, 1994). DAMPs can be secreted, released, and/or exposed on the outer leaflet of the plasma membrane, and can provide several kinds of signals: "find-me" (chemotactic), "eat-me" (phagocytic), and "activation" (immune stimulatory) factors. Physiological cell death, like regular cell turnover in tissues, is non-immunogenic, even tolerogenic, and hence does not provoke autoimmunity and adverse inflammatory reactions (Ravichandran, 2010). On the other hand, cell death in tumor tissues may lead to immune responses as the result of early cell surface exposure of calreticulin (CLR) and/or heat shock proteins (such as Hsp70, Hsp90), secretion of ATP, and late release of HMGB1 (Green *et al.*, 2009). These dangerous molecules can be recognized by macrophages and DCs via particular receptors, such as P_2X_7 for ATP, or TLR4 for HMGB1, and CD91, C1q, SR-A, or SREC1 for calreticulin (Tesniere *et al.*, 2008). The role of *secreted ATP* in inflammasome activation is discussed above.

Heat shock proteins (Hsps) are involved in protein folding and unfolding, intracellular trafficking of proteins, and regulation of proteins denatured by heat or other stresses, such as toxins, starvation, hypoxia, infection, or inflammation (Ma *et al.*, 2011). They play a role in protein–protein interactions, prevention of protein aggregation, and antigen binding and presentation. *Calreticulin* is a member of the Hsp family that usually localizes in the ER, where it assures proper conformation of the proteins, but it can also reside on the outer surface of the cells, in the cytosol and in the ECM, where it has important biological functions (Ma *et al.*, 2011). Treatment of cancer cells by anthracyclins and oxaliplatin causes activation of the CLR exposure pathway: pre-apoptotic ER stress causes phosphorylation of eIF2α, caspase 8-mediated proteolysis of ER proteins, and activation of the pro-apoptotic proteins Bax and Bak, which further leads to the transport of CLR from ER to Golgi, exocytosis of CLR-containing vesicles, and, finally, CLR translocation onto the plasma membrane. When colon cancer and fibrosarcoma cells are treated with anthracyclins or ionizing irradiation, they die and become immunogenic due to the exposure of CLR translocated from the ER to the cell surface (Ma *et al.*, 2011). Phagocytosis by DCs could be impaired and the immunogenicity in mice abolished when CLR exposure was prevented by blocking or knocking down CLR on dying cancer cells. In immunogenic dying cells, selective CLR exposure happens relatively earlier than PS exposure, and when cell morphology still looks normal. According to these findings, immunogenicity occurs in the earlier stages of cell death. It was also observed that several Hsps, such as Hsp90, Hsp70, Hsp74, and Hsc70, are secreted from necrotic dying cells, thereby suggesting that, during irreversible and slow release, Hsps can be a danger signal and thus candidates for "dying messages." Hsps including CLR can induce immunogenicity of dying tumor cells due to their interaction with antigen-presenting cell (APC) surface receptors, and facilitate cross-presentation of tumor antigens. Hsps can also promote DC maturation and activate natural killer cells (NK) cells as well as act as immunoadjuvants. *HMGB1* is a non-histone protein that has two functions: playing a role in transcriptional regulation in the nucleus, and serving as a cytokine outside the cell (e.g., a late mediator upon LPS treatment) (Green *et al.*, 2009). HMGB1 can be released from cells with sustained autophagy, late apoptosis, and necrosis (Ma *et al.*, 2011). Necrotic cells release HMGB1, whereas apoptotic cells keep HMGB1 in the nucleus during the apoptotic process. Later, it was also shown that apoptotic cells can release HMGB1 according to cell type (Green *et al.*, 2009). HMGB1 can activate the inflammatory response by acting as a chemotactic and/or activating factor for macrophages, neutrophils, and DCs (Ma *et al.*, 2011). Here, too, it is still not clear whether or not it causes inflammasome activation.

DAMPS FROM AUTOPHAGIC DYING CELLS CAN ACTIVATE THE INFLAMMASOMES

It is now broadly accepted that killing cancer cells by chemotherapy alone does not eradicate the tumor; the patient's immune response should also be stimulated. It has been reported that autophagy is not needed for chemotherapy-induced cell death, but is required for its immunogenicity (Michaud *et al.*, 2011). In response to chemotherapy, only autophagy-competent cancers could bring DCs and T lymphocytes into the tumor tissue. Autophagy was needed for the release of *ATP* from dying tumor cells, and, in autophagy-deficient tumors, increasing extracellular ATP resulted in an efficient immune response, supporting the conclusion that autophagy-deficient cancer cells may avoid immune surveillance because they cannot release ATP upon chemotherapeutic treatment (Michaud *et al.*, 2011). After anthracyclin treatment, protease activity is inhibited due to binding of anthracyclins to proteasomes; this proteasome inhibition can activate autophagy, which may lead to activation of caspase-8 in an autophagy-dependent manner (Zhu *et al.*, 2010) and immunogenic cell death with ATP release. There are several other cancer therapy conditions that may lead to similar cell death conditions. High doses of doxorubicin can induce both autophagy and poly (ADP-ribose) polymerase (PARP-1) activity, and it was concluded that autophagy plays a cytoprotective role against DNA damage via PARP-1 activation. DNA damage induced by the anticancer reagents could induce p53-dependent genes, which could also lead to autophagy induction (Munoz-Gomez *et al.*, 2009).

Autophagy can be induced in cancer cells not only by chemotherapeutic agents but also by withdrawal or blocking of survival factors, which leads to cell death. The question has been raised as to whether such cells can be immunogenic or not. We have recently demonstrated that autophagic dying MCF-7 tumor cells (treated by anti-estrogen) and Ba/F3 B cell lymphoma cells (after removal of IL-3) can initiate a proinflammatory cytokine response via NALP-3 inflammasome activation and IL-1β release in human and mouse macrophages, respectively (Petrovski *et al.*, 2011; Ayna *et al.*, 2012). Unlike apoptotic and anoikic-autophagic cells, autophagic dying cells can trigger proinflammatory cytokine release, such as Il-6 and TNF-α, as a result of the paracrine or autocrine action of the secreted IL-1β. There is limited information regarding candidate danger molecules derived from autophagic dying cells which may lead to inflammasome activation in macrophages and DCs. According to our recent data, ATP is the crucial DAMP trigger in such cases (Figure 14.1); during co-incubation of peritoneal macrophages and autophagic dying cells, the ATP released from the dying cells through pannexin-1 channels activates the P_2X_7 receptor and K^+ efflux pathway, resulting in NALP3 inflammasome formation and IL-1β secretion (Ayna *et al.*, 2012). Different PAMPs and DAMPs have been shown to lead to ATP release from macrophages, followed by an autocrine stimulation of the purinergic receptors. We also showed that human monocyte-derived macrophages (HMDMs) release ATP during their co-incubation with autophagic dying MCF-7 tumor cells, leading to subsequent inflammasome activation (Petrovski *et al.*, 2011).

We have also explored the possible contribution of the *cathepsin B* enzyme activity to inflammasome activation in mouse macrophages engulfing autophagic dying Ba/F3 cells. In our study, the incubation of macrophages with cathepsin B inhibitor before and during phagocytosis of autophagic dying Ba/F3 cells resulted in inhibition of inflammasome activation which was induced by exogenous ATP released from the dying cells and upon phagocytosis (unpublished data). Autophagic death may also produce activator molecules for the

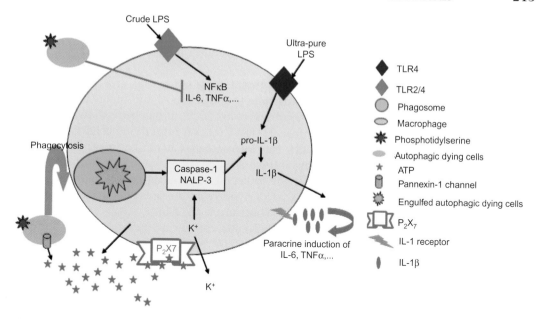

FIGURE 14.1 **Proposed model of inflammasome activation with autophagic dying cells.** Dying cells that carry autophagic features lead to NALP3 inflammasome activation in macrophages engulfing the dying cells. Upon phagocytosis, P_2X_7 purinergic receptor activation occurs by exogenous ATP released either from macrophages or autophagic dying cells. K^+ efflux from the cytosol leads to NALP3 inflammasome activation, and subsequent IL-1β maturation and secretion. In macrophages, priming with ultra-pure LPS is sometimes needed in order to achieve initial levels of inflammasome components including pro-IL-1β in the cells. Besides, it is also shown that the same autophagic dying cells can behave as apoptotic cells and can inhibit the TLR-dependent proinflammatory cytokine release through the classical NF-κB pathway (Ayna *et al.*, 2012; Petrovski *et al.*, 2011).

inflammasome system in the lysosomal compartment where the autophagic dying cells are eventually degraded after their phagocytosis. However, we did not observe loss of autophagic dying cells' induced inflammasome activation in cathepsin B-deficient peritoneal macrophages (unpublished data). It cannot be excluded, however, that cathepsin B, a known inflammasome activator, is released from the lysosomal compartment containing autophagic dead cell corpses and contributes to the activation process. A possible explanation could be the appearance of compensatory mechanisms in mice with deleted cathepsin B.

Regarding *calreticulin exposure* as a well-documented inducer of immunogenic cell death and autophagy or autophagic death induced by removal of survival mechanisms, we found that immunogenicity does not necessarily depend on CLR exposure on autophagic dying MCF-7 cells which have the capacity to induce inflammasome activation (Petrovski *et al.*, 2011). It is possible that anticancer chemotherapy-based treatments have the capacity to induce an immunogenic cell death which is different than the anti-estrogen treatment and estrogen depletion, as well as cell-type specific and independent of CLR exposure on the cellular membrane.

In an *in situ* auto-vaccination protocol, injection of autologous DCs was combined with localized tumor hyperthermia in order to increase expression of the Hsps on dying tumor cells (Mukhopadhaya *et al.*, 2007). The relationship between the immune system response and the dying cells which undergo thermal stress-induced autophagy has not yet been investigated. It has been shown that in traumatic brain injury (TBI), inflammasome activation occurs as an early innate inflammatory response to injury (Tomura *et al.*, 2012). Thus, it may be presumed that hyperthermia can lead to inflammasome activation and could possibly be utilized in future tumor therapy.

Epithelial and glioblastoma tumor cell treatment with epidermal growth factor receptor targeted diphtheria toxin (DT-EGF) leads to both induction of autophagy and cell death without rupture of the cell membrane (Thorburn *et al.*, 2009). It has been shown that when autophagy is induced by DT-EGF, it controls *HMGB1* release from dying cells. On the other hand, HMGB1 release from macrophages can be regulated by inflammasome activation upon exposure to known inflammasome inducers (such as ATP, monosodium urate, aluminium). As HMGB1 is known as a danger molecule for the induction of inflammatory response, it could be one of the DAMPs that derived from the autophagic dying cells and which may lead to inflammasome activation (Thorburn *et al.*, 2009).

Ceramide levels in autophagic dying MCF-7 cells can be an inflammasome inducing danger signal. In this estrogen-dependent cancer cell line, cell death induction through autophagy with estrogen-depleted charcoal-stripped-fetal calf serum and anti-estrogen tamoxifen treatment leads to NALP3 inflammasome activation upon engulfment by macrophages (Vandanmagsar *et al.*, 2011). It has been shown that tamoxifen increases the ceramide levels in cells, and eliminates the inhibitory effect of the class I PI3K pathway and upregulates Bcl-2-interacting protein-1 (Beclin 1) (Scarlatti *et al.*, 2004), which could be a possible method for how autophagic dying MCF-7 cells trigger inflammasome activation (Petrovski *et al.*, 2007, 2011). Danger molecules released from or exposed on dying apoptotic, necrotic, and autophagic cells that have capacity to induce inflammasome activation in DCs and macrophages are shown in Figure 14.2.

INTERFERON REGULATORY FACTORS (IRFS) PLAY A ROLE IN ACTIVATION OF THE INFLAMMATORY RESPONSE

Members of the IRF family can also activate IL-1β. Three key transcriptional activators, PU.1, C/EBP, and IRF4, are capable of rapidly inducing IL-1β during stimulation of monocytes (Zhang *et al.*, 2008). Autophagic dying MCF-7 cells upregulate expression of IRF4, and this upregulation is strongly present during their engulfment by non-professional (living MCF-7) and professional (macrophage) phagocytes (Figure 14.3). IRF8, another member of the IRF family, which is a key factor required for macrophage development, makes these cells responsive to IFN-γ-LPS signaling, thereby triggering expression of genes important for innate immunity. IRF8 interacts with partner proteins PU.1 and IRF1, allowing it to bind to the IFN-stimulated response element (Laricchia-Robbio *et al.*, 2005). The autophagic dying MCF-7 and not the anoikic-autophagic ones could induce the expression of IRF1 and IRF8 in macrophages engulfing them. On the contrary, the engulfment of anoikic-autophagic MCF-7 cells induced no change in the IRF1 and decreased the expression of IRF8 in the macrophages. Living MCF-7 cells engulfing autophagic or anoikic-autophagic MCF-7 cells seem not to be armed with the same IRF machinery that professional phagocytes have. Clearly, death through autophagy can differentially activate IL-1β activating transcription activators such as IRFs 1, 4 and 8 in macrophages (Figure 14.3).

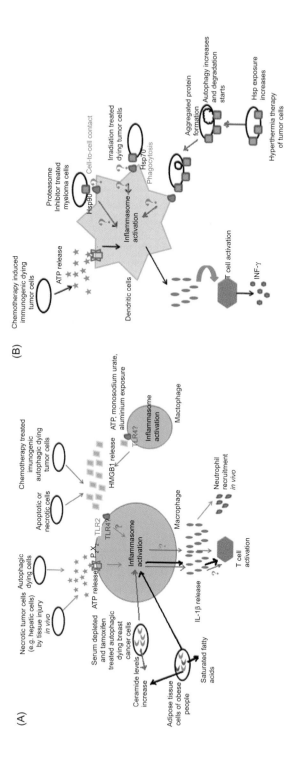

FIGURE 14.2 **Danger molecules from dying cells can induce inflammatory response and inflammasome activation.** Danger molecules released from or exposed on dying cells can have the capacity to induce inflammasome activation in macrophages (A) or dendritic cells (B). (A) Different types of cells can release (e.g., ATP, HMGB1) or contain (e.g., ceramide or saturated fatty acids) molecules, which can lead to immune response in macrophages. Colors of arrows represent results of different studies. (B) The different types of dying cells can release (e.g., ATP) or expose (e.g., Hsps) molecules in order to induce the inflammatory response in dendritic cells. It is known that ATP release from immunogenic dying tumor cells can lead to inflammasome activation. Besides, exposure of Hsps on dying cells can lead to immune response through T cell activation, thus playing a role in inflammasome activation as well. Question marks represent that a given pathway is not yet shown or explained in the literature. References for (A): black arrows, Vandanmagsar et al. (2011); green arrows, Petrovski et al. (2011); red arrows, Ayna et al. (2012), Iyer et al. (2009); blue arrows, Bell et al. (2006), Lu et al. (2012). References for (B): black arrows, Aymeric et al. (2010), Ghiringhelli et al. (2009); red arrows, Chan et al. (2007), Spisek et al. (2007); green arrows, Tomura et al. (2012).

Category	Gene description	Phagocytosing macrophages			Phagocyting MCF-7			Dying MCF-7	
		Control	+AU	+AN-AU	Control	+AU	+AN-AU	AU	AN-AU
IRFs	IRF1		++						
	IRF4		++	+		+++		+++	
	IRF5								
	IRF7								
	IRF8		+	−				−	−

Rel. expression level compared to ISS RNA:

$10^{-8} 10^{-7} 10^{-6} 10^{-5} 10^{-4} 10^{-3} 10^{-2}$ $10^{-8} 10^{-7} 10^{-6} 10^{-5} 10^{-4} 10^{-3} 10^{-2}$

FIGURE 14.3   **Gene expression levels in macrophages and MF-7 cells and their changes during phagocytosis.** The basal expression levels were determined in three independent biological samples, and each was analyzed in two parallel runs in which each gene had two technical replicates. Based on the average of the obtained result (the variation coefficient was less than 20% in each case), the relative expression of a particular gene in macrophages and MCF-7 cells is indicated. The increments of the horizontal bars represent one order of magnitude higher range of relative expression (related to 18S RNA), and the size of the bar at each gene indicates into which range the actual expression data (average of three repeated experiments) falls. In case of analyzing gene expression changes during phagocytosis, change of mRNA level was considered significant when it repeatedly (at least in two biological samples, both analyzed in two parallel runs each with two replicates per gene) exceeded 2.5 times the average expression level of the controls, either increasing or decreasing (+ or −). The table also indicates where the change of expression was more than 5 times (++ or −) and 10 times (+++ or − as compared to controls. The nomenclature of the genes studied is in compliance with the HUGO classification; AU, autophagic dying MCF-7 cells; AN-AU, anoikic-autophagic dying cells; IRFs, interferon regulatory factors.

IN VIVO EVIDENCE OF INFLAMMATORY RESPONSE TO AUTOPHAGIC DYING CELLS

A wide range of chemotherapeutic agents can induce ATP release, which is the endogenous inducer of inflammasome activation, from tumor cells. Mitoxantrone (MTX) anticancer chemotherapy when injected into the intratumoral area in mice and autophagy competent cancers can recruit DCs and T lymphocytes into the tumor area (Michaud et al., 2011), very likely as a result of ATP-induced inflammasome activation and IL-1β secretion. Additionally, autophagy-deficient tumor cells failed to induce T and dendritic cell-dependent immune response in vivo due to inhibition of ATP release from dying cells. When the tumor is autophagy-deficient and is itself treated chemically by inhibitors of ecto-ATPases, increasing intracellular ATP concentrations re-establishes the antitumoral T and dendritic cell-dependent immune response in vivo through the purinergic receptor-dependent way (Michaud et al., 2011). Pre-mortem autophagy can establish the immunogenicity of chemotherapy-induced cancer cell death by determining the level of extracellular ATP in balance with the activity of ecto-ATPases in tumor tissues (Martins et al., 2012). We have observed that doxorubicin-treated apoptotic cells can recruit high amounts of neutrophils to the peritoneal cavity of mice, which indicates the immunogenicity of the cells treated by this member drug of the anthracyclin type of anticancer agents (Ayna et al., 2012).

However, we have also demonstrated that not only the anthracyclin-treated dying cells but also the growth factor-depleted, ATP-releasing autophagic dying cells can be highly inflammatory, capable of recruiting high numbers of neutrophils in mice. This is in line with the fact that IL-1β, also known as lymphocyte-activating factor, can stimulate T cell proliferation and mediate repair responses such as angiogenesis and neutrophil influx to remove the cellular debris. Indeed, the released extracellular ATP from necrotic hepatic cells has been shown to further recruit blood neutrophils to the site of inflammation (McDonald, 2010). Another study recently demonstrated that doxorubicin-induced immunogenic apoptotic cells can be recognized, and responded to the TLR-2/TLR-9-Myeloid differentiation primary response gene (88) (Myd88) signaling pathway, which leads to acute neutrophil recruitment to the site of inflammation and release of IL-6 and monocyte chemotactic protein-1 (MCP-1) (Krysko et al., 2011).

CONCLUDING REMARKS

A general conclusion can be drawn from the many related studies that immunogenic cell death induction can be the most efficient way for cancer therapy, leading to conversion of the patient's own tumor cells to therapeutic vaccines. More and more evidence is emerging in support of the involvement of autophagy and inflammasome activation in this process. Immunogenic death of tumor cells may be evoked through various mechanisms, including induction of autophagy. Stimulation of immune-competent cells is mediated by several danger molecules released from the dying cells, and some of them, particularly ATP, lead to IL-1β release through inflammasome activation. IL-1β is a multifunctional and pivotal inflammatory cytokine of the innate immune system which is capable of initiating early and delayed elements of an effective antitumor immune response. Secreted IL-1β binds to IL-1 receptors in an autocrine and paracrine fashion (Petrovski et al., 2011), and triggers local effects (leukocyte infiltration and lymphocyte activation) as well as distant responses such as fever and acute phase protein induction (Kersse et al., 2011). Upon binding to the receptor, IL-1β leads to activation of the transcription factor NF-κB through different signaling molecules (Kersse et al., 2011). DNA-binding motifs for NF-κB are found in the promoters and enhancers of many genes (such as the proinflammatory IL-6, IL-8, etc.) that are known to be activated upon inflammation. Furthermore, it has been recently shown that the inflammasome activity can be regulated by autophagy via targeting and degrading inflammasomes in macrophages in order to limit their overactivation (Kersse et al., 2011). Therefore, different strategies to target autophagy via cancer-specific autophagy inducers should be developed to induce the immune response in order to fight cancers efficiently.

Acknowledgments

The authors have received research support from the Hungarian Scientific Research Fund (OTKA NK 105046, PD 101316), TÁMOP-4.2.2.A-11/1/KONV-2012-0023 "VÉD-ELEM" project implemented through the New Hungary Development Plan and co-financed by the European Social Fund, EU FP7 TRANSCOM IAPP 251506, TRANSPATH ITN 289964, and NKTH NTP Schizo08. We thank Dr Gábor Zahuczky for his help in the preparation of the gene expression results shown in Figure 14.3.

References

Aymeric, L., Apetoh, L., Ghiringhelli, F., et al., 2010. Tumor cell death and ATP release prime dendritic cells and efficient anticancer immunity. Cancer Res. 70 (3), 855–858.

Ayna, G., Krysko, D.V., Kaczmarek, A., et al., 2012. ATP release from dying autophagic cells and their phagocytosis are crucial for inflammasome activation in macrophages. PLoS ONE 7 (6-e40069), 1–14.

Bell, C.W., Jiang, W.W., Reich, C.F., et al., 2006. The extracellular release of HMGB1 during apoptotic cell death. Am. J. Physiol. Cell Physiol. 291 (6), C1318–C1325.

Casares, N., Pequignot, M.O., Tesniere, A., et al., 2005. Caspase-dependent immunogenicity of doxorubicin-induced tumor cell death. J. Exp. Med. 202 (12), 1691–1701.

Chan, T., Chen, Z., Hao, S., et al., 2007. Enhanced T-cell immunity induced by dendritic cells with phagocytosis of heat shock protein 70 gene-transfected tumor cells in early phase of apoptosis. Cancer Gene Ther. 14 (4), 409–420.

Chekeni, F.B., Elliott, M.R., Sandilos, J.K., et al., 2010. Pannexin 1 channels mediate "find-me" signal release and membrane permeability during apoptosis. Nature 467 (7317), 863–867.

Clayton, A.R., Prue, R.L., Harper, L., et al., 2003. Dendritic cell uptake of human apoptotic and necrotic neutrophils inhibits CD40, CD80, and CD86 expression and reduces allogeneic T cell responses – relevance to systemic vasculitis. Arthritis Rheum. 48 (8), 2362–2374.

Crotzer, V.L., Blum, J.S., 2009. Autophagy and its role in MHC-mediated antigen presentation. J. Immunol. 182 (6), 3335–3341.

Galluzzi, L., Vitale, I., Abrams, J.M., et al., 2012. Molecular definitions of cell death subroutines: recommendations of the nomenclature committee on cell death 2012. Cell Death Differ. 19 (1), 107–120.

Ghiringhelli, F., Apetoh, L., Tesniere, A., et al., 2009. Activation of the NLRP3 inflammasome in dendritic cells induces IL-1 beta-dependent adaptive immunity against tumors. Nat. Med. 15 (10), 1170–1178.

Green, D.R., Ferguson, T., Zitvogel, L., et al., 2009. Immunogenic and tolerogenic cell death. Nat. Rev. Immunol. 9 (5), 353–363.

Gregory, C.D., Devitt, A., 2004. The macrophage and the apoptotic cell: an innate immune interaction viewed simplistically? Immunology 113 (1), 1–14.

Halle, A., Hornung, V., Petzold, G.C., et al., 2008. The NALP3 inflammasome is involved in the innate immune response to amyloid-beta. Nat. Immunol. 9 (8), 857–865.

Iyer, S.S., Pulskens, W.P., Sadler, J.J., et al., 2009. Necrotic cells trigger a sterile inflammatory response through the Nlrp3 inflammasome. Proc. Natl Acad. Sci. USA 106 (48), 20388–20393.

Kersse, K., Bertrand, M.J., Lamkanfi, M., et al., 2011. NOD-like receptors and the innate immune system: coping with danger, damage and death. Cytokine Growth Factor Rev. 22 (5-6), 257–276.

Krysko, D.V., Kaczmarek, A., Krysko, O., et al., 2011. TLR-2 and TLR-9 are sensors of apoptosis in a mouse model of doxorubicin-induced acute inflammation. Cell Death Differ. 18 (8), 1316–1325.

Laricchia-Robbio, L., Tamura, T., Karpova, T., et al., 2005. Partner-regulated interaction of IFN regulatory factor 8 with chromatin visualized in live macrophages. Proc. Natl Acad. Sci. USA 102 (40), 14368–14373.

Lu, B., Nakamura, T., Inouye, K., et al., 2012. Novel role of PKR in inflammasome activation and HMGB1 release. Nature 488 (7413), 670–674.

Ma, Y., Conforti, R., Aymeric, L., et al., 2011. How to improve the immunogenicity of chemotherapy and radiotherapy. Cancer Metastasis Rev. 30 (1), 71–82.

Majai, G., Gogolak, P., Ambrus, C., et al., 2010. PPAR gamma modulated inflammatory response of human dendritic cell subsets to engulfed apoptotic neutrophils. J. Leukoc. Biol. 88 (5), 981–991.

Mantovani, A., Schioppa, T., Porta, C., et al., 2006. Role of tumor-associated macrophages in tumor progression and invasion. Cancer Metastasis Rev. 25 (3), 315–322.

Mariathasan, S., Weiss, D.S., Newton, K., et al., 2006. Cryopyrin activates the inflammasome in response to toxins and ATP. Nature 440 (7081), 228–232.

Marques-da-Silva, C., Burnstock, G., Ojcius, D.M., et al., 2010. Purinergic receptor agonists modulate phagocytosis and clearance of apoptotic cells in macrophages. Immunobiology 216 (1-2), 1–11.

Martins, I., Michaud, M., Sukkurwala, A.Q., et al., 2012. Premortem autophagy determines the immunogenicity of chemotherapy-induced cancer cell death. Autophagy 8 (3), 413–415.

Matzinger, P., 1994. Tolerance, danger, and extended family. Annu. Rev. Immunol. 12, 991–1045.

McDonald, B., 2010. Intravascular danger signals guide neutrophils to sites of sterile inflammation (2010). Science 331 (6024), 1517.

Michaud, M., Martins, I., Sukkurwala, A.Q., et al., 2011. Autophagy- dependent anticancer immune responses induced by chemotherapeutic agents in mice. Science 334 (6062), 1573–1577.

Michaud, M., Sukkurwala, A.Q., Martins, I., et al., 2012. Subversion of the chemotherapy-induced anticancer immune response by the ecto-ATPase CD39. Oncoimmunology 1 (3), 393–395.

Mukhopadhaya, A., Mendecki, J., Dong, X.Y., et al., 2007. Localized hyperthermia combined with intratumoral dendritic cells induces systemic antitumor immunity. Cancer Res. 67 (16), 7798–7806.

Munoz-Gomez, J.A., Rodriguez-Vargas, J.M., Quiles-Perez, R., et al., 2009. PARP-1 is involved in autophagy induced by DNA damage. Autophagy 5 (1), 61–74.

Petrovski, G., Zahuczky, G., Katona, K., et al., 2007. Clearance of dying autophagic cells of different origin by professional and non- professional phagocytes. Cell Death Differ. 14 (6), 1117–1128.

Petrovski, G., Ayna, G., Majai, G., et al., 2011. Phagocytosis of cells dying through autophagy induces inflammasome activation and IL-1 beta release in human macrophages. Autophagy 7 (3), 321–330.

Qu, Y., Misaghi, S., Newton, K., et al., 2011. Pannexin-1 is required for ATP release during apoptosis but not for inflammasome activation. J. Immunol. 186 (11), 6553–6561.

Ravichandran, K.S., 2010. Find-me and eat-me signals in apoptotic cell clearance: progress and conundrums. J. Exp. Med. 207 (9), 1807–1817.

Scarlatti, F., Bauvy, C., Ventruti, A., et al., 2004. Ceramide-mediated macroautophagy involves inhibition of protein kinase B and up-regulation of beclin 1. J. Biol. Chem. 279 (18), 18384–18391.

Spisek, R., Charalambous, A., Mazumder, A., et al., 2007. Bortezomib enhances dendritic cell (DC)-mediated induction of immunity to human myeloma via exposure of cell surface heat shock protein 90 on dying tumor cells: therapeutic implications. Blood 109 (11), 4839–4845.

Tassiulas, I., Park-Min, K.H., Hu, Y., et al., 2007. Apoptotic cells inhibit LPS-induced cytokine and chemokine production and IFN responses in macrophages. Hum. Immunol. 68 (3), 156–164.

Tesniere, A., Apetoh, L., Ghiringhelli, F., et al., 2008. Immunogenic cancer cell death: a key–lock paradigm. Curr. Opin. Immunol. 20 (5), 504–511.

Thorburn, J., Horita, H., Redzic, J., et al., 2009. Autophagy regulates selective HMGB1 release in tumor cells that are destined to die. Cell Death Differ. 16 (1), 175–183.

Tomura, S., de Rivero Vaccari, J.P., Keane, R.W., et al., 2012. Effects of therapeutic hypothermia on inflammasome signaling after traumatic brain injury. J. Cereb. Blood Flow Metab. 32 (10), 1939–1947.

Trabanelli, S., Ocadlikova, D., Gulinelli, S., et al., 2012. Extracellular ATP exerts opposite effects on activated and regulatory CD4+ T cells via purinergic P2 receptor activation. J. Immunol. 189 (3), 1303–1310.

Tschop, J., Schroder, K., 2010. NLRP3 inflammasome activation: the convergence of multiple signalling pathways on ROS production? Nat. Rev. Immunol. 10 (3), 210–215.

Vandanmagsar, B., Youm, Y.H., Ravussin, A., et al., 2011. The NLRP3 inflammasome instigates obesity-induced inflammation and insulin resistance. Nat. Med. 17 (2), 179–U214.

Zhang, Y., Saccani, S., Shin, H., et al., 2008. Dynamic protein associations define two phases of IL-1beta transcriptional activation. J. Immunol. 181 (1), 503–512.

Zhu, K., Dunner, K., McConkey, D.J., 2010. Proteasome inhibitors activate autophagy as a cytoprotective response in human prostate cancer cells. Oncogene 29 (3), 451–462.

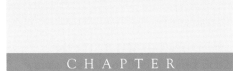

CHAPTER
15

Selenite-Mediated Cellular Stress, Apoptosis, and Autophagy in Colon Cancer Cells

Emil Rudolf

Abstract

Colorectal carcinoma (CRC) continues to be a major problem in developed countries, and successful preventive strategies concerning this malignancy are still missing. Sodium selenite has emerged as a potential chemopreventive agent due to a number of special effects which produce colon cancer cells, regardless of their status. Selenite has been able to decrease cell proliferation and induce cytotoxicity by several mechanisms. These include direct inhibition of several molecular targets, signaling pathways (p53-dependent, mTOR, p38, JNK), or subcellular compartments (mitochondria), as well as activation of apoptosis and autophagy. Our data combined with results of studies conducted by other research groups demonstrate a close connection between selenite-induced oxidative stress and apoptosis. In addition, the concurrent existence of autophagy and apoptosis in selenite-treated cells, their mutual relationship, and diverse regulatory patterns upon differing p53 status of cells suggest a multilevel regulation of both processes which warrants future studies.

M.A. Hayat (ed): Autophagy, Volume 1
DOI: http://dx.doi.org/10.1016/B978-0-12-405530-8.00015-7

© 2014 Elsevier Inc. All rights reserved.

INTRODUCTION

Colorectal carcinoma (CRC) continues to be among the leading causes of premature morbidity and mortality from cancers worldwide. Its development and progression are linked with the accumulation of acquired genetic as well as epigenetic changes that transform normal colonic epithelium first into aberrant crypt foci (ACF), which may later develop into a polypous or flat benign precursor lesion termed an adenoma. Over years, this adenoma can progress into an invasive adenocarcinoma which may penetrate the wall of colon and eventually disseminates locally as well as systemically.

The traditional model explaining a sequence of steps leading to the development of CRC assumed involvement of only a limited number of genetic alterations and genes in the context of one molecular pathway (Vogelstein *et al.*, 1988). Today, however, we know that at least three or even more different scenarios reflecting varying molecular events may drive polyp-cancer progression. In addition, it is now appreciated that thousands of genetic and possibly epigenetic alterations are found in the average colon cancer genome, which give rise to a considerable molecular heterogeneity. On the other hand, in the light of recent evidence it appears clear that only a subset of these alterations in a limited number of genes is important for formation of cancer (Sjoblom *et al.*, 2006).

One of the initial events, occurring as early as in ACF, is mutations in the tumor suppressing adenomatous polyposis coli (*APC*) gene. In migrating progenitor cells within the crypt of Lieberkühn, the product of this gene is, along with glycogen synthase kinase 3-beta (GSK-3β), responsible for sequestration of free intracellular β-catenine, which leads to inactivation of the Wingless/Wnt pathway. Mutations in *APC* or in gene coding for β-catenine arrest non-differentiated cells in the wall of the crypt, where they cannot be removed by apoptosis and thus have an increased chance to accumulate other changes. Concomitantly, deregulation of the epidermal growth factor (EGF) pathway takes place. Activation of the receptor for epidermal growth factor (EGFR) leads, via its downstream effector KRAS and BRAF, to stimulation of the MAPK signaling pathway, which further potentiates proliferation and survival of cells. Mutations in *KRAS* or *BRAF* occur in approximately 55–60% of colorectal cancers, and affect internal GTP-ase activity of the protein with subsequent constitutive signaling (Downward, 2003).

Mutations in the type II TGF-β receptor (*TGFBR2*) occur in approximately 30% of CRCs, and lead to inactivation of this receptor, depending upon the molecular subtype of the developing cancer cell. In addition, various genetic as well as epigenetic changes may affect other TGF-β signaling pathway members, such as *SMAD2*, *SMAD4*, *RUNX3*, and *TSP1* (Vogelstein *et al.*, 1988).

Defects in the phosphatidylinositol-3-kinase (PI3K) signaling pathway are found in up to 40% of CRC cases, and it is believed that they enable transition of the adenoma stage to carcinoma. The most commonly affected proteins are p110α (catalytical subunit of PI3K) and PTEN – a tumor suppressor protein negatively regulating PI3K signaling (Samuels and Velculescu, 2004).

Protein p53 is a transcription factor involved in many biological activities, including stress response, differentiation, migration, angiogenesis, etc. In response to various forms of stress, p53 specifically binds to the DNA and induces the expression of several genes regulating DNA repair, cell cycle arrest, senescence, or apoptosis (Kroemer *et al.*, 1995). In addition, protein p53 acts directly, and in the cytoplasm it may activate apoptosis or suppress autophagy in a transcription-independent way. Due to all these functions, p53 represents an important tumor suppressor protein. Mutations in the *p53* gene are present in more than half of all malignancies, and in the rest we find defects in the p53-dependent signaling pathway. Upon loss of function in p53, the malignant cell may escape apoptotic death and enhance its aggressive phenotype, including the development of multiple chemo- or radio-resistance. In CRC, the *p53* gene accumulates mutations at later developmental stages (4–6% of adenomas, 50% of invasive adenomas, and 50–75% of carcinomas).

To accumulate mutations, malignant cells have to be unstable. The majority of CRCs are positive for whole chromosome or chromosome arm changes, called chromosomal instability (CIN) (Pino and Chung, 2010). These changes can result in the overexpression of oncogenes, suppressed expression of tumor suppressor genes, or altered epigenetic mechanisms (micro-RNAs) which can contribute to tumor progression (Pino and Chung, 2010). Another form of instability is microsatellite instability (MSI), occurring in 10–15% of CRCs. The cause of MSI is defective DNA mismatch repair machinery leading to an accumulation of mutations (Boland and Goel, 2010). Cells of MSI tumors are diploid, unlike those of CIN tumors.

Various lines of evidence demonstrate that dietary habits and, in particular, food composition may play a role in the malignant conversion of cells in the alimentary tract. On the other hand, there are many food-borne chemicals that play protective roles and help in maintenance of the optimal functional state of these cells. Positive effects of these chemicals–nutrients include stimulation of antioxidant defense mechanisms or detoxification enzyme cascades in normal colonic cells, or active inhibition of proliferation and or autophagy, and stimulation of cell death in malignant cells. One of these chemicals is selenium, whose role in the pathogenesis of CRC has been investigated in a number of studies, often with ambiguous outcomes. This suggests the need for further studies aimed at elucidation of the molecular mechanisms of selenium action, and thorough characterization of the scope of selenium-dependent biological responses.

SELENIUM

Selenium Chemistry and Metabolism

Selenium is a chemical element existing in nature in both inorganic and organic forms at all major physical states – i.e., solid, liquid, and gas. Selenium enters the food chain via plants. These absorb mostly inorganic selenium (selenate or selenite) from the soil and convert it into selenomethionine, selenocysteine, and selenomethyl-selenocysteine, which are incorporated into their proteins (Combs, 2001). In dietary supplements freely available in the market, selenium exists in the form of inorganic selenite and selenate, or as selenium-enriched brewery yeasts containing mostly selenomethionine plus other selenium formulas.

Selenium enters human metabolic pathways in both chemical forms. Inorganic selenium (selenite and selenate) is reduced by glutathione into selenodiglutathione (GS-Se-SG), which is subsequently reduced to hydrogen selenide via glutathione reductase. Hydrogen selenide is toxic to cells, and therefore they use it as a precursor for the synthesis of selenoproteins (via phosphorylation and conversion into selenophosphate), or subject it to stepwise methylation to generate mono-, di-, or tri-methylated forms of selenium, which may interfere with various cellular functions (Ip *et al.*, 1991). Selenocysteine is cleaved by β-lyase into selenol and alanine. Selenomethionine undergoes a specific reaction which transforms it into selenocysteine; alternatively, it may release methylselenol by means of methionine-γ-lyase. In addition, selenomethionine may also be non-specifically incorporated into proteins instead of methionine. Selenomethyl-selenocysteine and other methylated forms of selenium are directly converted into methylselenol, which may be again demethylated into hydrogen selenide. Excretion of selenium proceeds via its highly methylated forms (Brigelius-Flohe, 2008).

The physiological role and importance of selenium are determined by its presence in selenium-containing proteins or selenoproteins, where it exists in the form of selenocysteine. Due to the mechanism of its synthesis and incorporation into protein structures, selenocysteine represents the 21st amino acid of the genetic code (Hatfield *et al.*, 2006). The cell does not contain any free selenocysteine, to prevent random incorporation of this very reactive amino acid instead of cysteine (Lu and Holmgren, 2009). So far, 25 selenoproteins expressed in humans have been described; however, the functions of some of these remain obscure. Some selenoproteins show cell- and tissue-specific expression while others seem to be expressed ubiquitously and to take part in key cellular processes, including synthesis of nucleotides, removal of harmful peroxides, reduction of oxidized proteins and membranes, regulation of redox signaling, and metabolism of thyroid gland hormones.

Selenium and Malignant Diseases

As early as the 1960s and 1970s, some reports correlated low selenium content in the diet with increased occurrence of malignant diseases (Shamberger and Frost, 1969). The first intervention studies reporting a decreased incidence of malignant diseases that was associated with selenium supplementation were carried out in China between 1985 and 1991 (Blot *et al.*, 1993). Their results, however, should be interpreted with caution, as selenium was supplemented along with other chemicals, and the target study population was undernourished.

An important milestone study on the anticarcinogenic effect of selenium was carried out in the 1980s and 1990s in the USA under the name of the Nutritional Prevention of Cancer Trial. It was a double-blind randomized study focusing on the prevention of recurrent skin tumors in participants dosed with 200 μg selenium/day in the form of selenium-enriched yeasts. The study did not demonstrate any positive effect of selenium supplementation on recurrent skin tumors, but yielded data on a significant reduction in the occurrence of prostate, lung, and colon cancers (Duffield-Lillico *et al.*, 2002). In 2001, one of the largest selenium intervention studies was launched in the USA. This randomized, prospective, double-blind study was named SELECT (the Selenium and Vitamin E Cancer Prevention Trial), and involved 36,000 participants. It was aimed primarily at prevention of prostate cancer, with secondary outcomes focusing on the frequency of lung and colon cancers, as well as other diseases. Participants in this study received L-selenomethionine at 200 μg/day alone or in combination with vitamin E (Klein *et al.*, 2003). Although the study was projected for 12 years, it had to be terminated after 7 years because of lack of any positive results; this "failure" led to a wave of scepticism regarding the plausibility of the concept of chemoprevention with selenium.

A number of studies addressed the relationship between the anticarcinogenic potential of selenium and colon cancer pathogenesis, but their results were often ambiguous, given the fact that associations between selenium intake and levels and colorectal adenomas and carcinomas have not been clearly determined (Fernandez-Banares et al., 2002; R. Nelson et al., 1995; M. Nelson et al., 2005). The strongest support for a possible preventive potential of selenium against colon cancer came from a large randomized controlled trial of selenium in the prevention of non-melanoma skin cancer (Clark et al., 1996), and from a pooled analysis of three randomized clinical trials of dietary interventions in the prevention of colorectal adenomas (Jacobs et al., 2004). Their results showed that higher selenium plasma levels were associated with a 34% decrease in development of new adenomas, which may constitute the basis for setting up new selenium trials with more specific designs and aims.

EFFECTS OF SELENITE IN COLON CANCER CELLS

The cellular and molecular effects of selenium in premalignant or malignant colonic cells depend on several variables, including its chemical form, its dosage, the type of model, and the stage of colon cancer. While organic selenium produces more specific effects in cells, as anticipated from its complex intracellular metabolism, inorganic selenium tends to be generally more toxic and its effects are rather more straightforward. Low to medium doses of both inorganic and organic selenium tend to protect normal cells against various forms of stress. This may occur by means of enhanced synthesis of selected antioxidant selenoproteins, suppression of DNA damage, interference with the metabolism of carcinogens, or via epigenetic regulation (Davis et al., 2000; El-Bayoumy and Sinha, 2005; Hu et al., 2005). Conversely, higher doses of selenium actively induce stress and toxicity, mostly in the case of inorganic selenium, due to oxidative stress. In line with the subject matter of this chapter, the protective effects of selenite on normal cells of the colon will not be discussed further here, and the focus will be on the cytostatic and cytotoxic activities of selenite in malignant colonocytes.

Stress Signaling

Treatment of various types of colon cancer cells with sodium selenite results in decreased cell growth, loss of proliferation activity, and induced differentiation, which in many cases precede terminal stages including apoptosis, autophagy, or senescence. These effects are likely to be due to non-specific oxidative stress activity, even though some more specific interactions may not be ruled out. Thus, selenite has been reported to suppress DNA cytosine methyltransferase (Mtase) in HT-29 cells, with subsequent differentiation and apoptosis (Stewart et al., 1997). In the same cells, selenite inhibited cell growth via activated AMP-activated protein kinase (AMPK), which led to a decrease in expression of cyclooxygenase-2 (Cox-2) and of prostaglandin E2 (PGE2) (Hwang et al., 2006). In addition, in HCT-116 and SW620 cells, selenite-dependent antiproliferative activities occurred via increased c-Jun NH2 terminal kinase (JNK1) phosphorylation and suppression of β-catenin signaling (Fang et al., 2010). Selenite is also known to activate the DNA damage response pathway, with subsequent cell cycle-specific changes, including cell cycle arrest. Moreover, our data also indicate that even mitochondria, or other possible subcellular compartments, could be among selenite's targets (unpublished observations).

Apoptosis

Nowadays, we understand apoptosis as a form of programmed cellular event acting to remove a particular cell from a multicellular organism in cases where the cell is defective, superfluous, or otherwise interfering with normal homeostasis. This applies to a host of physiological conditions as well as to situations where, for example, apoptosis is actively induced with the aim of selective destruction of a target cell population during cytotoxic chemotherapy or chemoprevention. Regulation of apoptosis is very complex, since each cell expresses numerous pro-apoptotic as well as anti-apoptotic signaling cascades, and the number of identified molecules directly or indirectly involved in this process is still growing. In addition, it appears that activation and suppression of apoptosis are not linear decisions, but rather a consequence of the prevalent type of signaling at the particular moment in a given cellular context.

Our interest in selenite and its ability to induce apoptosis was based on our previous studies with different cancer models, and earlier observations by other research groups. Selenite has been shown to induce oxidative stress and apoptosis in human adenocarcinoma HT-29 cells. The authors concluded that observed apoptosis, as evidenced by specific DNA fragmentation, is directly linked with depletion of reduced glutathione, which in turn is mediated by generation of the superoxide anion (Stewart *et al.*, 1997). The results of this study were further confirmed in SW480 cells, which represent an invasive metastasizing stage of CRC. In these cells, sodium selenite induced mitochondrial apoptosis associated with a loss of mitochondrial membrane potential. Still, unlike previous studies, glutathione levels in thus treated cells were unchanged, and the authors were able to demonstrate a significant increase in intracellular calcium levels with resulting mitochondrial calcium overload. These results led them to conclude that sodium selenite acts via calcium to increase mitochondrial-driven production of reactive oxygen species (ROS), with ensuing apoptosis (Wang *et al.*, 2003). A recent study comprising various colon cancer cell lines representing diverse stages of CRC (HCT-116, HT-29, and SW480) provided further, deeper insights into the mechanisms of selenite-dependent activation of apoptosis. Here, sodium selenite increased the output of ROS from mitochondria, which served as a putative redox signal to an exposure of the BH3 domain and C-terminal transmembrane domain of pro-apoptotic protein Bax. Conserved Cys 62/126 residues in these domains were then pinpointed as a critical target for activation of Bax, its translocation into mitochondrial outer membrane, and stimulation of selenite-specific, caspase-dependent apoptosis (Huang *et al.*, 2009). Further to this, in HCT-116 and SW620 cells as well as tumor xenographs, selenite inhibits activation of Akt and thus influences the localization as well as the activity of β-catenin, leading to apoptosis (Luo *et al.*, 2012).

The pro-oxidative potential of sodium selenite may alter calcium signaling or the redox balance in exposed cells, with specific activation of some pro-apoptotic proteins such as BAX or inhibition of survival signals (Akt/β-catenin axis), but some other crucial or canonical changes also may influence the final endpoints. These may include, for instance, DNA and the p53-dependent pathway, which are logical targets of selenite activities. We investigated possible differences in selenite-induced cellular stress and apoptosis in the colon cancer cell lines

HCT-116, with wild-type *p53*, and HCT-116-p53KO, where *p53* was knocked out. We used a range of techniques and markers to compare in detail the contribution of the p53 pathway to the apoptotic phenotype. Our data demonstrate that although sodium selenite induces comparative levels of oxidative stress in both models, the spectrum and activity of pro-apoptotic and anti-apoptotic signals differ considerably. We noted that HCT-116-p53KO cells are more resistant to selenite-dependent apoptosis compared to HCT-116 cells. The lower rate of apoptosis in these cells was linked with lower levels, and delayed expression, of DNA damage markers (such as phosphorylated histone H2A.X) (Figure 15.1). Furthermore, p53 expression, and caspase-2 and -3 activities, were also notably present in HCT-116 cells only. These results, together with Bax expression analyses, indicate that, in HCT-116 cells, p53 and a p53-dependent response might contribute to selenite-induced apoptosis.

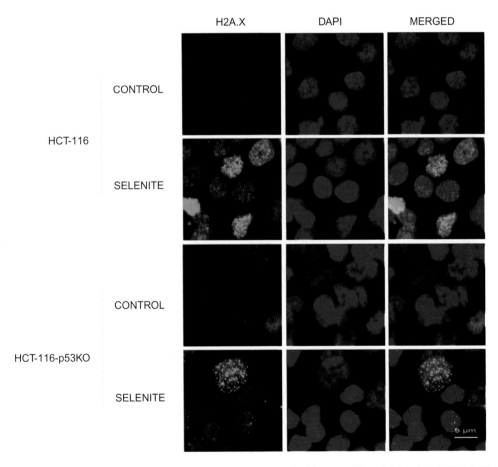

FIGURE 15.1 DNA damage in colon cancer cells HCT-116 (wild-type p53) and HCT-116-p53KO (p53 was deleted) in control conditions (no treatment) and after treatment with 10-µM sodium selenite at 12 hours of exposure. DNA damage was investigated using immunofluorescent detection of phosphorylated histone H2A.X with background use of DNA-specific DAPI at magnification 400×. Selenite induced in DNA breaks (H2A.X-positive foci) in both cell lines, but stronger response was observed in HCT-116 cells.

Another mechanism contributing to selenite-induced apoptosis is likely to be the activity of stress kinases, in particular p38 and JNK. These kinases are known to be involved in apoptosis in cancer cells, where they act via p53 or in a p53-independent manner. We detected elevated activities of p38 and JNK in both HCT-116 and HCT-116-p53KO cells, although with differing intensity and time frames. The use of specific pharmacological inhibitors and gene knockdown technology aimed at these kinases finally proved that, in HCT-116 cells, p38 kinase was actively involved in apoptosis activated by sodium selenite, while JNK activity most likely resulted from apoptosis rather then being its cause. Conversely, in HCT-116-p53KO cells, sodium selenite-dependent ROS mediated an increase in JNK activity and this could have been one of the crucial pro-apoptotic stimuli, whereas p38 was found to have a negligible role. These observations thus argue for disparate abilities of selenium to induce apoptosis in colon cancer cells with differing p53 genotypes, which also attests to the importance of p53 signaling in this type of model.

Autophagy

Autophagy is a highly conserved process which ensures survival of living systems (cells) upon stressful conditions via recycling of proteins and other cellular compartments. Autophagy pathways involve several sequential and regulated steps whose genesis, occurrence, and regulation differ depending on the particular setting. Most typically, autophagy begins with initiation and nucleation steps, where a cup-shaped membrane structure called a phagophore is formed, followed by its elongation and closure to generate a double-membrane vacuole termed an autophagosome. The entire process is completed by fusion of the autophagosome with a lysosome, and resulting degradation of sequestered material. Optimal functioning of the autophagic pathway is regulated by three different groups of proteins: Atg9, a phosphatidylinositol 3-OH kinase (PI3K) complex, and an ubiquitin-like protein system (Atg12 and Atg8) (Rubinsztein *et al.*, 2012).

The role of autophagy in the development and progression of malignancies remains controversial. On the one hand, autophagy seems vital for maintaining cellular homeostasis, and therefore it has been proposed to function as a tumor-promoting mechanism. Conversely, genetic evidence suggests that autophagy exerts tumor-suppressive functions. In CRC, autophagy is compromised at different levels. Its defects are associated with immune responses, bacterial clearance, and malfunctions in goblet as well as Pannet cells. Perhaps most importantly, autophagy defects accompany the malignant phenotype in colonic cells at different stages of their transformation. Here, several existing studies are focusing on the role of Beclin 1, which is an essential protein for autophagosome formation. It seems that loss of Beclin 1 expression in CRC, related to either allelic loss of the gene or microRNA activity, contributes to poor clinical prognosis of the disease. On the other hand, Beclin 1 overexpression, which is often linked to tumor hypoxia and acidity, may also influence tumor aggressiveness (Koukourakis *et al.*, 2010).

The effect of selenite on autophagy in malignant cells has been a focus of relatively few studies. Most of them report on either induced or suppressed autophagy in the context of apoptosis, with differing roles of particular proteins or signals, such as mTOR, Beclin 1 or heat shock protein 90 (Hsp90), relevant for both processes. For instance, in leukemic cells, sodium selenite decreased Hsp90 expression and attenuated its interaction with the protein inhibitor of nuclear factor κB (IKK). This signaling continued in suppressed Beclin 1 expression and, possibly, in expression of some anti-apoptotic genes, finally resulting in a signaling switch from autophagy to apoptosis. In addition, the authors also hypothesized that this observed Hsp90-mediated switch is under the influence of p53 activity (Jiang et al., 2011). Currently, the only study aimed at the investigation of autophagy and apoptosis in colon cancer cells treated with selenite has been conducted by our group (Kralova et al., 2012). We discovered that selenite induces differing levels of autophagy in HCT-116 and HCT-116-p53KO cells, as evidenced by specific cellular morphologies (Figure 15.2) as well as the expression of autophagy-relevant proteins and their cellular topography. In addition, we proved that the differing p53 status of malignant colonocytes plays a decisive role in selenite-induced autophagy, which is concordant with the study conducted in leukemic cells. Nevertheless, unlike the reported importance of the Hsp90–IKK axis, we found that

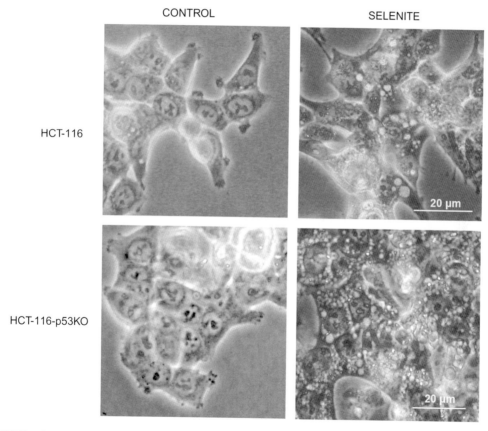

FIGURE 15.2   Morphological appearance of colon cancer cells HCT-116 (wild-type p53) and HCT-116-p53KO (p53 was deleted) in control conditions (no treatment) and after treatment with 10-μM sodium selenite at 24 hours of exposure. Changes in morphology were recorded using phase contrast microscopy at magnification 400×. Treatment with selenite resulted in both cell lines showing development of vacuolization, cell detachment, and nucleolar clarification. Vacuolization was more extensive in HCT-116-p53KO cells.

in the presence of normal (wild-type) p53 in the cells, the mTOR pathway does not seem to be primarily regulated by selenite and thus responsible for autophagy. Conversely, p38 stress kinase activity in the same cells proved to be of significant importance in selenite-induced autophagy, as evidenced by decreasing autophagy rates in cells where p38 activity was blocked. Moreover, when p53 is deleted, as in HCT-116-p53KO cells, selenite-induced autophagy tended to proceed via a suppressed mTOR pathway, with a significant role being played by JNK.

DISCUSSION

Our work on selenite and its effects in malignant colon cancer cells shows varying response rates in terms of activated or suppressed signaling pathways, as well as final phenotypes. We conclude that this plethora of responses most probably reflects the mechanisms whereby sodium selenite exerts biological effects. Due to its intracellular metabolism, sodium selenite may interact with individual targets (molecules, signaling circuits, compartments) either directly or indirectly. While most reports on direct selenite activity concern individual molecules or signaling pathways (see section on Stress Signaling), we demonstrated that, in certain circumstances, selenite may damage chromatin structure or change mitochondrial topography, as well as their viability, in some colon cancer cells. Since these phenomena may be clearly separated from indirect selenite effects in a given experimental model, we hypothesize that both of them act synergistically to strengthen particular signaling towards a selected biological response.

The most agreed-upon indirect mechanism of selenite is the much researched oxidative stress. Oxidative stress results from the shifting balance of the intracellular redox environment towards a pro-oxidative state, which typically occurs after depletion of redox-balancing antioxidant systems and increased generation of ROS. As mentioned in previous sections, the intracellular presence of selenite and its metabolite hydrogen selenide leads to overproduction of superoxide ions, and possibly other ROS, which ultimately interact with different targets and activate or suppress respective signaling pathways or activities in the cell. What is not clear at the moment is the exact mechanism whereby selenite-dependent ROS are generated in the context of a particular biological response. Limited available evidence suggests that in colon cancer cells, selenite mobilizes free calcium stores, which in turn leads to mitochondria-dependent ROS overproduction (Wang et al., 2003). Another potential scenario entails depletion of antioxidant systems, such as reduced glutathione, during the course of intracellular selenite metabolism, and subsequent graduated effects of ROS, which are naturally produced by functional mitochondria. Whether these two or possibly other mechanisms are truly responsible for ROS generation is in this case impossible to state, but it is reasonable to believe that it could be their combination. So far, no systematic study or review of changes in redox balance of cells at different stages of CRC has been conducted. Also, responses to oxidative stressors such as sodium selenite are likely to change not only vertically (premalignant→metastatic stages of CRC) but also horizontally (heterogeneity of malignant cell population at given stage). Thus, individual reported data might simply reflect the changing nature of exposed malignant cells. This is typically seen when one compares identical doses of sodium selenite and their effects on different cell lines.

ROS have many potential targets within the cell, including some of the most important intracellular compartments, such as the nucleus, mitochondria, and endoplasmic reticulum. Signals from these compartments are crucial for cellular homeostasis, stress response, cell survival, and/or cell death. The fact that sodium selenite exposure in malignant cells results in their apoptosis is widely acknowledged. In view of our knowledge on apoptosis regulation, it may be concluded that selenite induces this type of cell death via an inner or mitochondrial pathway. Nevertheless, existing reports demonstrate plasticity of this process. First, selenite activates apoptosis via acetylation of Bax, which leads to mitochondrial, caspase-dependent apoptosis in colon cancer cell lines representing various stages of CRC (Huang et al., 2009). In invasive SW480 cells, mitochondria are also a target of selenite pro-apoptotic activity, albeit not via Bax but throughout calcium overload (Wang et al., 2003). In the same cells, however, selenite inhibits Akt/β-catenin signaling too, which was proposed to lead to apoptosis (Luo et al., 2012). Furthermore, our data suggest that, in HCT-116 cells, p53 may represent a key player in selenite-induced apoptosis by mediating direct p53-dependent pro-apoptotic communication as well as by modulating the expression and activities of several stress kinases such as p38 and JNK (Kralova et al., 2012). Taken together, the above-mentioned reports on apoptosis of colon cancer cells induced by selenite clearly illustrate the heterogeneity of the respective signaling in particular colon cancer cell types. Rather than being contradictory, this heterogeneity might actually reflect multiple circuit signal regulation and final amplification which is necessary to activate and execute a given biological response.

Basal levels of autophagy exist in all human cells, regardless of their status, differentiation state, or age. Upon malignant transformation, autophagy may increase, decrease, or become erratic, and this occurs in most malignancies, including CRC. Many studies in CRC as well as in other malignancies demonstrated that autophagy increases in response to treatment, and suppression of autophagy contributed to better treatment results. Autophagy may exist alongside apoptosis, and both processes could act in a coordinated, cooperative, or antagonistic fashion. This functional linkage of autophagy and apoptosis is made obvious in light of fact that many recognized apoptotic or autophagy proteins are involved in regulation of both processes. Known examples include Bcl-2 and its phosphorylation, which has been proposed to regulate the switch between the two pathways, JNK, Beclin 1, or mTOR. A complex role at the intersection of both autophagy and apoptosis is played by p53, which regulates both apoptosis and autophagy in a positive or in a negative fashion, depending on its subcellular localization, expression, and interacting partners. Autophagy and apoptosis may be activated by common upstream signals, which would possibly explain the concurrent presence of both processes in selenite-treated cells. At this point, and with respect to autophagy, it is necessary to mention and explain one more term: autophagic cell death. This type of death has been reported in diverse experimental settings, including selenite-treated malignant cells. Since its inception, the existence of autophagic cell death has been a matter of discussion and controversy because of its often confusing features and lack of clear distinguishing criteria. It has been proposed that autophagic cell death as an independent cell death modality occurs in a system which shows no features of apoptosis, while an increase of autophagic flux is clearly present in dying cells, and, finally, suppression of autophagy is able to rescue or prevent cell death (Shen and Codogno, 2011). In light of our own results, autophagic cell death did not occur in colon cancer cells treated with selenite.

On the other hand, apoptosis as well as autophagy were induced by selenite in HCT-116 cells, and the use of autophagy inhibitors such as 3-methyadenine (3-MA) reduced autophagy while increasing apoptosis, thereby proving that in this case autophagy played the survival role. Subsequent experiments then showed that the molecule responsible for autophagy induction is p38; this was surprising, as the same molecule also actively regulated apoptosis. Thus, since p38 is known to regulate both processes, its respective role in CRC in relation to selenite treatment needs to be studied further (Kralova et al., 2012).

The absence of p53 in colon cancer cells exposed to selenite leads to activation of apoptosis and autophagy, too, but inhibition of autophagy has a similar effect on apoptosis. In this case it appears that apoptosis and autophagy act synergistically and key signaling pathways, unlike in wild-type p53 cells, depend on mTOR and JNK (Kralova et al., 2012). These data represent a first report on the role of p53 and stress kinases in selenite-induced autophagy in colon cancer cells. Our discovered patterns of signaling circuits influenced by sodium selenite treatment reveal the complex role autophagy plays in the stress response in CRC models, and call for more thorough profiling of the molecules and pathways involved.

In summary, the role of selenium in the development and progression of malignant diseases, and in particular CRC, is now acknowledged. Sodium selenite might be considered as a potential chemopreventive compound showing significant cytotoxicity against colon cancer cells at all stages of malignant transformation, where it targets, indirectly or directly, a number of molecules, signaling pathways, and compartments, resulting in apoptosis and autophagy. Relationships between these two forms of cellular response to stress are complex in the case of selenite and CRC, and we are only now beginning to understand their nature and mutual interactions. In future, more mechanistic studies into the role of autophagy induced by selenite in colon cancer cell lines are needed to evaluate the potential of this chemical form of selenium for its potential use as a chemopreventive agent in humans.

Acknowledgment

This work was supported by the program PRVOUK P37/01.

References

Blot, W.J., Li, J.Y., Taylor, P.R., et al., 1993. Nutrition intervention trials in Linxian, China: supplementation with specific vitamin/mineral combinations, cancer incidence, and disease-specific mortality in the general population. J. Natl. Cancer Inst. 85, 1483–1492.
Boland, C.R., Goel, A., 2010. Microsatellite instability in colorectal cancer. Gastroenterology 138, 2073–2087.
Brigelius-Flohe, R., 2008. Selenium compounds and selenoproteins in cancer. Chem. Biodivers. 5, 389–395.
Clark, L.C., Combs Jr, G.F., Turnbull, B.W., et al., 1996. Effects of selenium supplementation for cancer prevention in patients with carcinoma of the skin. A randomized controlled trial. Nutritional Prevention of Cancer Study Group. JAMA 276, 1957–1963.
Combs Jr, G.F., 2001. Selenium in global food systems. Br. J. Nutr. 85, 517–547.
Davis, C.D., Uthus, E.O., Finley, J.W., 2000. Dietary selenium and arsenic affect DNA methylation in vitro in Caco-2 cells and in vivo in rat liver and colon. J. Nutr. 130, 2903–2909.
Downward, J., 2003. Targeting RAS signalling pathways in cancer therapy. Nat. Rev. Cancer 3, 11–22.
Duffield-Lillico, A.J., Reid, M.E., Turnbull, B.W., et al., 2002. Baseline characteristics and the effect of selenium supplementation on cancer incidence in a randomized clinical trial: a summary report of the Nutritional Prevention of Cancer Trial. Cancer Epidemiol. Biomarkers Prev. 11, 630–639.
El-Bayoumy, K., Sinha, R., 2005. Molecular chemoprevention by selenium: a genomic approach. Mutat. Res. 591, 224–236.

Fang, W., Han, A., Bi, X., et al., 2010. Tumor inhibition by sodium selenite is associated with activation of c-Jun NH2-terminal kinase 1 and suppression of beta-catenin signaling. Int. J. Cancer 127, 32–42.

Fernandez-Banares, F., Cabre, E., Esteve, M., et al., 2002. Serum selenium and risk of large size colorectal adenomas in a geographical area with a low selenium status. Am. J. Gastroenterol. 97, 2103–2108.

Hatfield, D.L., Carlson, B.A., Xu, X.M., et al., 2006. Selenocysteine incorporation machinery and the role of seleno-proteins in development and health. Prog. Nucleic Acid Res. Mol. Biol. 81, 97–142.

Hu, Y., Benya, R.V., Carroll, R.E., et al., 2005. Allelic loss of the gene for the GPX1 selenium-containing protein is a common event in cancer. J. Nutr. 135, 3021S–3024S.

Huang, F., Nie, C., Yang, Y., et al., 2009. Selenite induces redox-dependent Bax activation and apoptosis in colorectal cancer cells. Free Radic. Biol. Med. 46, 1186–1196.

Hwang, J.-T., Kim, Y.M., Surh, Y.-J., et al., 2006. Selenium regulates cyclooxygenase-2 and extracellular signal-reg-ulated kinase signaling pathways by activating AMP-activated protein kinase in colon cancer cells. Cancer Res. 66, 10057–10063.

Ip, C., Hayes, C., Budnick, R.M., et al., 1991. Chemical form of selenium, critical metabolites, and cancer prevention. Cancer Res. 51, 595–600.

Jacobs, E.T., Jiang, R., Alberts, D.S., et al., 2004. Selenium and colorectal adenoma: results of a pooled analysis. J. Natl. Cancer Inst. 96, 1669–1675.

Jiang, Q., Wang, Y., Li, T., et al., 2011. Heat shock protein 90-mediated inactivation of nuclear factor-kappaB switches autophagy to apoptosis through becn1 transcriptional inhibition in selenite-induced NB4 cells. Mol. Biol. Cell 22, 1167–1180.

Klein, E.A., Thompson, I.M., Lippman, S.M., et al., 2003. SELECT: the selenium and vitamin E cancer prevention trial. Urol. Oncol. 21, 59–65.

Koukourakis, M.I., Giatromanolaki, A., Sivridis, E., et al., 2010. Beclin 1 over- and underexpression in colorectal cancer: distinct patterns relate to prognosis and tumour hypoxia. Br. J. Cancer 103, 1209–1214.

Kralova, V., Benesova, S., Cervinka, M., et al., 2012. Selenite-induced apoptosis and autophagy in colon cancer cells. Toxicol. In Vitro 26, 258–268.

Kroemer, G., Petit, P., Zamzami, N., et al., 1995. The biochemistry of programmed cell death. FASEB J. 9, 1277–1287.

Lu, J., Holmgren, A., 2009. Selenoproteins. J. Biol. Chem. 284, 723–727.

Luo, H., Yang, Y., Huang, F., et al., 2012. Selenite induces apoptosis in colorectal cancer cells via AKT-mediated inhi-bition of beta-catenin survival axis. Cancer Lett. 315, 78–85.

Nelson, M., Goulet, A.-C., Jacobs, E., et al., 2005. Studies into the anticancer effects of selenomethionine against human colon cancer. Ann. N. Y. Acad. Sci. 1059, 26–32.

Nelson, R.L., Davis, F.G., Sutter, E., et al., 1995. Serum selenium and colonic neoplastic risk. Dis. Colon Rectum. 38, 1306–1310.

Pino, M.S., Chung, D.C., 2010. The chromosomal instability pathway in colon cancer. Gastroenterology 138, 2059–2072.

Rubinsztein, D.C., Codogno, P., Levine, B., 2012. Autophagy modulation as a potential therapeutic target for diverse diseases. Nat. Rev. Drug Discov. 11, 709–730.

Samuels, Y., Velculescu, V.E., 2004. Oncogenic mutations of PIK3CA in human cancers. Cell Cycle. 3, 1221–1224.

Shamberger, R.J., Frost, D.V., 1969. Possible protective effect of selenium against human cancer. Can. Med. Assoc. J. 100, 682.

Shen, H.M., Codogno, P., 2011. Autophagic cell death: Loch Ness monster or endangered species? Autophagy 7, 457–465.

Sjoblom, T., Jones, S., Wood, L.D., et al., 2006. The consensus coding sequences of human breast and colorectal can-cers. Science 314, 268–274.

Stewart, M.S., Davis, R.L., Walsh, L.P., et al., 1997. Induction of differentiation and apoptosis by sodium selenite in human colonic carcinoma cells (HT29). Cancer Lett. 117, 35–40.

Vogelstein, B., Fearon, E.R., Hamilton, S.R., et al., 1988. Genetic alterations during colorectal-tumor development. N. Engl. J. Med. 319, 525–532.

Wang, H., Yang, X., Zhang, Z., et al., 2003. Both calcium and ROS as common signals mediate Na2SeO3-induced apoptosis in SW480 human colonic carcinoma cells. J. Inorg. Biochem. 97, 221–230.

Enhancement of Cell Death in High-Grade Glioma Cells: Role of N-(4-Hydroxyphenyl) Retinamide-Induced Autophagy

Meenakshi Tiwari, Lokendra K. Sharma, and Madan M. Godbole

OUTLINE

M.A. Hayat (ed): Autophagy, Volume 1
DOI: http://dx.doi.org/10.1016/B978-0-12-405530-8.00016-9

© 2014 Elsevier Inc. All rights reserved.

Abstract

Despite clinical advancements, high-grade glioma continues to remain incurable in the majority of patients, largely due to recurrence of the tumor caused by resistance towards the conventional therapies. The therapeutic goal of cancer treatment has been to trigger cancer cell death through apoptosis; however, the cancer cells develop resistance to apoptosis induction. This underscores the need to identify newer chemotherapeutic strategies that can maximize apoptosis or induce alternate mode of cell death in apoptosis-resistant cells. For these reasons, autophagy, which can play a role in cell survival or cell death, is receiving scientific attention as a target to modulate the cell death response of cancer cells. Of interest, autophagy has been shown to be induced by a number of current and experimental glioma therapies. Further, a better understanding of the link between apoptosis and autophagy might allow development of more effective therapies for high-grade gliomas. N-(4-hydroxyphenyl) retinamide (4-HPR) is a potent synthetic retinoid with anticancer activity in a variety of tumors, which is largely dependent on its ability to engage apoptotic pathways in transformed cells, and its relative lack of adverse side effects *in vivo*. We have identified a novel role for 4-HPR in high-grade glioma cell lines: the ability to induce autophagy at a lower concentration and apoptosis at a higher concentration, leading to elimination of cancer cells. Notably, inhibition of autophagy at a lower concentration sensitizes high-grade glioma cells to 4-HPR-induced apoptosis, suggesting a survival-promoting role for 4-HPR-induced autophagy. These findings propose further evaluation of autophagy inhibition in combination with 4-HPR in high-grade gliomas to achieve higher efficacy and prevent recurrence of these malignancies.

INTRODUCTION

Primary brain tumors are among the top 10 causes of cancer-related deaths in the United States. Gliomas, or glial tumors, are the most common type of primary brain tumor. Gliomas develop in glial cells and are named after the types of glial cell with which they share histological features. The main forms of glioma are ependymomas, astrocytomas (of which glioblastoma multiforme is the most common), oligodendrogliomas, and mixed gliomas, such as oligoastrocytomas, which contain cells from different types of glia. Gliomas are further categorized according to their grade, as determined by pathologic evaluation of the tumor. They include low-grade gliomas (World Health Organization (WHO) grades I–II), which are non-anaplastic, i.e., well differentiated, and high-grade gliomas (WHO grades III–IV), which are anaplastic, i.e. undifferentiated, and have a poor prognosis (Tabatabai *et al.*, 2012). The majority of high-grade glial tumors are malignant, accounting for approximately 70% of new cases of malignant primary brain tumors diagnosed in adults each year. Despite considerable advances in multimodality treatment of tumors, malignant gliomas are still associated with high morbidity and mortality. The median survival is 12–15 months for patients with glioblastoma, and 2–5 years for those with anaplastic glioma (Wen and Kesari, 2008).

Treatment for gliomas depends on the location, the cell type, and the grade of malignancy. The treatment requires a multidisciplinary approach, which involves the surgical removal of solid tumor masses usually combined with a series of chemical (chemotherapy) or physical (radiotherapy) treatments (Butowski and Chang, 2006). Following surgery, a variety of chemotherapeutic options are currently available that are given in an adjuvant setting with radiation therapy. These agents include nitrosourea-based regimen, the imidotetrazine analogue, temozolomide, platinum-based regimens, and procarbazine (Spinelli *et al.*, 2012). However, high-grade gliomas are still associated with a very poor prognosis. Causative factors for the poor survival rate include the highly invasive nature of high-grade gliomas, making them intractable to complete surgical resection. Also, the response of tumors to chemotherapy, radiotherapy, or other adjuvant therapies depends at least in part on their propensity to undergo cell death mediated by apoptosis. However, resistance to apoptosis is considered a characteristic of many diverse cancer cells, and defects in apoptosis underlie not only tumorigenesis but also resistance to cancer treatments (Okada and Mak, 2004). Further, due to their aggressiveness, ability to form secondary tumors, and metastatic potential, these tumors recur after surgery. To prevent recurrence, they require adjuvant therapy that includes radiation and chemotherapy, which may overcome the resistance offered by the cancer cells. Currently available chemotherapeutic agents are associated with limitations including side effects, drug delivery, and drug resistance. The difficult clinical situation associated with most types of primary brain tumors has fostered significant interest in defining novel therapeutic modalities for this heterogeneous group of neoplasms. In order to identify novel therapeutics, a better understanding of molecular mechanisms underlying cancer development, the chemotherapeutic action of drugs, and drug resistance is required.

CELL DEATH INDUCED BY CHEMOTHERAPEUTIC AGENTS

The therapeutic goal of cancer treatment has been to trigger tumor-selective cell death. Although the death of cancer cells by therapeutic agents can be achieved not only by apoptosis (type 1 programmed cell death) but also by necrosis and senescence, apoptosis remains the preferred pathway of induction of cell death (Chaabane et al., 2012). Apoptotic cell death acts as part of a quality control and repair mechanism by elimination of unwanted, genetically damaged, or senescent cells. Apoptosis may occur via death receptor-dependent (extrinsic) or independent (intrinsic or mitochondrial) pathways. Mitochondria play an important role in apoptosis by releasing pro-apoptotic molecules leading to caspase-dependent or caspase-independent apoptosis. The major biochemical features of apoptosis are the activation of intracellular proteases that mainly include caspases, and internucleosomal DNA fragmentation (Hotchkiss et al., 2009). Changes in several cell surface molecules ensure that apoptotic cells are immediately recognized and phagocytosed by neighboring cells in tissues, so that these apoptotic cells can be deleted from tissues in a relatively short time. Therefore, apoptosis results in the orderly elimination of cells without generating an inflammatory response, and is thus the preferred pathway for the majority of therapeutic targets. However, cancer cells, in their relentless drive to survive, hijack cell processes, resulting in apoptosis resistance, which underlies not only tumorigenesis but also the inherent resistance of certain cancers to radiotherapy and chemotherapy. Thus, newer targets that can overcome the resistance of cancer cells to undergo apoptosis, or that induce alternative modes of cell death alone or in combination with known agents, are under investigation. More recently, modulation of autophagy has emerged as a potential novel mechanism for cancer therapies to induce cell death (Carew et al., 2012). Macroautophagy (hereafter referred to autophagy) is a eukaryotic, evolutionarily conserved homeostatic process in which organelles and bulk proteins are turned over by lysosomal activity (Mizushima, 2007). Autophagy is a stress-induced response that may promote cell survival or may lead to cell death, depending on a variety of factors, including cell type, stressor, and duration of stress. In periods of metabolic stress, autophagy recycles molecules and provides ATP and other macromolecules as energy sources to enable cell survival; however, if the intensity or duration of metabolic stress is excessive, cells may progress to autophagic programmed cell death, which is distinct from apoptosis. Many signaling pathways, including mammalian target of rapamycin (mTOR), class I phosphatidylinositol 3-kinase (PI3KC1)/PKB, GTPases, and protein synthesis, play important roles in regulating autophagy. The kinase mTOR is a critical regulator of autophagy induction, with activated mTOR (Akt and mitogen-activated protein kinase (MAPK) signaling) suppressing autophagy, and negative regulation of mTOR (AMP-activated protein kinase (AMPK) and p53 signaling) promoting it. The class III PI3K complex, containing hVps34, Beclin 1, p150, and autophagy related protein (Atg) or ultraviolet irradiation resistance-associated gene (UVRAG), is required for the induction of autophagy. Also, important roles for autophagy-related gene (Atg) (1–12) proteins (essential proteins of the autophagic machinery) have been well characterized in the regulation of autophagy. Further, autophagy and apoptosis may be interconnected, and even simultaneously regulated by the same trigger in tumor cells.

Various agents are being evaluated in high-grade glioma cells for their efficacy to induce autophagy and to modulate autophagy as a combinational agent to improve the apoptosis-inducing capacity of a variety of available chemotherapeutic agents (Kaza et al., 2012). Once such agent is 4-HPR, a synthetic retinoid that, depending upon its concentration, has shown an ability to induce autophagy as well as apoptosis in glioma cells (Tiwari et al., 2008). Interestingly, inhibition of autophagy enhances the sensitivity of glioma cells towards 4-HPR-induced apoptosis. In the following sections of the chapter, we discuss the potential use of 4-HPR in combination with autophagy inhibitors to enhance apoptosis and thus improve its efficacy in high-grade glioma cells.

RETINOIDS AS CHEMOTHERAPEUTIC AGENTS

N-(4-hydroxyphenyl) retinamide is a retinoid analogue. Retinoids (the collective term for vitamin A and its natural and synthetic congeners) are fat-soluble molecules that exert pleiotropic effects in a variety of biologic systems, including embryogenesis, differentiation, and maintenance of normal growth, as well as neoplastic transformation (Theodosiou et al., 2010). The use of retinoids in the treatment of cancer began with the observation that the flattened, keratinized epithelial cells in lung cancer tissue were similar to those seen in vitamin A deficiency. Retinoid signaling is often compromised early in carcinogenesis, which has suggested a role for reduced vitamin A in tumor development. Hence, supplementation with pharmacologic doses of retinoids was thought to provide an effective treatment by correcting an underlying deficiency (Tang and Gudas, 2011).

Retinoids exert most of their effects via multiple nuclear receptors that are members of the nuclear steroid/thyroid hormone superfamily, and function as ligand-dependent transcriptional regulators. Retinoids bind to specific nuclear retinoic acid receptors (RARs) and retinoid X receptors (RXRs), each of which is encoded by three separate genes designated as α, β, and γ. An important source of diversity in transducing the retinoid signal is generated through the existence of two families of receptors, RAR and RXR, and their binding as an

RAR/RXR heterodimer to the polymorphic cis-acting response element of retinoic acid (RA) target genes (Theodosiou *et al.*, 2010).

Retinoids and their analogues have also been extensively evaluated as chemopreventive agents in a variety of cancers (Tang and Gudas, 2011). Further, in glioma and/or cell lines they have shown beneficial antineoplastic actions, such as inducing morphological alterations, inhibiting growth, and increasing the doubling time (Mawson, 2012). Human gliomas express all the isoforms of RAR, and two of the three isoforms of RXR. Clinical trials with all trans-retinoic acid (ATRA) for recurrent malignant glioma suggest modest but significant clinical benefit.

However, the ability of natural retinoids to regulate cellular processes *in vivo* is unfortunately associated with a high incidence of undesirable side effects. In general, supplementary vitamin A using retinyl esters or synthetic retinoids has only temporary benefits in cancer treatment, and these appear to be outweighed over time by toxic effects – notably the occasionally fatal "retinoic acid syndrome," characterized by respiratory distress, pulmonary infiltrates, fever, hypotension, weight gain, renal failure, and leg edema (Mawson, 2012). As a result of the quest for new retinoid-related compounds capable of selectively activating the mechanisms for apoptosis in cancer cells but devoid of undesirable side effects, some structural features have been developed that seem to be important in conferring ring apoptosis vs differentiation activity to well-known and newly built molecules.

Two classes of synthetic retinoids have important implications in the biology of various normal and neoplastic cells: the arotinoids (aromatic retinoids), in which the retinoic acid structure is fixed in the cisoid geometric structure, and retinamides, in which the terminal carboxyl group has been substituted with a single amide group. More than 1500 retinoids have been tested so far, but very few of them have been entered into clinical trials because of their side effects.

N-(4-HYDROXYPHENYL) RETINAMIDE, A SYNTHETIC RETINOID

N-(4-hydroxyphenyl) retinamide (4-HPR) is one synthetic retinoid that has been entered into clinical trials. 4-HPR is a synthetic analogue of ATRA that was first produced by R. W. Johnson Pharmaceuticals in the late 1960s, with a modification of the carboxyl end of retinoic acid with an N-4 hydroxyphenyl group (the structure is depicted in Figure 16.1). It is reported to have fewer side effects and better efficacy compared to naturally occurring retinoids such as ATRA and 9-cis retinoic acid (RA). Furthermore, it lacks the ability to induce point mutations or chromosomal aberrations, and is therefore not genotoxic. Based on clinical and preclinical data, 4-HPR has shown potent anticancer activity, which may be largely dependent on its ability to engage apoptotic pathways in transformed cells, and its relative lack of adverse side effects *in vivo* (reviewed by Hail *et al.*, 2006). Moreover, a review of the results from ongoing clinical trials for 4-HPR has suggested that its anti-angiogenic property, anti-invasive activity, ability to induce apoptosis, and enhancement of ROS production as possible molecular bases for its chemopreventive action in patients (Sogno *et al.*, 2010). Many of the apoptogenic pathways triggered by 4-HPR are almost certainly cell-type dependent, and complex. It has become important to better understand its mechanism of action for its use as a chemotherapeutic agent, either alone or in combination.

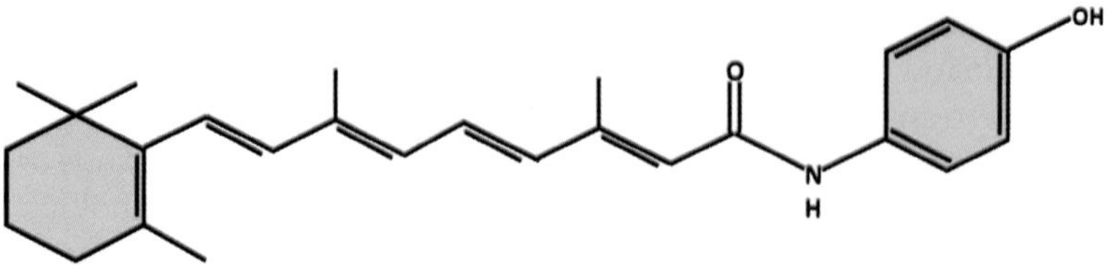

N-(4-hydroxyphenlyl) retinamide (4-HPR) ($C_{26}H_{33}NO_2$)

FIGURE 16.1   Structure of 4-HPR that contains a modification of the carboxyl end of retinoic acid with an N-4 hydroxyphenyl group.

N-(4-HYDROXYPHENYL) RETINAMIDE: MECHANISM OF ACTION

N-(4-hydroxyphenyl) retinamide is a synthetic retinoid that was developed as a retinoic acid receptor (RAR)-β- and RAR-γ-selective agonist and has emerged as a potential chemo-therapeutic agent owing to its effectiveness relative to toxicity in a variety of malignancies (see review by Hail *et al.*, 2006). In cancer cells, 4-HPR induces cytotoxicity through induction of apoptosis, which mainly involves at least three different complex mechanisms that may overlap in the same cell line: mechanisms (1) involving RARs, (2) involving 4-HPR-induced reactive oxygen species (ROS); and (3) independent of ROS or RARs, and remaining unclear.

An essential role for ROS and oxidative stress has been identified in 4-HPR-induced cytotoxicity. Besides ROS levels, 4-HPR treatment also enhances cellular ceramide and ganglioside (GD)3 levels during apoptosis. In 4-HPR-treated cancer cells, signals such as enhanced ROS, ceramide, and/or GD3 may trigger the activation of cellular stress response pathways. Many proteins, including transcription factors p53, GADD153, and nuclear factor-kappa B (NF-κB), have been implicated in apoptotic regulatory mechanisms associated with oxidative and/or genotoxic stress induced by 4-HPR in various cell systems. Once active, these proteins can determine a cell's fate through the initiation of apoptosis. Further, 4-HPR-induced apoptosis also involves activation of MAPK, namely c-jun N-terminal kinases (JNKs), extracellular signal-regulated protein kinases 1 and 2 (ERK1/2), and p38-MAPK, which are downstream of 4-HPR-induced ROS generation. Induction of 4-HPR-induced ROS can further modulate Bcl-2 family protein and can lead to rapid dissipation of mitochondrial membrane potential (ΔΨm) and mitochondrial membrane permeabilization (MMP). Moreover, mitochondria play a central role in initiating the 4-HPR-induced intrinsic pathway of apoptosis by releasing cytochrome c from the intermembrane space, leading to apoptosome formation and thereby initiating apoptosis by activating executioner caspases. Besides the intrinsic pathway, 4-HPR can also lead to activation of caspase-8, leading to cell death by the extrinsic pathway of apoptosis. Further, 4-HPR can also induce caspase-independent cell death involving apoptosis inducing factor (AIF) and endonuclease G. More interestingly, growing evidences also suggest that besides apoptosis-induction 4-HPR can also induce autophagy in a variety of cancer cells (Armstrong *et al.*, 2011; Liu *et al.*, 2010; Messner and Cabot, 2011; Tiwari *et al.*, 2008). Thus, 4-HPR can mediate its cytotoxic effects via targeting multiple pathways of programmed cell death, depending upon the cell type.

N-(4-HYDROXYPHENYL) RETINAMIDE IN GLIOMAS

Given its lipophilicity, results from animal studies and Phase II clinical trials on high-grade glioma together suggest that 4-HPR can not only cross the blood–brain barrier and accumulate in brain tissue, but may also have a prolonged half-life in brain tissue (Puduvalli *et al.*, 2004). Furthermore, a Phase II clinical study on glioma, performed using a lower dose of 4-HPR, raised the possibility that it may have activity in a subset of patients with gliomas, and higher doses of the agent may be needed for anti-tumor efficacy due to the overall lack of major adverse events and lack of activity (Puduvalli *et al.*, 2004). However, the complex biologic effects of 4-HPR are difficult to evaluate in a clinical trial as a measure of the agent's therapeutic activity. Therefore, we and others have performed studies to understand the molecular mechanism involved in 4-HPR-induced cytotoxicity in high-grade glioma cells.

N-(4-Hydroxyphenyl) Retinamide-Induced Apoptosis in High-Grade Glioma Cells

Initial studies performed in high-grade glioma cell lines identified apoptosis as a primary mechanism of 4-HPR-mediated cytotoxicity (Puduvalli *et al.*, 1999). We performed studies to gain a better insight into the molecular pathway involved in 4-HPR-induced cytotoxicity in high-grade glioma cells (Tiwari *et al.*, 2006). We utilized two different glioma cell lines, U87MG (p53-wild type) and U373MG (p53-mutant), both representing malignant high-grade glioma. Our studies demonstrated that at inhibitory concentration $(IC)_{50}$, 4-HPR induced apoptosis in glioma cells but not in normal astrocytes, suggesting its cancer cell-specific action as shown previously (Asumendi *et al.*, 2000). Moreover, in comparison with 4-HPR, apoptosis was not induced with ATRA and 9-cisRA, even at higher concentrations at which they showed growth inhibitory action in glioma cells. Our data further contributed in delineating part of the apoptotic pathway induced by 4-HPR in high-grade glioma cell lines. Our study to delineate apoptotic pathways demonstrated an involvement of multiple pathways in 4-HPR-mediated cytotoxicity in glioma cells. In glioma cells, the pro-oxidant capacity of 4-HPR was sustained and hydroperoxide production was associated with apoptosis induction. Further, 4-HPR also led to a loss of $\Delta\Psi m$ leading to MMP as a subsequent event to ROS generation, and both were associated events (positive feedback loop) that led to apoptosis in glioma cells. Under various conditions ROS and MMP are often associated with Ca^{2+} homeostasis, and all three are cohort events (Duchen, 1999). Our data suggested an important role of 4-HPR in mediating the disruption of intracellular Ca^{2+} homeostasis and/or ER stress induction in glioma cells. N-(4-hydroxyphenyl) retinamide-induced rise in free cytosolic Ca^{2+} played an important role in apoptosis induction. An association between 4-HPR-induced Ca^{2+} increase, ROS generation, and MPT was also identified in glioma cell lines.

Further, involvement of the intrinsic pathway was observed in 4-HPR-induced apoptosis in glioma cells. 4-HPR mediated upregulation of Bax (a pro-apoptotic protein of the Bcl-2 family) as well as its translocation to mitochondria, leading to release of cytochrome c and AIF in glioma cells. The release of cytochrome c from mitochondria and its interaction with cytosolic factors including Apaf-1 and dATP can activate caspase-9 and then caspases-3 and caspase-7 (Hotchkiss *et al.*, 2009). Accordingly, an activation of caspase-3 and caspase-7 was observed in glioma cells upon 4-HPR treatment. Interestingly, in the presence of pan-caspase inhibitor, oligonucleosomal fragmentation was prevented but peripheral chromatin condition still took place, suggesting that 4-HPR also triggers the caspase-independent pathway. It was further identified that 4-HPR induced AIF nuclear translocation in the presence of caspase inhibitors, which leads to peripheral chromatin condensation in the absence of nuclear fragmentation. AIF nuclear translocation was inhibited by antioxidants and MMP inhibitors, suggesting a role for 4-HPR-induced ROS generation and MMP in AIF-mediated apoptosis. Thus, our study identified that 4-HPR induces parallel pathways of chromatin processing in glioma cells, where nuclear fragmentation is governed by caspases and peripheral chromatin condensation by AIF.

Given the pro-apoptotic role of 4-HPR and its ability to induce apoptosis via multiple pathways in high-grade glioma cells, further studies were performed to evaluate 4-HPR as a combinatorial agent to improve efficacy against glioma cells. Combination of 4-HPR has been studied with a variety of agents to enhance its apoptotic effect, including IFN-gamma (Janardhanan et al., 2008), inhibition of survivin (George et al., 2010), and paclitaxel (Janardhanan et al., 2009). Further studies are warranted to evaluate the potential of these agents in combination with 4-HPR in clinical trials.

N-(4-Hydroxyphenyl) Retinamide-Induced Autophagy in High-Grade Glioma Cells

As discussed previously, we identified that 4-HPR (10 μM, IC$_{50}$) induces apoptosis in high-grade glioma cell lines via a mitochondrial-mediated pathway and generation of endoplasmic reticulum stress (Tiwari et al., 2006). However, we noticed that (1) the IC$_{50}$ concentration of 4-HPR was higher in high-grade glioma cell lines as compared with other cancer cell lines; and (2) an inability of 4-HPR to initiate apoptosis at a lower cytotoxic concentration. These observations led us to investigate why high-grade glioma cell lines show resistance to 4-HPR treatment. Thus, we further performed studies in glioma cells U373MG and U87MG to study the correspondence of 4-HPR-induced cell death with apoptosis in a concentration-dependent manner (Tiwari et al., 2008). Our study demonstrated that even though apoptosis was absent at a lower concentration (5–7 μM), a significant number of cells were still dying. Further, with an increase in concentration of 4-HPR (~10 μM), apoptosis was identified as a primary mode of cell death. These results suggested the existence of an alternative mode of cell death at low doses of 4-HPR in glioma cells. More interestingly, it was observed that the glioma cell lines treated with a lower concentration of 4-HPR could recover and proliferate again when the drug was removed and replaced with the normal media, whereas when the cells were treated with a higher concentration of 4-HPR followed by its removal and replacement with normal growth media the cells could not recover and continued to die. These results suggest that, at a lower concentration, cells could overcome the stress-induced by 4-HPR once it is removed. On the other hand, at a higher concentration of 4-HPR, cells undergo irreversible damage and cannot recover (Figure 16.2).

We further studied the mode of cell death at a lower concentration. U373MG cells were chosen because they are less sensitive to 4-HPR-induced apoptosis as compared with U87MG cells. Results from electron microscopy revealed characteristic features of autophagy with an absence of apoptotic features in the cells treated with a lower concentration (5 μM) of 4-HPR. Numerous autophagic vacuoles, empty vacuoles, and secondary lysosomes with an absence

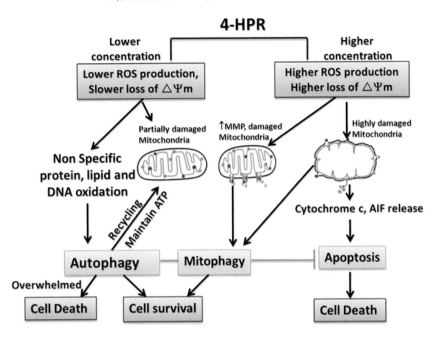

FIGURE 16.2 **4-HPR induces autophagy and apoptosis in a concentration-dependent manner in high-grade glioma cells.** Lower concentration of 4-HPR results in lower ROS generation and loss of $\Delta\Psi$m. Autophagy is activated at a lower concentration that leads to removal of damaged mitochondria and macromolecules. Autophagy also promotes survival of 4-HPR stressed cells by recycling the macromolecules and maintaining ATP levels. At a higher concentration of 4-HPR, a higher level of ROS is produced, leading to higher loss of $\Delta\Psi$m, thus causing mitochondrial membrane permeabilization (MMP), leading to release of pro-apoptotic proteins from mitochondria and thus induction of apoptosis. Autophagy induction at a lower concentration inhibits apoptosis.

of nuclear condensation or fragmentation were observed in cells treated with a 5-µM concentration of 4-HPR. On the other hand, at a higher concentration (10 µM) it was interesting to note the coexistence of autophagy and apoptosis features in 4-HPR-treated cells, as determined by electron microscopy analysis. In the same cell, typical morphological features of apoptosis, such as cell shrinkage, margination, and condensation of chromatin as well as autophagy (e.g., autophagosomes and autophagic vacuoles) were observed. These observations were further confirmed by quantifying acidic vacuoles (AVO) (by acridine orange staining, which increased during autophagy) as well as by performing microtubule-associated protein light chain 3 (LC3) immunocytochemistry (an increase in LC3 puncta due to its association with autophagosomes and/or autophagolysosomes indicates an increase in autophagy). An increase in AVO staining as well as LC3 punctuation was observed at both lower and higher concentrations of 4-HPR in high-grade glioma cells. These findings further confirmed 4-HPR-induced autophagy activation at a lower concentration, and coexistence of autophagy with apoptosis at a higher concentration. Although we reported a dose-dependent response of 4-HPR in inducing autophagy and apoptosis, the molecular switch remains unidentified.

Autophagy is a stress-induced adaptation process in eukaryotic cells. It results in degradation of damaged and unnecessary macromolecules and cellular organelles by lysosomes, thus recycling and proving energy for the survival of the cells (Mizushima, 2007). In the case of cancer cells, chemotherapy-induced autophagy can serve as an adaptive stress response that can promote survival, or as an alternate mode of cell death (Carew et al., 2012). Thus, to understand the role of 4-HPR-induced autophagy in high-grade glioma cells, further studies were performed. Autophagy was inhibited at an early stage, using 3-methyl adenine (3-MA), or at a late stage, using Bafilomycin-A1 (Baf-A1), and 4-HPR-induced cell death was studied. It was observed that inhibition of autophagy at either an early stage or a late stage significantly enhanced cell death induced by 4-HPR, at autophagic as well as apoptotic concentrations. These results suggested a survival role for autophagy induction by 4-HPR in glioma cells.

Our study also demonstrated that 4-HPR-induced autophagy was associated with slow/lower ROS production and loss of $\Delta\Psi$m, whereas apoptosis was associated with rapid and higher enhancement of ROS production and rapid loss of $\Delta\Psi$m. Further, when autophagy was inhibited, enhanced apoptosis was coupled with an increase in mitochondrial depolarization and ROS generation. Thus, these findings indirectly indicated that inhibiting autophagy prevents the removal of damaged mitochondria and may promote MMP and ROS generation, thereby initiating apoptosis (discussed further below). Moreover, mitochondrial dysfunction may be a point of overlap between apoptotic and autophagocytic processes (Thorburn, 2008).

Further, we investigated the molecular mechanisms that were involved in 4-HPR-induced autophagy and apoptosis. Preference for a particular pathway may depend on the intensity of the stimulus, and the cells may choose between the autophagic and the apoptotic execution pathways. Several studies point out that apoptosis and autophagy may be interconnected in some settings, and apoptosis–autophagy interaction may manifest itself in various ways (Thorburn, 2008). Plenty of overlaps of signaling networks are found between autophagy and apoptosis, including various kinases such as MAPKs. Families of MAPKs play a role in complex cellular programs such as proliferation, differentiation, development, transformation, and apoptosis (Widmann et al., 1999). Mainly, three MAPK families have been characterized: JNK, p38-MAPK, and ERK. JNK and p38-MAPK are mainly involved in cell death, and ERK plays a role in survival (Widmann et al., 1999). Our study further identified a role for MAPK in 4-HPR-induced cytotoxicity. It was observed that JNK and p38-MAPK were involved in 4-HPR-induced cytotoxicity at both concentrations (higher and lower); however, ERK1/2 activation was only observed at a lower concentration. Interestingly, inhibition of ERK1/2 enhanced 4-HPR-induced cell death, suggesting a role for ERK1/2 activation in promoting cell survival at a lower concentration.

In our study we also demonstrated that 4-HPR treatment led to activation of NF-κB at a lower concentration but not at a higher concentration. Interestingly, it has been identified that NF-κB is mainly a survival pathway that plays a role in chemoresistance of the cancer cells (Aggarwal, 2004; Béraud et al., 1999). Further, to gain a better insight of the mechanisms of 4-HPR-induced autophagy, a role for Beclin 1 was studied. Beclin 1 is part of a PI3KC3 complex that is essential in mediating the localization of other autophagy proteins to autophagic vesicles; its expression correlates directly with autophagosome formation (Mizushima, 2007). Moreover, Beclin 1 has been identified as a Bcl-2-interacting protein that acts as an anti-autophagy protein via its inhibitory interaction with Beclin 1. Our data demonstrated a considerable upregulation of Beclin 1 and downregulation of Bcl-2 protein expressions in

U373MG cells after 5-µM 4-HPR treatment, which was consistent with the autophagy induction at this concentration. However, the role of Beclin 1 and Bcl-2 family protein in modulating 4-HPR-induced autophagy remains to be investigated. Furthermore, it will be interesting to study the pathways that are involved in 4-HPR-induced autophagy. Since 4-HPR can induce autophagy at a lower concentration and apoptosis at a higher concentration, it is important to identify the molecules involved in the switch between autophagy and apoptosis. Identification of these molecular mechanisms is required for developing therapeutics to improve cancer treatments.

DISCUSSION

The poor response of high-grade glioma to current treatment modalities based on apoptosis induction underscores the need to target non-apoptotic death pathways as well as prosurvival signaling mechanisms that add resistance to conventional therapies. For these reasons, autophagy, which can be either survival-promoting or death-inducing, depending on cellular context, has received increasing scientific attention (Carew et al., 2012; Yang et al., 2011). Autophagy, a cellular homeostatic and recycling mechanism involving lysosome-mediated degradation, is being explored in multiple cancers, including glioma, and is a promising avenue for further therapeutic development. Of interest, autophagy has been shown to be induced by a number of current and experimental glioma therapies (Kaza et al., 2012; Lefranc et al., 2007). It has been identified that high-grade gliomas have lower expression of autophagy-related proteins when compared with low-grade gliomas, and that the progression of gliomas to a high grade is associated with a decrease in autophagic capacity. On the other hand, autophagy has been recognized as an adaptive stress response in high-grade gliomas that helps them maintain their survival in a setting of increased metabolic demands, a hypoxic microenvironment, or cancer therapy. Of interest, several studies have shown that modulation of autophagy sensitizes high-grade glioma cells to standard chemotherapy- and radiotherapy-induced death, but the relevance of these findings in regard to the *in vivo* situation is unknown. Thus, the increasingly recognized relevance of autophagy to tumorigenesis, tumor progression, tumor suppression, and, ultimately, tumor therapy make it an extremely important investigative focus. Currently, the role of promoting autophagy in tumor cells is incompletely understood and may depend on multiple factors, including the extent of induction and duration, and the cellular context. While autophagy mediates tumor cell resistance and survival in some therapies, in other therapies it contributes to the cytotoxic and/or cytostatic response. The specific role of autophagy in promoting survival or death in various therapeutic settings is yet to be clearly elucidated, and this would play a crucial role in designing effective therapeutic combinations (Carew et al., 2012). Thus, in order to target autophagy in glioma cells alone or in combination, researchers are aiming to understand the autophagic process and its potential utility as a therapeutic agent in glioma cells.

In our previous study, we identified that 4-HPR induces apoptosis at a higher concentration (10–15 µM) in high-grade glioma cells, independent of their p53 status, through a mitochondrial-mediated pathway and endoplasmic reticulum stress (Tiwari et al., 2006). However, Phase II clinical trial studies conducted at a lower concentration of 4-HPR (600 mg/m^2 b.i.d.) were associated with a lack of activity, whereas when used at a higher doses (900 mg/m^2 b.i.d.) patients showed a durable radiologic response and remained progression-free, with no substantial toxicity after 13 cycles of therapy (Puduvalli *et al.*, 2004). This finding raised the question of whether glioma cells acquire resistance to the pro-apoptotic effect of 4-HPR at a lower concentration. Incidentally, in our subsequent study on 4-HPR-induced cytotoxicity in glioma cells, we identified that high-grade glioma cells used in our study were comparatively resistant to 4-HPR-induced apoptosis at lower concentrations that were sufficient to induce apoptotic cell death in a variety of other cancer cell lines (Tiwari *et al.*, 2008). Interestingly, we observed that 4-HPR induces survival autophagy at a lower concentration and inhibits apoptosis (summarized in Figure 16.2). To our knowledge, this was the first report that identified the potential of 4-HPR as a pro-autophagic agent. This finding becomes important because high-grade glioma showed resistance to 4-HPR-induced therapy at lower dosage in a clinical trial (Puduvalli *et al.*, 2004). In our study, the high-grade glioma cells had the capacity to undergo apoptosis in response to 4-HPR treatment, suggesting the presence of intact apoptotic machinery; still, the cells showed resistant to apoptosis due to activation of autophagy. Thus, our study proposed targeting autophagy inhibition in combination with 4-HPR to enhance its apoptosis-inducing effect in glioma therapy. Including our study, a growing weight of evidence is suggesting that autophagy, a stress-induced pathway, is important in cell death decisions and can protect cells by preventing them from undergoing apoptosis (Carew *et al.*, 2012).

In regard to autophagy inhibition as a target for combination therapy, to promote the apoptotic potential of existing anticancer agents, it is very important to consider that inhibition of autophagy at different stages, as well as timing, may lead to varied outcome. It has been shown that in the case of imatinib mesylate and temozolomide, chemotherapeutic agents used in glioma, suppression of autophagy at an early stage attenuated cytotoxicity, whereas late-stage inhibition of autophagy enhanced the cytotoxicity through induction of apoptosis (Kanzawa *et al.*, 2004; Shingu *et al.*, 2009). Furthermore, it has been suggested that autophagy inhibition at an early stage by 3-MA, when used concurrently with temozolomide, rescued the tumor cells from death, whereas use of 3-MA after temozolomide treatment enhanced tumor cell death (Kaza *et al.*, 2012). Thus it has been suggested that differing outcomes of autophagy inhibition in various therapies might depend on the nature of the autophagy initiator, the combination therapy used, and other factors that are not yet clearly understood. Currently, several groups are exploring the potential use of combining autophagy inhibition to synergize with the effect of known chemotherapeutic agents to induce tumor cell death by apoptosis induction. Unfortunately, at least from the perspective of a simple explanation, things are not so straightforward, because autophagy can also do the opposite – it can also kill a cell, and can be a prerequisite for apoptosis induction. Various agents that have been implicated in eliciting autophagy-dependent cell death in malignant glioma cell lines include arsenic trioxide, ceramide, temozolomide, sodium selenite, and BH3 mimetic, and radiation has been reported to induce autophagic cell death in malignant glioma cells through mitochondrial and ER-mediated pathways. In these cases, autophagy activation has proven beneficial from therapeutic point of view (Kaza *et al.*, 2012; Lefranc *et al.*, 2007; Yang *et al.*, 2011).

An additional layer of complexity is added by the genetic makeup of the high-grade glioma cells. It has been identified that the genetic makeup of a particular cancer cell determines how the cell responds to autophagy modulation, and this knowledge is critical when formulating therapeutic strategies targeting the autophagy lysosomal pathway. This becomes increasingly important in the context of glioma cells, which display immense genetic heterogeneity.

Returning to understanding how autophagy inhibition can be beneficial as a potential combinatorial approach to enhance the apoptotic potential of 4-HPR and other chemotherapeutic agents, it is not clear how autophagy prevents cells from undergoing apoptosis. However, based on existing evidence it is hypothesized that, during chemotherapeutic stress, autophagy promotes sequestration and lysosome-mediated degradation of the damaged mitochondria, preventing cytochrome c from being released from damaged mitochondria and the formation of functional apoptosomes in the cytoplasm, thus inhibiting apoptosis (Thorburn, 2008). During stress, autophagy also recycles damaged molecules and provides ATP and other macromolecules as energy sources to enable cell survival, thus delaying cell death. Furthermore, since damaged mitochondria are an important source of ROS generation, removal of damaged mitochondria by autophagy prevents accumulation of ROS and oxidative damage, and thus prevents the positive feedback loop that further enhances mitochondrial damage and apoptosis. Interestingly, in our study we observed that inhibition of 4-HPR-induced autophagy led to an increase in apoptosis that was associated with enhanced loss of $\Delta\Psi$m and ROS generation, supporting the proposed hypothesis (Tiwari et al., 2008).

In our study, we also observed that at a higher concentration of 4-HPR at which apoptosis was induced, glioma cells displayed the features of autophagy along with apoptosis, suggesting coexistence of autophagy with apoptosis in glioma cells (Tiwari et al., 2008). It has been observed that dying cells may present features of both autophagy and apoptosis, or the programs may run in parallel (Thorburn, 2008). In some cases, cells may choose between the autophagic and apoptotic execution pathways. Moreover, the complementarity of apoptosis and autophagy suggests mutual interconnections between both programmed cell death pathways; however, the molecular switch remains unidentified. Interactions between autophagy and apoptosis are complex and not yet defined in glioma models. Are the two processes polarized, or are they cooperative? Looking from a different prospective, it is plausible that both apoptotic and autophagic mechanisms underlie the toxicity resulting from 4-HPR-mediated cytotoxicity, with apoptosis being a more critical and dominant mediator of 4HPR-induced cell death. Conversely, apoptosis may negatively regulate autophagy; however, this notion implicates autophagy as a cell survival mechanism in response to 4-HPR treatment. An interesting and novel study would investigate the effects of blocking certain apoptotic regulators on autophagic events in 4-HPR-treated glioma cells. This notion becomes important, since there is a variety of genetic mutations that result in defective apoptotic machinery in glioma cells; in these cases 4-HPR-induced autophagic cell death may have a beneficial role.

Further, in search for the activation of survival pathways that lead to chemoresistance, our study identified a role for NF-κB and ERK1/2 activation, and their role in promoting survival against 4-HPR at autophagic concentration but not at apoptosis-inducing concentration. NF-κB and ERK1/2 are mainly survival pathways that play a role in chemoresistance of the cancer cells (Aggarwal, 2004; Widmann et al., 1999). Thus, specific activation of the survival pathways NF-κB and ERK1/2 at a lower concentration of 4-HPR but not at a higher concentration may explain (1) why the cell shows less sensitivity at a lower concentration and

(2) why, when the drug is removed, the cell starts proliferating again at lower concentration of 4-HPR. Thus, our study also suggests targeting NF-κB and ERK1/2 pathways to inhibit autophagy and enhance 4-HPR-induced apoptosis in high-grade glioma cells.

To our knowledge, we were the first to report the autophagy-inducing ability of 4-HPR (Tiwari *et al.*, 2008). It is encouraging to note that an increasing amount of preclinical evidence validates 4-HPR-induced autophagy in glioma cells as well as other tumor cells, establishing its role as a pro-autophagic drug (Armstrong *et al.*, 2011; Liu *et al.*, 2010; Messner and Cabot, 2011). These studies further confirm the survival role for 4-HPR-induced autophagy in other cancer cell types. Thus, the basis for a combinatorial approach for autophagy inhibition with 4-HPR is further strengthened. Currently, chloroquine, an antimalarial drug that inhibits autophagy at a late stage, is the most widely tested in preclinical models. Also, multiple ongoing Phase I and II clinical trials are evaluating hydroxy-chloroquine for its autophagy inhibitory potential, alone or in combination with cytotoxic chemotherapy or targeted agents, mostly in patients with solid tumors (see review by Yang *et al.*, 2011). However, it is important to note that, presently, there is no existing consensus on how to manipulate autophagy to improve clinical outcomes, and most of the available anti-autophagic drugs lack specificity and antitumor activity.

Targeting autophagy in high-grade gliomas along with 4-HPR may provide new opportunities for drug development. However, more potent and specific inhibitors of autophagy are clearly needed. Thus, newer agents to inhibit autophagy and their evaluation in therapeutic models are required for use as a combinational agent. Biomarkers to measure autophagy modulation during treatment should be an important component of drug development efforts. Although significant strides have been made, several key issues remain unresolved, including how autophagy is regulated in tumor cells, the interplay between autophagy and apoptosis, and the specific mechanism by which autophagy confers treatment resistance. An increased understanding of autophagy in cancer is important for its optimal exploitation for therapeutic advantage. Thus, future studies are warranted to describe the role of autophagy in cancer therapeutics and newer approaches for its modulation.

Taken together, it is now recognized that 4-HPR can target multiple sites of cell death pathways in chemoresistant high-grade glioma cells. Our studies provided additional mechanistic information regarding 4-HPR's mode of action, which involves activation of autophagy and apoptosis in a concentration-dependent manner. This information may contribute to future studies of possible synergism between 4-HPR and other candidate chemotherapeutic agents that can inhibit autophagy for eradication of cancer cells. We believe that continued characterization of the mechanism(s) associated with 4-HPR-induced cytotoxicity are relevant, considering the possible usefulness of 4-HPR in high-grade glioma therapy. This will contribute to the development of mechanism-based strategies for the chemoprevention of cancer.

Acknowledgments

The work was supported by Council for Scientific Industrial Research, New Delhi, India (9/590(33)/2001-EMR-I to MT); Department of Science and Technology, New Delhi, India, through fund for improvement of S&T infrastructure (SR/SO/HS/17/2003 to MMG).

References

Aggarwal, B.B., 2004. Nuclear factor-kappa B: the enemy within. Cancer Cell 6, 203–208.

Armstrong, J.L., Corazzari, M., Martin, S., et al., 2011. Oncogenic B-RAF signaling in melanoma impairs the therapeutic advantage of autophagy inhibition. Clin. Cancer Res. 17, 2216–2226.

Asumendi, A., Morales, M.C., Alvarez, A., et al., 2002. Implication of mitochondria-derived ROS and cardiolipin peroxidation in N-(4-hydroxyphenyl)retinamide-induced apoptosis. Br. J. Cancer 86, 1951–1956.

Béraud, C., Henzel, W.J., Baeuerle, P.A., 1999. Involvement of regulatory and catalytic subunits of phosphoinositide 3-kinase in NF-kappaB activation. Proc. Natl Acad. Sci. USA 96, 429–434.

Butowski, N.A., Chang, S.M., 2006. Glial tumors: the current state of scientific knowledge. Clin. Neurosurg. 53, 106–113.

Carew, J.S., Kelly, K.R., Nawrocki, S.T., 2012. Autophagy as a target for cancer therapy: new developments. Cancer Manag. Res. 4, 357–365.

Chaabane, W., User, S.D., El-Gazzah, M., et al., 2012. Autophagy, apoptosis, mitotosis and necrosis: interdependence between those pathways and effects on cancer. Arch. Immunol. Ther. Exp. (Warsz) Dec 11 (Epub ahead of print).

Duchen, M.R., 1999. Contributions of mitochondria to animal physiology: from homeostatic sensor to calcium signaling and cell death. J. Physiol. 516, 1–17.

George, J., Banik, N.L., Ray, S.K., 2010. Survivin knockdown and concurrent 4-HPR treatment controlled human glioblastoma *in vitro* and *in vivo*. Neuro. Oncol. 12, 1088–1101.

Hail Jr, N., Kim, H.J., Lotan, R., 2006. Mechanisms of fenretinide-induced apoptosis. Apoptosis 11, 1677–1694.

Hotchkiss, R.S., Strasser, A., McDunn, J.E., et al., 2009. Cell death. N. Engl. J. Med. 361, 1570–1583.

Janardhanan, R., Banik, N.L., Ray, S.K., 2008. N-(4-Hydroxyphenyl)retinamide induced differentiation with repression of telomerase and cell cycle to increase interferon-gamma sensitivity for apoptosis in human glioblastoma cells. Cancer Lett. 261, 26–36.

Janardhanan, R., Butler, J.T., Banik, N.L., et al., 2009. N-(4-Hydroxyphenyl) retinamide potentiated paclitaxel for cell cycle arrest and apoptosis in glioblastoma C6 and RG2 cells. Brain Res. 1268, 142–153.

Kanzawa, T., Germano, I.M., Komata, T., et al., 2004. Role of autophagy in temozolomide-induced cytotoxicity for malignant glioma cells. Cell Death Differ. 11, 448–457.

Kaza, N., Kohli, L., Roth, K.A., 2012. Autophagy in brain tumors: a new target for therapeutic intervention. Brain Pathol. 22, 89–98.

Lefranc, F., Facchini, V., Kiss, R., 2007. Proautophagic drugs: a novel means to combat apoptosis-resistant cancers, with a special emphasis on glioblastomas. Oncologist 12, 1395–1403.

Liu, X.W., Su, Y., Zhu, H., et al., 2010. HIF-1α-dependent autophagy protects HeLa cells from fenretinide (4-HPR)-induced apoptosis in hypoxia. Pharmacol. Res. 62, 416–425.

Mawson, A.R., 2012. Retinoids in the treatment of glioma: a new perspective. Cancer Manag. Res. 4, 233–241.

Messner, M.C., Cabot, M.C., 2011. Cytotoxic responses to N-(4-hydroxyphenyl)retinamide in human pancreatic cancer cells. Cancer Chemother. Pharmacol. 68, 477–487.

Mizushima, N., 2007. Autophagy: process and function. Genes Dev. 21, 2861–2873.

Okada, H., Mak, T.W., 2004. Pathways of apoptotic and non-apoptotic death in tumour cells. Nat. Rev. Cancer 4, 592–603.

Puduvalli, V.K., Saito, Y., Xu, R., et al., 1999. Fenretinide activates caspases and induces apoptosis in gliomas. Clin. Cancer Res. 5, 2230–2235.

Puduvalli, V.K., Yung, W.K., Hess, K.R., et al., 2004. North American brain tumor consortium. Phase II study of fenretinide (NSC 374551) in adults with recurrent malignant gliomas: a North American brain tumor consortium study. J. Clin. Oncol. 22, 4282–4289.

Shingu, T., Fujiwara, K., Bögler, O., et al., 2009. Inhibition of autophagy at a late stage enhances imatinib-induced cytotoxicity in human malignant glioma cells. Int. J. Cancer 124, 1060–1071.

Sogno, I., Venè, R., Ferrari, N., et al., 2010. Angioprevention with fenretinide: targeting angiogenesis in prevention and therapeutic strategies. Crit. Rev. Oncol. Hematol. 75, 2–14.

Spinelli, G.P., Miele, E., Lo Russo, G., et al., 2012. Chemotherapy and target therapy in the management of adult high-grade gliomas. Curr. Cancer Drug Targets 12, 1016–1031.

Tabatabai, G., Hegi, M., Stupp, R., et al., 2012. Clinical implications of molecular neuropathology and biomarkers for malignant glioma. Curr. Neurol. Neurosci. Rep 12, 302–307.

Tang, X.H., Gudas, L.J., 2011. Retinoids, retinoic acid receptors, and cancer. Annu. Rev. Pathol. 6, 345–364.

Theodosiou, M., Laudet, V., Schubert, M., 2010. From carrot to clinic: an overview of the retinoic acid signaling pathway. Cell Mol. Life Sci. 67, 1423–1445.

Thorburn, A., 2008. Apoptosis and autophagy: regulatory connections between two supposedly different processes. Apoptosis 13, 1–9.

Tiwari, M., Kumar, A., Sinha, R.A., et al., 2006. Mechanism of 4-HPR-induced apoptosis in glioma cells: evidences suggesting role of mitochondrial-mediated pathway and endoplasmic reticulum stress. Carcinogenesis 27, 2047–2058.

Tiwari, M., Bajpai, V.K., Sahasrabuddhe, A.A., et al., 2008. Inhibition of N-(4-hydroxyphenyl)retinamide-induced autophagy at a lower dose enhances cell death in malignant glioma cells. Carcinogenesis 29, 600–609.

Wen, P.Y., Kesari, S., 2008. Malignant gliomas in adults. N. Engl. J. Med. 359, 492–507.

Widmann, C., Gibson, S., Jarpe, M.B., et al., 1999. Mitogen-activated protein kinase: conservation of a three-kinase module from yeast to human. Physiol. Rev. 79, 143–180.

Yang, Z.J., Chee, C.E., Huang, S., et al., 2011. The role of autophagy in cancer: therapeutic implications. Mol. Cancer Ther. 10, 1533–1541.

Cisplatin Exposure of Squamous Cell Carcinoma Cells Leads to Modulation of the Autophagic Pathway

Rafael Guerrero-Preston and Edward A. Ratovitski

Abstract

Platinum chemotherapy is beneficial for human epithelial cancers because the platinum agents induce DNA damage signaling, leading to initiation of cell cycle arrest and apoptosis, and ultimately to tumor cell death. However, tumor cells often develop chemoresistance to platinum anticancer drugs, because of the initiation of autophagic pathways serving as a cell-protective mechanism against these chemical stresses. Although the molecular events underlying these events are not yet completely understood, the critical role of tumor protein (TP)-p53 family members, as key players in guarding the genome and proteome integrity under stress, is very much appreciated. As transcriptional factors, TP53 members exert their functions through the transcriptional regulation of genes encoding the autophagic intermediates, while also affecting the transcription of microRNA by inducing or reducing their expression in tumor cells sensitive or resistant to chemotherapeutic anticancer drugs. These microRNAs subsequently modulate the expression of

© 2014 Elsevier Inc. All rights reserved.

autophagic proteins and are very likely to change the molecular landscape of tumor-cell response to the anticancer drugs. Thus, a clear and in-depth understanding of molecular pathways leading to modulation of autophagic intermediates through transcription, microRNA modulation, and protein–protein interactions would lead to potentially beneficial adjustments of existing chemotherapeutics supplemented with small molecule- or microRNA-based regimens.

INTRODUCTION

An optimal cellular response to DNA damage/stress (ionizing radiation, oxidative stress, chemotherapeutic drugs, ultraviolet (UV) irradiation, nutrient deprivation, and hypoxia) requires repair of damage and coordination of critical cellular processes such as transcription, translation, and metabolism, and control of cell survival through apoptosis or autophagy (Kroemer *et al.*, 2010).

Platinum-based drugs (cisplatin or cis-diamminedichloridoplatinum-II, as well as carboplatin and oxaliplatin) are often used in the treatment of human epithelial cancers because of their ability to dramatically induce the programmed cell death of neoplastic cells (Borst *et al.*, 2008). After uptake by the cells, cisplatin mediates its toxicity toward tumor cells through binding to DNA, triggering the apoptotic response, and by inducing endoplasmic reticulum stress. Almost all tumors, however, eventually become resistant to platinum chemotherapy

The fate of cisplatin between its uptake and binding to the DNA has recently become centered on the copper transporters (CTR1, ATOX1, and ATP7B), which play a role in the metabolism of copper and cisplatin, as well as in developing cell resistance to them (Blair *et al.*, 2009; Leonhardt *et al.*, 2009; Palm *et al.*, 2011). A few studies report that cancer cells overexpressing ATP7B show higher tolerance to the increasing concentration of cisplatin, thereby suggesting a role for ATP7B in cisplatin resistance. However, siRNA silencing of ATP7B leads to an increase in cancer cell sensitivity to cisplatin. Furthermore, the downregulation of ATP7B in an ovarian cancer mouse model decreases the size of growing tumors by 40% upon cisplatin therapy in an additive manner. Cu-ATPases were suggested to control (directly or indirectly) the availability of the drug in the cytosol rather than directly mediating transport of the cisplatin.

Cisplatin is known to induce DNA damage and leads to the accumulation of activated tumor protein (TP)-p53 family members (Riley *et al.*, 2008; Ryan, 2011). The TP53 transcriptional factors (TP53, TP63, and TP73) respond to DNA damage through the induction of cell cycle checkpoints, cell death, or cellular senescence (Riley *et al.*, 2008). When induced, TP53, TP63, and TP73 alter the expression of a large set of downstream target genes encoding mRNAs and microRNAs, which leads to cell cycle arrest, programmed cell death, and increased DNA repair (Hermeking, 2012). MicroRNA (miR) species, which act through the RNA interference pathway, repress target gene expression at the post-transcriptional and translational levels. Altered expression of microRNA genes has been found in a variety of tumor types, and several functional studies have shown the oncogenic, tumor-suppressive, or apoptotic potential of specific microRNAs (Hermeking, 2012).

Emerging evidence supports the notion that cisplatin-induced autophagy plays a central role in tumor cell resistance to platinum-based therapy (Borst *et al.*, 2008). A dose- and time-dependent induction of autophagy observed in tumor cells following cisplatin treatment is evidenced by upregulation of BECN1 and cisplatin-triggered activation of the AMPK pathway leading to subsequent suppression of mTOR activity (Furuya *et al.*, 2005; Harhaji-Trajkovic *et al.*, 2009). Autophagy is also shown to delay or even inhibit apoptosis in renal tubular epithelial cells exposed to cisplatin cytotoxicity (Kaushal *et al.*, 2008).

Accumulating evidence suggests that induction of autophagy mounts an adaptive cell response preceding or delaying apoptosis mediated by cisplatin exposure, and is likely contributing to chemoresistance in various cancers (Borst *et al.*, 2008; O'Donovan *et al.*, 2011; Rikiishi, 2012). Furthermore, several oncogenes and tumor suppressors, including TP53 family members, were shown to be involved in certain pathways leading to an autophagic outcome (Sui *et al.*, 2011). Although the essential autophagy-like genes (*Atg*) have been identified, the molecular mechanisms through which Atg proteins control autophagy in mammalian cells remain poorly understood (Kroemer *et al.*, 2010).

We previously observed that squamous cell carcinoma (SCC) cells exposed to cisplatin displayed a dramatic downregulation of ΔNp63α through an ATM-dependent phosphorylation mechanism (Huang and Ratovitski, 2010). We also showed that phosphorylated (p)- ΔNp63α is critical for the transcriptional regulation of downstream mRNA and microRNA gene targets in SCC cells (Huang *et al.*, 2011). Finally, we found that p-ΔNp63α regulates autophagic gene expression in cisplatin-treated SCC cells through both transcriptional and post-transcriptional mechanisms (Y. Huang *et al.*, 2012). In this review, we will attempt to summarize the role that TP53 family members play in the transcriptional and post-transcriptional regulation of autophagy and tumor cell response to cisplatin exposure.

THE AUTOPHAGY PATHWAY CONFERS CISPLATIN CHEMORESISTANCE

Autophagy is an intrinsic tightly controlled catabolic cellular process in which proteins and organelles are eliminated through delivery to lysosomes, while preserving cell function and survival (Kroemer *et al.*, 2010). The core pathway of mammalian autophagy begins with the formation of the isolation membrane, and comprises defined molecular steps including: autophagy induction, regulated by the Atg1/unc51-like kinase (ULK) complex; vesicle nucleation, involving the BECN1/class III PI3K complex; vesicle elongation, controlled by two ubiquitin-like conjugation systems (Atg12 and Atg8/LC3); retrieval, in which the transmembrane Atg9 and associated proteins provide lipids and recruit other Atg proteins; and fusion between autophagosomes and lysosomes, involving proteins such as lysosomal-associated membrane protein 2 and Ras-related protein-7, resulting in vesicle breakdown and cargo degradation by lysosomal hydrolases (Frankel and Lund, 2012).

Autophagic pathways can be stimulated by multiple forms of cellular stress, including nutrient or growth factor deprivation, hypoxia, reactive oxygen species, DNA damage, protein aggregates, damaged organelles, or intracellular pathogens. Autophagy is thus a central component of the integrated stress response, which can serve as a cell survival pathway by suppressing apoptosis or just delaying apoptotic cell death (Kroemer *et al.*, 2010).

Emerging evidence supports the notion that cisplatin-induced autophagy plays a central role in tumor cell resistance to platinum-based therapy (Borst *et al.*, 2008). A dose- and time-dependent induction of autophagy observed in tumor cells following cisplatin treatment is evidenced by upregulation of BECN1 and cisplatin-triggered activation of the AMPK pathway leading to a subsequent suppression of mTOR activity (Furuya *et al.*, 2005; Harhaji-Trajkovic *et al.*, 2009). Autophagy is also shown to delay apoptosis in renal tubular epithelial cells exposed to cisplatin cytotoxicity (Kaushal *et al.*, 2008). The switch from autophagy to apoptosis suggests that autophagy induction mediates a pre-apoptotic lag phase observed in renal tubular cells exposed to cisplatin, supporting the idea that autophagy mounts an adaptive cell response that delays apoptosis and might contribute to cisplatin resistance in other cellular systems, including head/neck and ovarian cancers (O'Donovan *et al.*, 2011; Zhang *et al.*, 2012).

Deregulation of autophagy under stress leading to a malfunction of autophagic regulatory mechanisms contributes to cancer- and tumor-cell response to chemotherapy (Kroemer *et al.*, 2010). Pharmacologic or genetic inhibition of autophagy was shown to result in increased cell death, suggesting a protective role of autophagy induced by chemotherapeutic agents (doxorubicin, cisplatin, paclitaxel, tamoxifen, etc.), indicating that autophagy might increase cell survival in the response to DNA damage via BECN1 induction, PARP1 activation, or HMGB1 release (J. Huang *et al.*, 2012; O'Donovan *et al.*, 2011; Wyrsch *et al.*, 2012). Other studies uncovered a significant contribution of the reactive oxygen species-induced ATM activation of TSC2 to regulate mTORC1 signaling and subsequently to autophagy, thereby supporting the cross-talk between the cellular damage response and key pathways involved in metabolism, protein synthesis, and cell survival (Alexander *et al.*, 2010). Prior reports showed that cisplatin exposure leads to an autophagic flux in various pathophysiologic conditions, including tumor cell chemoresistance, nephrotoxicity, and tubular cell injury, shown by available techniques such as immunofluorescence and electron microscopy, LC3B-I/-II conversion, and SQSTM1 degradation (Harhaji-Trajkovic *et al.*, 2009; Huang and Ratovitski, 2010; Y. Huang *et al.*, 2012; Kaushal *et al.*, 2008; Zhang *et al.*, 2012).

We employed the unique cellular models of SCC cells expressing either ΔNp63α -wt (also referred as p-ΔNp63α) or mutated ΔNp63α -S385G (also referred to as non-p-ΔNp63α) proteins, as described elsewhere (Huang and Ratovitski, 2010; Y. Huang *et al.*, 2011, 2012). The advantage of these SCC clones is that, upon cisplatin exposure, ΔNp63α-wt protein undergoes ATM-dependent phosphorylation at serine 385, leading to its subsequent degradation, while mutated ΔNp63α -S385G protein is not phosphorylated and remains fairly stable under cisplatin pressure. In our experimental settings, p-ΔNp63α was shown to activate expression of numerous genes involved in cell death via apoptosis and cell cycle arrest, while non-p-ΔNp63α displayed the characteristics of a prosurvival regulator contributing to tumorigenesis and chemoresistance, and failed to induce either apoptosis or autophagy. We have previously shown that cisplatin exposure of sensitive ΔNp63α-wt cells led to the autophagic flux features assessed by immunofluorescence microscopy and LC3B-I conversion into LC3B-II in the presence of lysosomal inhibitor (Huang and Ratovitski, 2010). However, resistant ΔNp63α -S385G cells, which do not support the ATM-dependent phosphorylation of ΔNp63α, failed to display autophagic characteristics in response to cisplatin treatment. We re-examined this process in more detail, showing that cisplatin exposure induced autophagic flux in ΔNp63α-wt cells, as evidenced by electron microscopy, LC3B-I/LC3B-II conversion, and SQSTM1 degradation in the presence and absence of autophagic/lysosomal inhibitor (Y. Huang *et al.*, 2012).

Using a systems biology approach, previous studies specifically emphasized the role of E2F1, TP53, TP63, SREBP1, USF, AP-1, FOXO1, NFE2, and NAC1 in the regulation of autophagic gene promoters, while miR-10b, 30a, 98, 101, 124, 130, 142, and 204 were shown to act as putative post-transcriptional regulators of the autophagic-lysosomal genes (Jegga *et al.*, 2011; Kusama *et al.*, 2009).

TP53 FAMILY MEMBERS MODULATE AUTOPHAGIC SIGNALING THROUGH TRANSCRIPTIONAL REGULATION

Cisplatin is the most applicable drug for treating various human cancers; however, its efficiency is limited due to development of drug resistance by tumor cells (Ryan, 2011). Cisplatin-induced programmed cell death is associated with expression of specific "cell death" genes and downregulation of "survival" genes (Ryan, 2011). Failure of cancer cells to maintain expression of the former genes may be an important factor in cisplatin resistance (Ryan, 2011). A few oncogenes (e.g., phosphatidylinositol 3-kinase, activated AKT1) inhibit autophagy, while numerous tumor suppressors (e.g., BH3-only proteins, death-associated protein kinase-1, DAPK1, PTEN, tuberous sclerosis complexes 1 and 2, TSC1 and TSC2, and LKB1/STK11) induce autophagy (Kroemer *et al.*, 2010; Ryan, 2011).

As known guardians of genome integrity, p53 and p73 were shown to be involved in autophagic processes (Ryan, 2011). However, there was no evidence that TP63 plays a role in the autophagic pathway. Accumulating evidence clearly suggests that TP53 family transcription factors regulate a network of genes implicated in cell death, and may enhance or fine-tune the autophagic response upon stress stimuli. To date, over 125 protein-coding genes and non-coding RNAs have been shown to be direct transcriptional targets of p53 – i.e., ones defined as genes that contain specific sequences to which p53 binds, leading to activation of their transcription on induction of p53 (Riley *et al.*, 2008). TP53 as a tumor suppressor protein has been implicated in multiple aspects of biological processes, including apoptosis, cell cycle arrest, senescence, metabolism, differentiation, and angiogenesis (Ryan, 2011; Sui *et al.*, 2011). Several studies have shown that TP53 can regulate autophagy in both transcription-dependent and -independent manners (Ryan, 2011; Sui *et al.*, 2011). In addition, p53 participates in homeostatic regulation of energy metabolism, oxidative stress, and amino acid metabolism (Ryan, 2011; Shen *et al.*, 2012). The tumor suppressor TP53 has a well-recognized role in the induction of tumor cell death via transcription of pro-apoptotic genes, or by activating mitochondrial pro-apoptotic molecules (Ryan, 2011). Despite recognition of the roles played by TP53 in both autophagy and apoptosis, little is known about the mechanism that governs the dual roles and the potential switch (Ryan, 2011; Sui *et al.*, 2011).

TP53 can modulate autophagy in a dual fashion, depending on its subcellular localization. TP53 functions as a nuclear transcription factor and transactivates pro-apoptotic, cell cycle-arresting and pro-autophagic genes (Crighton *et al.*, 2006; Eby *et al.*, 2010; Maiuri *et al.*, 2009; Ryan, 2011; Sui *et al.*, 2011). However, cytoplasmic TP53 can trigger a mitochondrial mechanism to promote cell death, and can repress autophagy (Sui *et al.*, 2011; Tasdemir *et al.*, 2008). Genotoxic stress can induce autophagy in a TP53-dependent fashion through transcriptional activation of autophagy-inducing genes. The critical regulators of autophagy, *Dram1* (damage-regulated autophagy modulator) and *Atg1/Ulk1* (autophagy-initiation kinase), are transcriptionally activated by TP53 and subsequently induce autophagic pathways (Ryan, 2011).

TP53 regulates autophagy through two distinct mechanisms. On the one hand, TP53 promotes BCL2 phosphorylation, resulting in dissociation of the BECN1–BCL2 complex (Maiuri *et al.*, 2010). The liberation of BECN1, an essential autophagy modulator, thereby stimulates autophagy. On the other hand, TP53 leads to the upregulation of *Dram1*, which can stimulate the accumulation of autophagosomes by regulating autophagosome–lysosome fusion to generate autolysosomes (Crighton *et al.*, 2006; Eby *et al.*, 2010; Maiuri *et al.*, 2009; Ryan, 2011). In some cases TP53-induced autophagy may lead to cell death, and this can be blocked by *Dram1* siRNA (Crighton *et al.*, 2006). However, p53-mediated autophagy increases cell survival, as blockade of autophagosomal maturation enhances p53-mediated tumor regression and tumor-cell death (Ryan, 2011). Recently, AEN/ISG20L1 was also identified as a TP53- dependent, genotoxic stress-induced modulator of autophagy (Eby *et al.*, 2010). Transcription of *Aen* can be regulated by all three TP53 family members (TP53, TP63, and TP73), and *Aen* knockdown decreases levels of autophagic vacuoles and LC3-II after genotoxic stress, strengthening the connection between TP53 signaling and autophagy (Eby *et al.*, 2010). Several pro-apoptotic genes, such as PUMA (TP53-upregulated modulator of apoptosis) and Bax (Bcl-2-associated X protein), are also positive regulators of autophagy (e.g., mitochondrial autophagy), as reviewed elsewhere (Ryan, 2011). Activated p53 may downregulate the negative regulator of autophagy mTOR (mammalian target of rapamycin) through transcriptional regulation of *Sesn1* and *Sesn2* (Maiuri *et al.*, 2009). The central signaling molecules in determining the levels of autophagy in cancer cells are AMPK, a positive regulator of autophagy, and mTOR, a negative autophagic regulator, which lies upstream of the autophagy core pathway (Alexander *et al.*, 2010). AMPK may also inhibit mTOR by activating TSC1/TSC2. TP53 was shown to regulate various targeted genes in order to activate AMPK, a positive regulator of autophagy, or inhibit mTOR, subsequently inducing autophagy (Alexander *et al.*, 2010).

Recent studies have reported the ability of TP53 to regulate the expression of several cell metabolism-related genes (GAMT, TIGAR, SCO2, PGM, GLUT-1 and -4, and GLS2) with roles in mitochondrial respiration, glycolysis, and oxidative stress. These reports link the TP53 protein with energy metabolism, and provide a novel mechanism through which TP53 might play an important role as a "guardian of metabolic balance" (Cheung and Vousden, 2010). For example, the TP53-target TIGAR (TP53-induced glycolysis and apoptosis regulator) lessens fructose-2, 6-bisphosphate levels in cells, resulting in inhibition of glycolysis and a decrease in intracellular levels of reactive oxygen species. Thus, the regulation of autophagy by p53 is multifaceted: stress-induced activation of p53 promotes autophagy, whereas physiological levels of p53 repress autophagy. The dual effects of p53 reflect the coordinated regulation of cellular metabolism, including autophagy, which can be subverted by nuclear p53 or capitalized on by cytoplasmic p53 during malignant transformation.

TP63 and TP73 share similar structure with TP53, and have both unique and coordinated roles during development and tumorigenesis. Recently, the interplay of mTOR and TP53 was shown. The inhibition of mTOR activated TP73, resulting in TP73-dependent modulation of genes involved in mTOR-induced metabolism and autophagy (Rosenbluth and Pietenpol, 2009). While TP73 transcriptionally regulates the p53 target gene *Dram1*, TP73-dependent autophagy does not require DRAM1 (Crighton *et al.*, 2007). Using ChIP analysis, the endogenous TP73 was shown to bind the regulatory regions of specific autophagic genes, such as *Atg5*, *Atg7*, and *Uvrag* (Rosenbluth and Pietenpol, 2009). Although TP73 was found to induce expression of *Atg5* and *Atg7*, *Tp73* knockdown increased the *Uvrag* expression levels, suggesting that, by binding to a region upstream of the *Uvrag* transcriptional start site, TP73 represses its expression through recruitment of histone deacetylases (Rosenbluth and Pietenpol, 2009).

The TP53 homologue TP63 is a novel transcription factor implicated in regulation of genes involved in the DNA damage response and chemotherapeutic stress in tumor cells (Huang and Ratovitski, 2010). Due to the existence of two independent promoters, the *Tp63* gene encodes two types of protein isotypes: those with the long transactivation (TA) domain, and those with the short TA domain. The latter is designated as ΔNp63α, which is the longest and most predominant isotype expressed in SCC cells. Due to several alternative-splicing events, p63 produces three isotypes with various lengths of the carboxyl terminus (α, β, and γ).

Ataxia-telangiectasia mutated (ATM) protein is a biosensor that coordinates cellular response with various damaging signals to preserve genomic integrity. ATM has been recently implicated in cellular response to elevated reactive oxygen species, and is therefore involved in redox homeostasis (Alexander *et al.*, 2010). The Cheryl Walker research team showed that ATM import to the cytoplasm activates the specific phosphorylation of LKB1 at the threonine 366 position, leading to subsequent TSC2 activation via the LKB1/AMPK metabolic pathway and a reduction in mTOR level, in turn promoting autophagy (Alexander *et al.*, 2010). Moreover, ATM was shown to translocate to cytoplasm, where it phosphorylates LKB1 kinase, subsequently leading to an autophagic process through the AMPK/mTOR signaling pathway (Alexander *et al.*, 2010).

Our previous observations showed that the cisplatin exposure induced the ATM-dependent phosphorylation of ΔNp63α, resulting in the p-ΔNp63α modification and subsequently leading to a proteasome-dependent degradation of ΔNp63α in SCC cells (Huang and Ratovitski, 2010). Our later studies emphasized the role for p-ΔNp63α in transcriptional regulation of numerous gene targets involved in tumor cell response to cisplatin, some of them with pro-apoptotic functions and some with cell survival functions (Y. Huang *et al.*, 2011, 2012). Recent observations defined ΔNp63α as a novel regulator of p53 activation through ATM kinase transcription, thereby supporting a feedback regulatory mechanism (Huang and Ratovitski, 2010). They further reported that the ΔNp63α protein interacts with the ATM promoter-derived CCAAT sequence, previously shown to be critical for the p-ΔNp63α transcription function in SCC upon cisplatin exposure. Intriguingly, these investigators showed that ΔNp63α activates the ATM gene transcription, whereas TAp63α does not, highlighting an essential role for the TA2 domain in mediating ΔNp63α function.

We found that p-ΔNp63α binds the ATM promoter, induces ATM promoter activity, and activates ATM cytoplasmic accumulation (Huang and Ratovitski, 2010). We further found that the p-ΔNp63α protein interacts with the Rpn13 protein, leading to a proteasome-dependent degradation of p-ΔNp63α. We next observed that ATM triggers the LKB1–AMPK–tuberin pathway leading to a downregulation of mTOR and subsequently enhancing the cisplatin-dependent autophagy in wild-type ΔNp63α cells upon cisplatin exposure (Huang and Ratovitski, 2010). Using the SCC cells with an altered ability to support ATM-dependent ΔNp63α phosphorylation, non-p-ΔNp63α failed to form protein complexes with RPN13 and allowed the latter to bind and target LKB1 into a proteasome-dependent degradation pathway, thereby modulating a cisplatin-induced autophagy (Huang and Ratovitski, 2010). SCC cells with the innate resistant/impaired response to cisplatin-induced cell death displayed a greater ratio of non-p-ΔNp63α/p-ΔNp63α than did cells that are sensitive to cisplatin-induced cell death (Huang and Ratovitski, 2010). Based on our findings so far, we suggest that the choice made by RPN13 between targeting p-ΔNp63α or LKB1 for degradation is critical for the cell death decision made by cancer cells in response to chemotherapy. The discovery that the ΔNp63 promoter is subject to both TP53-mediated activation and repression by ΔNp63α, and that ATM-dependent phosphorylation mediates ΔNp63α degradation, suggests that activity in the damage-response ΔNp63α–ATM–TP53 pathway is finely modulated by complex feedback mechanisms (Huang and Ratovitski, 2010).

ΔNp63α was shown to activate *Atm* transcription, thereby contributing to the ATM–TSC2–mTORC1-dependent autophagic pathway (Alexander *et al.*, 2010; Huang and Ratovitski, 2010). However, direct evidence of TP63 involvement in regulation of autophagic flux markers was missing. To fill this gap, we examined the role of p-ΔNp63α versus non-p-ΔNp63α in transcriptional and post-transcriptional regulation of autophagic genes such as *Atg1/Ulk1*, *Atg3*, *Atg4A*, *Atg5*, *Atg6/Becn1*, *Atg7*, *Atg9A*, and *Atg10* in SCC cells upon cisplatin exposure. We found that, in contrast to non-p-ΔNp63α, p-ΔNp63α activated the transcription of specific autophagic promoters and increased the protein levels of tested autophagic proteins after cisplatin treatment (Y. Huang *et al.*, 2012).

Distinct members of autophagic flux exert their specific roles through physical and functional interactions between one another and components of the apoptotic and cell cycle arrest machinery; therefore, the final outcome of cellular response to stress might lead to a variety of choices (Kroemer *et al.*, 2010). During chemotherapy- and UV-induced apoptosis, the UV-resistance-associated gene product, UVRAG, activates the BECN1/PI3KC3 complex, which promotes autophagosome formation. UVRAG also interacts with BAX, thereby inhibiting mitochondrial translocation of the BAX, reducing cytochrome c release, and caspase-9 and -3 activation, and ultimately suppressing apoptosis (Maiuri *et al.*, 2010). BECN1 was shown to interact with several cell death regulators, including Atg14L, UVRAG, BIF1, RUBICON, AMBRA1, HMGB1, etc. BECN1 binds to BIF1 through UVRAG, while activating autophagy (Maiuri *et al.*, 2010). However, BECN1 binds to either Atg14L or UVRAG while forming complexes with PI3KC3 (Maiuri *et al.*, 2010). Interestingly, *Becn1*-specific miR-30a inhibiting BECN1 protein expression was shown to reduce autophagic flux (Zhu *et al.*, 2009). In addition, SQSTM1 was found to associate with Atg8 and LC3B and facilitate degradation of ubiquitinated protein aggregates by autophagy, while cisplatin-resistant tumor cells express much higher levels of SQSTM1 than do cisplatin-sensitive tumor cells (Yu *et al.*, 2011).

Furthermore, the switch from autophagy to apoptosis was shown by downregulation of autophagic proteins BECN1 and Atg7, calpain-mediated cleavage of Atg5, and caspase-8-mediated cleavage of BECN1 (Kroemer *et al.*, 2010). This functional network supports an idea of intricate interplay between autophagic and apoptotic pathways, between cell life and cell death (Kroemer *et al.*, 2010). Although the execution of cell death is usually attributed to apoptosis, cell cycle arrest, and necrosis, autophagic flux signaling plays a critical role in delaying cell death, thereby generating the conditions for temporary cell survival under stress pressure (Kroemer *et al.*, 2010).

Our observations suggest that p-ΔNp63α, along with TP53 and TP73, positively regulates autophagic flux in SCC cells upon cisplatin exposure (Figure 17.1), while non-p-ΔNp63α

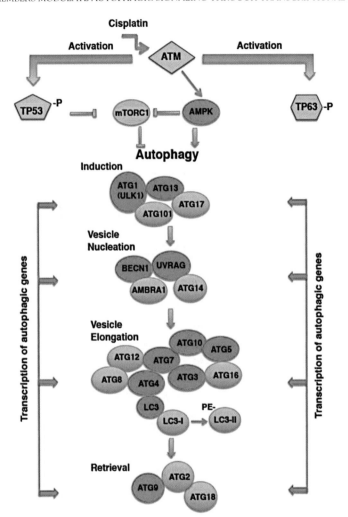

FIGURE 17.1 Cisplatin-induced and ATM-dependent activation (phosphorylation) of TP53 and TP63 leads to regulation of the autophagic intermediates through direct transcription. At the same time, p-TP63 was shown to induce transcription of the ATM gene (Huang and Ratovitski, 2010). As overviewed by Frankel and Lund (2012), the protein complex composed of Atg1 (ULK1/2), Atg101, and Atg13 regulates induction of autophagy; this complex is activated by upstream AMPK and inhibited by upstream mTORC1 signaling pathways, respectively. Both ULK1 and Atg13 are induced by TP53. Vesicle nucleation involves the BECN1 protein complex. BECN1 is induced by both TP53 and TP63, while UVRAG is upregulated by TP63 (Y. Huang *et al.*, 2012). Vesicle elongation is controlled by two ubiquitin-like conjugation systems. LC3 is cleaved by Atg4 to expose a C-terminal glycine allowing conjugation to phosphatidyl-ethanolamine (PE) by Atg7 and Atg3. Atg5 is conjugated to Atg12 by Atg7 and Atg10. Atg5–Atg12 forms a large multimeric complex with Atg16, which functions as the E3 ligase for LC3 isoforms. TP53 induces LC3B transcription, while TP63 was shown to induce Atg4, Atg5, Atg7, and Atg10 expression (Y. Huang *et al.*, 2012). During retrieval the Atg9–Atg2–Atg18 complex participates in recruiting lipids and other regulatory proteins to the growing phagophore. TP63 was found to induce Atg9 transcription in SCC cells upon cisplatin exposure (Y. Huang *et al.*, 2012). All induced proteins are highlighted in red, while reduced proteins (mTORC) are highlighted in green in SCC cells exposed to cisplatin treatment. Red arrows indicate the transcription activation by TP53 and TP63.

plays the role of prosurvival regulator activating *Akt1* transcription (Sen *et al.*, 2011). In contrast to non-p-ΔNp63α, the cisplatin-induced p-ΔNp63α activates key components leading to autophagic flux and is subsequently implicated in the response of cancer cells to chemotherapeutic drugs (Y. Huang *et al.*, 2012).

TP53 PROTEINS REGULATE MicroRNAs THAT CONTROL AUTOPHAGIC SIGNALING

Emerging evidence shows that specific non-coding microRNAs are involved in the regulation of autophagy and play a role in modulating the cross-talk between autophagy and apoptosis (Frankel and Lund, 2012; Xu *et al.*, 2012). microRNAs are engaged in modulation of numerous signaling intermediates of the autophagic pathway (e.g., miR-30a and miR-519a-3p for Atg6/BECN1; miR-17, -20, -93a and -106 for SQSTM1; miR-885-3p for ULK2; miR-630 and miR-374a-5p for UVRAG; miR-30a, miR-181a-5p and miR-374a-5p for Atg5; miR-630 for Atg12; miR-375 for Atg7; miR-519a-3p for Atg10 and Atg16; miR-885-3p for Atg16; miR-101a for Atg4 and RAB5A; and miR-34a for Atg9), as reviewed elsewhere (Frankel and Lund, 2012; Xu *et al.*, 2012).

By modulating BECN1, miR-30a leads to the suppression of the autophagic phenotype in cancer cells, thereby contributing to cancer progression (Zhu *et al.*, 2009; Zou *et al.*, 2012). Atg4–Atg8 conjunction is a crucial step in the autophagosome biogenesis pathway, thereby underscoring the importance of miR-101a-dependent regulation (Frankel *et al.*, 2011). SQSTM1 (p62), a multiple domain protein that acts as a signaling hub, was identified as a key target for multiple microRNAs (Mathew *et al.*, 2009). SQSTM1 can interfere with autophagy via binding to the autophagic regulator Atg8/MAP1LC3 (Mathew *et al.*, 2009). Thus, elimination of SQSTM1 through microRNA modulation may potentially inhibit proliferation of these tumor cells (Mathew *et al.*, 2009).

Intriguingly, several confirmed targets of microRNAs are also important mediators in the cross-regulation between autophagy and apoptosis. For example, the physical interaction between BECN1 and proteins in the anti-apoptotic family (e.g., BCL2) is pivotal for the interplay between the autophagic and apoptotic pathways (Maiuri *et al.*, 2007, 2010). Normally, BECN1 and anti-apoptotic BCL2 proteins can bind to each other to maintain cellular homeostasis (Maiuri *et al.*, 2007, 2010). However, upon stress, BECN1 and BCL2 proteins disassociate, thereby promoting autophagy and inhibiting apoptosis, respectively (Maiuri *et al.*, 2007, 2010). Both proteins have been shown to be modulated by microRNAs: miR-30a reduces the cytoplasmic level of BECN1, while miR-15a and -16 decrease the BCL2 levels (Zhu *et al.*, 2009; Zou *et al.*, 2012). As reviewed by Kroemer *et al.* (2010), SQSTM1 was recently shown to modulate the polyubiquitination and aggregation of CASP8, which is essential for the extrinsic apoptotic pathway, while Atg5, in addition to the promotion of autophagy, enhances susceptibility towards apoptotic stimuli. Enforced expression of *Atg5* renders tumor cells sensitive to chemotherapy, whereas silencing *Atg5* with short interfering RNA results in partial resistance to anticancer drugs. This tumor cell response was associated with calpain-mediated Atg5 cleavage resulting in cytochrome c release and caspase activation, suggesting a molecular link between autophagy and apoptosis and hereby reinforcing new venues in clinical anticancer therapies (Kroemer *et al.*, 2010).

As a transcription factor, TP53 mainly exerts its function through transcriptional regulation of target genes encoding proteins involved in cellular responses (Cheung and Vousden, 2010; Riley *et al.*, 2008; Shen *et al.*, 2012). In addition, accumulating evidence shows that TP53 induces the expression of specific microRNAs, which show tumor suppressive functions (Feng *et al.*, 2011; Hermeking, 2012). As reviewed by Hermeking (2012), TP53 can directly regulate the expression of miR-34 family members. TP53 binds to its specific consensus element in miR-34a and miR-34b/c promoters, and activates transcription of the miR-34 family (Raver-Shapira *et al.*, 2007). Ectopic expression of miR-34a promotes TP53-mediated apoptosis, cell cycle arrest, and senescence, whereas inactivation of endogenous miR-34a strongly inhibits TP53-dependent apoptosis in cells, suggesting a role for miR-34 downstream of TP53 (Raver-Shapira *et al.*, 2007). Studies have shown that miR-34 family members directly repress the expression of several targets involved in the regulation of the cell cycle and in the promotion of cell proliferation and survival, including cyclin E2, cyclin-dependent kinases 4 and 6 (CDK4 and CDK6), and BCL2 (Feng *et al.*, 2011; Hermeking, 2012).

In addition to the miR-34 family, TP53 also directly regulates the transcriptional expression of several additional microRNAs, including miR-107, miR-145, miR-149-3p, miR-192 and miR-215, through binding to their promoters, thereby modulating the multiple signaling pathways that contribute to tumor suppression and cell death (Hermeking, 2012). For example, negative regulation of c-Myc by the TP53-dependent miR-145 accounts partially for the miR-145-mediated inhibition of tumor cell growth both *in vitro* and *in vivo* (Sachdeva *et al.*, 2009), while TP53-dependent miR-192 and miR-215 modulate the expression of regulators of DNA synthesis and the G1 and G2 cell cycle checkpoints, resulting in cell cycle arrest and suppression of tumor cell colony formation (Georges *et al.*, 2008).

It was recently reported that, in response to DNA damage, TP53 promotes the DROSHA-mediated processing of certain microRNAs with growth-suppressive functions, including miR-16-1, miR-143, and miR-145 (Suzuki *et al.*, 2009). These microRNAs are decreased in various human cancers, and overexpression of them reduces tumor cell proliferation. These microRNAs negatively regulate some important regulators of the cell cycle and cell proliferation, such as K-Ras (as a target of miR-143) and CDK6 (as a target of miR-16-1 and miR-145). TP53 was further shown to interact with DROSHA and mediate the interaction of pri-microRNAs with DROSHA in the presence of p68 and p72 RNA helicases, supporting a role for TP53 in the microRNA maturation process (Suzuki *et al.*, 2009). Recently, Elsa Flores' research team elegantly showed that p63 coordinately regulates DICER1 and miR-130b transcription, while suppressing the tumor cell metastatic potential (Su *et al.*, 2010).

We previously found that the exposure of ΔNp63α-wt SCC cells to cisplatin induced the expression of DICER1, which is a critical component of the RNA-induced silencing complex (RISC) implicated in microRNA maturation (Huang *et al.*, 2011). We also showed that p-ΔNp63α induces DICER1 transcription in ΔNp63α-wt SCC cells upon cisplatin exposure. We further found that p-ΔNp63α deregulated (upregulated and downregulated) a number of microRNAs in ΔNp63α-wt SCC cells upon cisplatin exposure (Huang *et al.*, 2011). These data supported a cisplatin-induced and p-ΔNp63α-dependent mechanism of the profound effect of DICER1 expression on microRNA expression and maturation in SCC cells (Huang *et al.*, 2011).

Among the many microRNAs differentially regulated by p-ΔNp63α, a few (181a-5p, 519a-3p, and 374a-5p) showed the highest degree of inhibition, while miR-630 showed the highest degree of activation (Huang *et al.*, 2011). These observations support the cumulative effect of DICER1 on the p-ΔNp63α-dependent upregulated microRNAs and the antagonistic effect of DICER1 on the p-ΔNp63α-dependent downregulated microRNAs (Huang *et al.*, 2011). We then showed that p-ΔNp63α directly affects microRNA transcription by binding to the specific microRNA promoters and regulating microRNA expression levels accordingly (Huang *et al.*, 2011). Finally, we observed that the downstream targets affected by the p-ΔNp63α-dependent modulation of microRNA expression in ΔNp63α-wt SCC cells include critical regulators of TP53-dependent and TP53-independent apoptotic genes (Huang *et al.*, 2011).

There are two potential mechanisms by which p-ΔNp63α can regulate microRNA expression: through DICER1 transcriptional upregulation and subsequent maturation of microRNAs, and/or by direct transcriptional regulation of microRNA gene promoters via formation of protein complexes with other transcriptional and chromatin-associated factors (Huang *et al.*, 2011). On the one hand, the expression of mRNA target genes is maintained through a coupling mechanism that includes transcription factors and microRNA-mediated post-transcriptional machinery (Huang *et al.*, 2011). On the other hand, the microRNA expression levels in cells under various experimental conditions are controlled by dual regulation through transcription factors and by post-transcriptional regulation by RISC components (Huang *et al.*, 2011). It is likely that both mechanisms play specific roles in the cisplatin-induced microRNAome deregulation in SCC cells (Huang *et al.*, 2011).

Our previous report showed that a set of specific microRNAs was also affected by the cisplatin-induced p-ΔNp63α transcription factor leading to a downregulation of miR-181a-5p, miR-519a-3p and miR-374a-5p and upregulation of miR-630 in SCC cells (Huang *et al.*, 2011). We further found that mimics for these microRNAs (miR-181a-5p, miR-519a-3p, miR-374a-5p, and miR-630) downregulated the Atg5, Atg6/ BECN1, Atg10, Atg12, Atg16L1, and UVRAG protein levels, while tested microRNA inhibitors upregulated protein levels of specific autophagic proteins, thereby adding another level of expression control for autophagic pathways in SCC cells upon cisplatin exposure (Y. Huang *et al.*, 2012). Interestingly, some autophagic proteins (e.g., UVRAG) appeared to be targeted by several microRNAs – ones that are downregulated upon cisplatin exposure (e.g., miR-374a-5p) and ones that are upregulated by cisplatin treatment (e.g., miR-630).

Since p-ΔNp63α induced transcription of specific autophagic proteins, while the p-ΔNp63α-dependent microRNAs were set to negatively regulate these proteins (if they are cisplatin-induced, as in miR-630) and positively regulate these proteins (if they are cisplatin-reduced, as in miR-181a-5p, miR-519a-3p, and miR-374a-5p), it was important to show the final outcome of these molecular processes on cell survival upon treatment with cisplatin, and microRNA-specific mimics and inhibitors. Our prior study showed that miR-181a-5p, miR-519a-3p, miR-374a-5p, and miR-630 dramatically reduced levels of cell cycle arrest and pro-apoptotic regulators, such as CDKN1A and 1B, PARP1 and 2, TP73, and YES, and anti-apoptotic regulators, such as BCL2 and BCL2L2 (Huang *et al.*, 2011). Cisplatin treatment of ΔNp63α-wt SCC cells was shown to reduce the levels of miR-181a-5p, miR-519a-3p, and miR-374a-5p, and to concomitantly induce miR-630 levels, thereby leading to drastic changes in the survival of SCC cells (Huang *et al.*, 2011).

We found that cisplatin-sensitive ΔNp63α-wt SCC cells displayed a low viability while treated with cisplatin. However, cisplatin-resistant ΔNp63α-S385G SCC cells showed much greater ability to survive under cisplatin exposure (Huang and Ratovitski, 2010). When the cisplatin pressure was applied to SCC cells in the presence of BAF A$_1$, both ΔNp63α-wt and

ΔNp63α-S385G SCC cells displayed the enhanced cell death phenotype, further supporting that autophagy induced by cisplatin in these experimental settings is likely to protect SCC cells against apoptosis (Y. Huang *et al.*, 2012). miR-519a-3p inhibitor, as well as miR-630 mimic, were shown to reduce the viability of ΔNp63α-wt SCC cells treated with cisplatin (Y. Huang *et al.*, 2012).

We further observed that the exposure of SCC-11 cells to cisplatin led to p-ΔNp63α-dependent modulation of numerous microRNAs potentially implicated in the regulation of autophagic signaling intermediates (Figure 17.2). Although most of the autophagic proteins appeared to be induced, since their corresponding microRNAs are downregulated in SCC-11 cells upon cisplatin exposure, a few proteins are likely to be reduced by upregulated microRNAs (miR-194-5p, miR-297, and miR-630). However, all protein targets (Atg2B, Atg4A, Atg4C, Atg5, Atg10, Atg12, Atg16L1, DRAM1, GABARAPL1, MAP1LC3B, SQSTM1, and UVRAG1) seem to be affected by both downregulated and upregulated microRNAs. In summary, p-ΔNp63α also contributes to regulation of cell cycle arrest, apoptosis, and autophagy through regulation of microRNA expression and processing, ultimately leading to a specific tumor cell response to chemotherapeutic stresses.

DISCUSSION

Accumulating data support the idea that autophagy limits tumor initiation; however, once the neoplastic process is initiated, the autophagic processes play a role in malignant progression and subsequent tumor maintenance (Kroemer *et al.*, 2010; Rikiishi, 2012). Autophagy is also induced in response to cancer therapies, functioning as a survival mechanism for tumor cells and thereby limiting drug efficacy (Rikiishi, 2012). Recently, anti-autophagy therapies emerged as an entirely new approach to cancer treatment, emphasizing that aberrant control of autophagy is among the key hallmarks of cancer (Kroemer *et al.*, 2010).

Emerging evidence supports the notion that TP53 family members regulate tumor cell response to cancer therapies through direct transcriptional control of protein-encoding targets (Figure 17.1) and through microRNA-dependent modulation (Figure 17.2) of levels of proteins involved in cell cycle arrest, apoptosis, or autophagy (Feng *et al.*, 2011; Hermeking, 2012; Ryan, 2011; Sui *et al.*, 2011). Recent studies have demonstrated that the interplay between TP53 family members and microRNAs occurs at multiple levels in tumor cells exposed to chemical, biological, or radiation therapies, as reviewed by Sui *et al.* (2011) and Hermeking (2012).

First, both TP53 and TP63 induce or reduce the expression levels of numerous autophagic intermediates (Figure 17.1), as well as an intricate network of microRNAs, which in turn modulate autophagic proteins (Figure 17.2) in tumor cells affected by anticancer drugs (Hermeking, 2012; Y. Huang *et al.*, 2011, 2012; Iguchi *et al.*, 2010). TP53 induces the transcription expression of miR-34a/b/c, miR-107, miR-145, miR-149, miR-192, and miR-215, while TP63 induces the expression of miR-630 and miR-885-3p, and reduces the levels of miR-181a-5p, miR-374-5p, miR-519a-3p, and others (Figure 17.2). TP53-dependent microRNAs have been shown to be able to mediate the role of TP53 in tumor suppression through inducing apoptosis, cell cycle arrest, and/or senescence (Hermeking, 2012). Second, both TP53 and TP63 promote maturation of certain microRNAs with growth-suppressive function via DROSHA- and DICER-dependent RISC functions, respectively

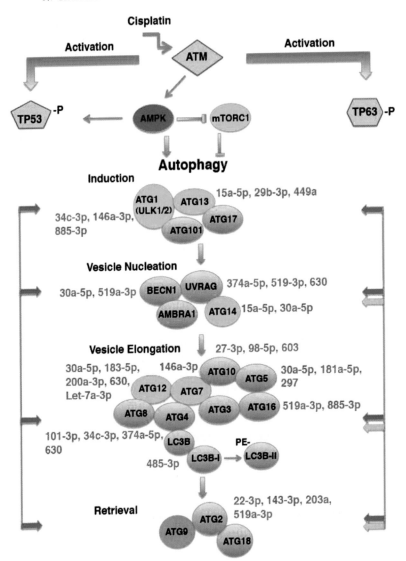

FIGURE 17.2   TP53- and TP63-dependent microRNAs regulate autophagic signaling via microRNA modulation. After being activated by a cisplatin-induced ATM-dependent phosphorylation, both TP53 and TP63 induce or repress the transcription of specific microRNA genes. TP53 induces the following microRNA genes: Let-7a-3p, 15a-5p, 29b-5p, 16a-5p, 30a-5p, 34a-3p, 34b-3p, 101a, 143-3p, 146-p, 200a-3p, and 449a-5p. TP63 induces microRNA genes for 297, 630, and 885-3p, and reduces microRNA genes for 22-3p, 27-3p, 98-5p, 181a-5p, 183-5p, 203a, 374a-5p, 485-3p, and 519a-3p. Induced microRNAs are highlighted in red, while reduced microRNAs are highlighted in green. All microRNAs predicted and tested are depicted next to their corresponding targets. The proteins affected by upregulated microRNAs are repressed and highlighted in green. Red arrows indicate the transcription activation of microRNA genes by TP53 and TP63, while green arrows indicate the transcription repression of microRNA genes by TP63.

(Huang *et al.*, 2011; Su *et al.*, 2010; Suzuki *et al.*, 2009). Third, microRNAs can negatively regulate the function of TP53 members through direct repression of the TP53 or TP63 proteins, or can positively regulate TP53 activity through regulation of some negative regulators of the TP53 protein (Kumar *et al.*, 2011). For example, TP53 can be negatively regulated by specific microRNAs (miR-125b and miR-504), which can directly downregulate TP53 protein levels and function (Hu *et al.*, 2010; Le *et al.*, 2009). At the same time, specific microRNAs positively regulate TP53 through the direct repression of SIRT1 (by miR-34a), p85α (by miR-29), or cyclin G1 (by miR-122), as reviewed by Hermeking (2012). We showed that the TP63 level is modulated by miR-181a-5p, miR-374a-5p, miR-519a-3p, miR-630, and miR-885-3p (Huang *et al.*, 2013).

These findings demonstrated that TP53 family members could mediate the fate of tumor cells toward cell survival or cell death in response to anticancer drugs through the regulation of transcription expression and/or maturation of specific microRNAs (Feng *et al.*, 2011; Hermeking, 2012; Y. Huang *et al.*, 2011, 2012; Iguchi *et al.*, 2010; Ryan, 2011; Sui *et al.*, 2011). At the same time, microRNAs could be a new group of regulators for TP53 proteins, joining a panel of kinases (e.g., ATM, ATR), ubiquitin ligases, and phosphatases that tightly regulate the levels and activity of TP53 members. Deregulation of TP53- and TP63-dependent microRNAs might serve as a key molecular mechanism underlying tumor cell response to anticancer therapies. The relative chemical simplicity of microRNA molecules (mimics or inhibitors) increases the enthusiasm about a potential reverse of the drug-resistant tumor phenotypes and restoration of the tumor-suppressive effects of TP53 or TP63, raising exciting possibilities for novel tumor therapeutic approaches (Rikiishi, 2012). Further studies are needed to understand how to restore TP53 or TP63 function and induce tumor regression by introducing specific mimics for TP53/TP63-dependent microRNAs downregulated in tumors, or by introducing inhibitors for microRNAs upregulated in cancer. These future studies will provide new insights into the interactions between microRNAs and the TP53/TP63 pathway, and open a new window for therapeutic intervention in cancer.

Acknowledgments

This study was supported in part by the Flight Attendant Research Institutions grant (#082469 to EAR), and by National Cancer Institute grants K01-CA164092 and U01-CA84986 (RG-P).

References

Alexander, A., Cai, S.L., Kim, J., et al., 2010. ATM signals to TSC2 in the cytoplasm to regulate mTORC1 in response to ROS. Proc. Natl. Acad. Sci. U.S.A. 107, 4153–4158.

Blair, B.G., Larson, C.A., Safaei, R., et al., 2009. Copper transporter 2 regulates the cellular accumulation and cytotoxicity of cisplatin and carboplatin. Clin. Cancer Res. 15, 4312–4321.

Borst, P., Rottenberg, S., Jonkers, J., 2008. How do real tumors become resistant to cisplatin? Cell Cycle 7, 1353–1359.

Cheung, E.C., Vousden, K.H., 2010. The role of p53 in glucose metabolism. Curr. Opin. Cell Biol. 22, 186–191.

Crighton, D., Wilkinson, S., O'Prey, J., et al., 2006. DRAM, a p53-induced modulator of autophagy, is critical for apoptosis. Cell 126, 121–134.

Crighton, D., O'Prey, J., Bell, H.S., et al., 2007. p73 regulates DRAM-independent autophagy that does not contribute to programmed cell death. Cell Death Differ. 14, 1071–1079.

Eby, K.,G., Rosenbluth, J.M., Mays, D.J., et al., 2010. ISG20L1 is a p53 family target gene that modulates genotoxic stress-induced autophagy. Mol. Cancer 9, 95.

Feng, Z., Zhang, C., Wu, R., et al., 2011. Tumor suppressor p53 meets microRNAs. J. Mol. Cell Biol. 3, 44–50.

Frankel, L.B., Lund, A.H., 2012. MicroRNA regulation of autophagy. Carcinogenesis 33, 2018–2025.

Frankel, L.B., Wen, J., Lees, M., et al., 2011. microRNA-101 is a potent inhibitor of autophagy. EMBO J. 30, 4628–4641.

Furuya, D., Tsuji, N., Yagihashi, A., et al., 2005. Beclin 1 augmented cis-diamminedi-chloroplatinum induced apoptosis via enhancing caspase-9 activity. Exp. Cell Res. 307, 26–40.

Georges, S.A., Biery, M.C., Kim, S.Y., et al., 2008. Coordinated regulation of cell cycle transcripts by p53-Inducible microRNAs, miR-192 and miR-215. Cancer Res. 68, 10105–10112.

Harhaji-Trajkovic, L., Vilimanovich, U., Kravic-Stevovic, T., et al., 2009. AMPK-mediated autophagy inhibits apoptosis in cisplatin-treated tumour cells. J. Cell. Mol. Med. 13, 3644–3654.

Hermeking, H., 2012. MicroRNAs in the p53 network: micromanagement of tumour suppression. Nat. Rev. Cancer 12, 613–626.

Hu, W., Chan, C.S., Wu, R., et al., 2010. Negative regulation of tumor suppressor p53 by microRNA miR-504. Mol. Cell 38, 689–699.

Huang, J., Liu, K., Yu, Y., et al., 2012. Targeting HMGB1-mediated autophagy as a novel therapeutic strategy for osteosarcoma. Autophagy 8, 275–277.

Huang, Y., Ratovitski, E.A., 2010. Phospho-ΔNp63α /Rpn13-dependent regulation of LKB1 degradation modulates autophagy in cancer cells. Aging 2, 959–968.

Huang, Y., Chuang, A., Hao, H., et al., 2011. Phospho-ΔNp63α is a key regulator of the cisplatin-induced microRNAome in cancer cells. Cell Death Differ. 18, 1220–1230.

Huang, Y., Guerrero-Preston, R., Ratovitski, E.A., 2012. Phospho-ΔNp63α-dependent regulation of autophagic signaling through transcription and micro-RNA modulation. Cell Cycle 11, 1247–1259.

Huang, Y., Kesselman, D., Kizub, D., et al., 2013. Phospho-ΔNp63α/microRNA feedback regulation in squamous carcinoma cells upon cisplatin exposure. Cell Cycle 12, 684–697.

Iguchi, H., Kosaka, N., Ochiya, T., 2010. Versatile applications of microRNA in anti-cancer drug discovery: from therapeutics to biomarkers. Curr. Drug Discov. Technol. 7, 95–105.

Jegga, A.G., Schneider, L., Ouyang, X., et al., 2011. Systems biology of the autophagy-lysosomal pathway. Autophagy 7, 477–489.

Kaushal, G.P., Kaushal, V., Herzog, C., et al., 2008. Autophagy delays apoptosis in renal tubular epithelial cells in cisplatin cytotoxicity. Autophagy 4, 710–712.

Kroemer, G., Mariño, G., Levine, B., 2010. Autophagy and the integrated stress response. Mol. Cell 40, 280–293.

Kumar, M., Lu, Z., Takwi, A.A., et al., 2011. Negative regulation of the tumor suppressor p53 gene by microRNAs. Oncogene 30, 843–853.

Kusama, Y., Sato, K., Kimura, N., et al., 2009. Comprehensive analysis of expression pattern and promoter regulation of human autophagy-related genes. Apoptosis 14, 1165–1175.

Le, M.T., Shyh-Chang, C., Xie, N., et al., 2009. MicroRNA-125b is a novel negative regulator of p53. Genes Dev. 23, 862–876.

Leonhardt, K., Gebhardt, R., Mössner, J., et al., 2009. Functional interactions of Cu-ATPase ATP7B with cisplatin and the role of ATP7B in the resistance of cells to the drug. J. Biol. Chem. 284, 7793–7802.

Maiuri, M.C., Malik, S.A., Morselli, E., et al., 2009. Stimulation of autophagy by the p53 target gene Sestrin2. Cell Cycle 8, 1571–1576.

Maiuri, M.C., Criollo, A., Kroemer, G., 2010. Crosstalk between apoptosis and autophagy within the Beclin 1 interactome. EMBO J. 29, 515–611.

Mathew, R., Karp, C.M., Beaudoin, B., et al., 2009. Autophagy suppresses tumorigenesis through elimination of p62. Cell 137, 1062–1075.

O'Donovan, T.R., O'Sullivan, G.C., McKenna, S.L., 2011. Induction of autophagy by drug-resistant esophageal cancer cells promotes their survival and recovery following treatment with chemotherapeutics. Autophagy 7, 509–524.

Palm, M.E., Weise, C.F., Lundin, C., et al., 2011. Cisplatin binds human copper chaperone Atox1 and promotes unfolding *in vitro*. Proc. Natl. Acad. Sci. U.S.A. 108, 6951–6956.

Raver-Shapira, N., Marciano, E., Meiri, E., et al., 2007. Transcriptional activation of miR-34a contributes to p53-mediated apoptosis. Mol. Cell 26, 731–743.

Rikiishi, H., 2012. Autophagic action of new targeting agents in head and neck oncology. Cancer Biol. Ther. 13, 978–991.

Riley, T., Sontag, E., Chen, P., et al., 2008. Transcriptional control of human p53-regulated genes. Nat. Rev. Mol. Cell Biol. 9, 402–412.

Rosenbluth, J.M., Pietenpol, J.A., 2009. mTOR regulates autophagy-associated genes downstream of p73. Autophagy 5, 114–116.

Ryan, K.M., 2011. p53 and autophagy in cancer: guardian of the genome meets guardian of the proteome. Eur. J. Cancer 47, 44–50.

Sachdeva, M., Zhu, S., Wu, F., et al., 2009. p53 represses c-Myc through induction of the tumor suppressor miR-145. Proc. Natl Acad. Sci. U.S.A. 106, 3207–3212.

Sen, T., Sen, N., Brait, M., et al., 2011. DeltaNp63alpha confers tumor cell resistance to cisplatin through the AKT1 transcriptional regulation. Cancer Res. 71, 1167–1176.

Shen, L., Sun, X., Fu, Z., et al., 2012. The fundamental role of the p53 pathway in tumor metabolism and its implication in tumor therapy. Clin. Cancer Res. 18, 1561–1567.

Su, X., Chakravarti, D., Cho, M.S., et al., 2010. TAp63 suppresses metastasis through coordinate regulation of Dicer and miRNAs. Nature 467, 986–990.

Sui, X., Jin, L., Huang, X., et al., 2011. p53 signaling and autophagy in cancer: a revolutionary strategy could be developed for cancer treatment. Autophagy 7, 565–571.

Suzuki, H.I., Yamagata, K., Sugimoto, K., et al., 2009. Modulation of microRNA processing by p53. Nature 460, 529–533.

Tasdemir, E., Maiuri, M.C., Galluzzi, L., et al., 2008. Regulation of autophagy by cytoplasmic p53. Nat. Cell Biol. 10, 676–687.

Wyrsch, P., Blenn, C., Bader, J., et al., 2012. Cell death and autophagy under oxidative stress: roles of poly (ADP-Ribose) polymerases and Ca (2+). Mol. Cell. Biol. 32, 3541–3553.

Xu, J., Wang, Y., Tan, X., et al., 2012. MicroRNAs in autophagy and their emerging roles in crosstalk with apoptosis. Autophagy 8, 873–882.

Yu, H., Su, J., Xu, Y., et al., 2011. p62/SQSTM1 involved in cisplatin resistance in human ovarian cancer cells by clearing ubiquitinated proteins. Eur. J. Cancer 47, 1585–1594.

Zhang, Y., Cheng, Y., Ren, X., et al., 2012. NAC1 modulates sensitivity of ovarian cancer cells to cisplatin by altering the HMGB1-mediated autophagic response. Oncogene 31, 1055–1064.

Zhu, H., Wu, H., Liu, X., et al., 2009. Regulation of autophagy by a beclin 1-targeted microRNA, miR-30a, in cancer cells. Autophagy 5, 816–823.

Zou, Z., Wu, L., Ding, H., et al., 2012. MicroRNA-30a sensitizes tumor cells to cis-platinum via suppressing beclin 1-mediated autophagy. J. Biol. Chem. 287, 4148–4156.

PART III

TUMORS

Autophagy, Stem Cells, and Tumor Dormancy

David A. Gewirtz

Abstract

There is currently a great deal of interest in autophagy, a process whereby a cell digests its constituents to generate energy and metabolic precursors under conditions of stress such as nutrient deprivation. Autophagy may serve as a mechanism for protection of the tumor cell from the effects of radiation and chemotherapy, but may also mediate tumor cell death in response to these challenges. Accumulating evidence indicates that autophagy is also a fundamental characteristic of stem cells, including tumor stem cells. As tumor stem cells are likely to play a central role in tumor dormancy, it appears that autophagy could contribute to the capacity of tumor stem cells to survive for extended periods of time in a dormant state and eventually give rise to recurrent tumors that are primary determinants of morbidity and mortality in cancer patients.

INTRODUCTION

One of the primary factors limiting the effectiveness of current cancer therapies is thought to be the existence of tumor stem cells that are resistant to chemotherapy and radiation through multiple mechanisms, including multidrug resistance, enhanced DNA repair, and the fact that the cells are relatively quiescent. Another factor is the capacity of small subpopulations of tumor cells to remain dormant either at the original site

© 2014 Elsevier Inc. All rights reserved.

of the malignancy or in a metastatic niche, and eventually to recover proliferate capacity, leading to disease recurrence, morbidity, and mortality in cancer patients. It is likely that dormant tumor cells have stem cell properties and, furthermore, that one element that contributes to stemness as well as tumor dormancy is the capacity to carry out autophagy, a process whereby the cell degrades internal constituents to generate energy and metabolic precursors to maintain and prolong survival in a state of quiescence or senescence.

AUTOPHAGY

The recent decade has been marked by recognition of the multiple roles of autophagy in various elements of cancer development and treatment. During the course of autophagy (literally, self-eating), the cell forms double-membraned vesicles that encompass cellular constituents such as mitochondria and endoplasmic reticulum, which are then digested upon fusion of these vesicles (autophagosomes) with lysosomes, with the consequent generation of energy and metabolic precursors (Kundu and Thompson, 2008). Historically, autophagy has long been recognized as a protective response to stress such as nutrient deprivation. With reference to tumor development, autophagy is thought to suppress tumorigenesis, in part, by limiting cytoplasmic damage, genomic instability, and inflammation (Liu and Ryan, 2012) – a premise that is supported by the fact that the loss of certain autophagy genes, such as Beclin, appears to be permissive for cancer development (Yue *et al.*, 2003).

Given that autophagy reflects a cytoprotective response in the face of external or internal stress, it is understandable that tumor cells frequently appear to undergo autophagy as a strategy to evade the impact of exogenously induced stress from cancer chemotherapeutic drugs or radiation therapy, in part by preventing apoptotic cell death from occurring (Abedin *et al.*, 2007; Amaravadi *et al.*, 2007). Conversely, there is convincing evidence indicating that autophagy serves to mediate cell death in response to both radiation and cancer chemotherapeutic drugs, at least in laboratory studies of tumor cells in culture (Bristol *et al.*, 2012; Eisenberg-Lerner and Kimchi, 2009; Kim *et al.*, 2011; Lin *et al.*, 2012; Wilson *et al.*, 2011). Intuitively, this might occur from extended and extensive autophagy that is quantitatively or qualitatively different from cytoprotective autophagy; however, this compelling hypothesis has yet to be clearly supported by data in the literature.

In further evaluating the role of autophagy in cancer chemotherapy and radiotherapy, recent studies using tumors grown in animal models have suggested that tumor cell autophagy generates signals (primarily release of ATP) that alert the immune system to the presence of the tumor, thereby mediating the antitumor action of at least some chemotherapeutic drugs (Michaud *et al.*, 2011). Finally, one study has suggested interdependence between autophagy and oncogene-induced senescence (Young *et al.*, 2009), although a careful analysis of this report clearly indicates that senescence can occur independently of autophagy and is delayed but not abrogated when autophagy is compromised. A similar relationship between chemotherapy-induced autophagy and senescence has recently been observed in our laboratory (Goehe *et al.*, 2012).

TUMOR DORMANCY

In a previous commentary, we proposed that autophagy and senescence may represent dual and complementary efforts of the tumor cell to evade the impact of chemotherapy and/or radiation, allowing the cell to survive for an extended period of time in a state of dormancy (Gewirtz, 2009). In this context, it should be recognized that there is a relatively limited understanding of the nature of tumor dormancy, despite the fact that dormancy is likely to be a central element of tumors that arise either at the primary site or at distant metastatic sites after prolonged periods of apparent remission (Allan *et al.*, 2006–2007). One explanation that has been proposed for tumor dormancy is that tumors in the dormant state have escaped immune surveillance. Although this clearly must be the case if disease is to recur, it is entirely unclear which factor or factors act as stimuli to promote tumor regrowth. In this context, tumor-associated stroma have been implicated in both dormancy and exit from the dormant state (Capparelli *et al.*, 2012).

The relevance of tumor dormancy to the effectiveness of cancer treatment, or lack thereof, is incontrovertible. Schewe and Aguirre-Ghiso (2008) discuss minimal residual disease as a potential source of tumor recurrence that can develop decades after treatment of the original primary tumor, proposing that minimal residual disease might be related to the "existence of survival programs that allow dormant tumor cells to resist therapy and survive for extended periods of time." This latter phrase could be a virtual definition of autophagy. Brackstone *et al.*, (2007) discuss breast cancer recurrence that can occur up to 20 years after diagnosis, and the difference between "solitary dormancy," which is defined as lack of proliferation or apoptosis, generally thought to be in single cells, and "micrometastatic dormancy," which is thought to involve a balance between proliferation and apoptosis. In this context, Trumpp and Wiestler (2008) have proposed that cancer stem cells exist in a state of relative dormancy; cancer stem cells are also characterized by efficient DNA repair, high expression of multidrug resistance phenotypes, and, perhaps most importantly, protection by a hypoxic niche environment, which would be a critical factor that promotes a state of autophagy (Hu *et al.*, 2012).

AUTOPHAGY AND STEM CELLS

A number of studies appear to support the premise that autophagy is a critical factor contributing to "stemness" in the tumor cell. This is a reasonable premise since one generally accepted characteristic of tumor stem cells is their tendency to be slow-growing or quiescent within the general tumor population, at least until the bulk of the population has been eliminated by conventional therapeutic approaches of surgery, chemotherapy, or radiation therapy. This might explain the observation that dormant tumors are apparently stimulated to grow in patients who have undergone tumor resection (Retsky *et al.*, 2008).

It is important to note that there is evidence for recovery of tumor growth from senescent cell populations, and that senescence is likely to be a central component of the dormant state of tumors (Gewirtz *et al.*, 2008; Gewirtz, 2009). Although yet unproven, cells that recover from the senescent state may be derived from a stem cell subpopulation in that stem cells are generally slow-growing or quiescent, and are considered to be relatively resistant to the cytotoxicity of chemotherapy or radiation. Given the evidence (presented below) for the occurrence of autophagy in stem cell populations, it appears reasonable to propose that autophagy is a strategy utilized by tumor stem cells for prolonged survival under conditions of exogenous stress, and that tumor stem cells could be responsible for tumor dormancy and ultimately disease recurrence.

Only a limited number of studies have addressed the presence of autophagy in stem cells. Oliver *et al.* (2012) reported that human mesenchymal stem cells exhibit a high level of constitutive autophagy based on staining with MDH (a dye that identifies autophagic vesicles), studies complemented by the detection of GFP-LC3 labeled vesicles (where LC3 is a component of the autophagic vesicular membrane). These studies were also suggestive of autophagic flux based on accumulation of LC3 in the presence of the autophagy inhibitor Bafilomycin, as well as the degradation of long-lived proteins – a hallmark of autophagic function. However, the protein degradation was apparently observed only with serum starvation, and it is not clear that autophagic flux is an underlying property of the stem cells, particularly given the lack of co-localization of the autophagic vesicles with lysosomes in this paper. Nevertheless, the fact that basal autophagy decreased markedly during the process of cellular differentiation is consistent with a potential contribution of autophagy to maintenance of the stem cell phenotype.

Similar to the studies by Oliver *et al.* (2012), Salemi *et al.* (2012) reported on the relative absence of the p62 protein in adult stem cells, indicative of high autophagic activity, as well as downregulation of autophagy in differentiated cells. Furthermore, Mortensen *et al.* (2011) indicated that autophagy is necessary for maintenance of adult hematopoietic stem cells and for protection against malignant transformation. Again, the fact that these cells were maintained in a hypoxic niche is consistent with the induction of autophagy in a hypoxic environment (Dohi *et al.*, 2012).

Additional support for the involvement of autophagy in stem cell survival is provided by Rausch *et al.* (2012), who reported that stem cell markers, markers of hypoxia, and markers of autophagy (specifically LC3-I conversion to LC3-II, the form associated with autophagic vesicle formation, and GFP-LC3 puncta formation) are co-expressed in patient-derived tissues of pancreatic cancer. Inhibition of autophagy also sensitized pancreatic tumor cells to apoptosis, and diminished clonogenicity, expression of cancer stem cell related genes, and tumorigenicity in mice – findings consistent with the premise that autophagy promotes tumor stem cell survival and tumorigenicity.

Studies in breast cancer also support the premise that autophagy and stem cells are factors in tumor dormancy. Cufí *et al.* (2011) reported that the residual breast tumor cell population surviving after radiation, chemotherapy, and endocrine therapy is enriched in a CD44 high/CD24 low (stem cell markers) cell subpopulation with both tumor initiating and mesenchymal features; complementary studies indicated that genetic and pharmacological ablation of autophagy regulatory genes reduced the number of cells with breast tumor stem cell characteristics.

Similarly, Gong *et al.* (2013) reported high levels of autophagic flux in breast tumor cells that are CD44 high, CD24 low, which express ALDH (aldehyde dehydrogenase), another stem cell marker, and which can regenerate tumors in mammary fat pads of immunodeficient mice as well as form mammospheres in serum-free medium. More specifically, these cells demonstrated increases in LC3 puncta formation, p62 degradation, and levels of LC3-II.

Furthermore, the number and size of mammospheres and *in vivo* tumorigenicity was reduced when the autophagy regulatory gene, Beclin 1, was silenced, and secondary mammosphere formation was abolished with pharmacological autophagy inhibition or genetic silencing.

Finally, studies by Lu *et al.* (2008) have demonstrated that the ras homolog ARHI induces autophagy, which appears to enable ovarian tumor cells to remain dormant when grown as xenografts in mice. Inhibition of autophagy with chloroquine reduced regrowth upon reduction of ARHI levels, suggesting that autophagy contributed to survival of dormant ovarian tumor cells.

SUMMARY

The relative dearth of information relating to autophagy and tumor dormancy is in large part a consequence of the absence of appropriate and generally accepted model systems of tumor dormancy. Despite the fact that the eventual escape from tumor dormancy and recurrence of disease, either at the primary site or at distant sites to which the tumor cells have metastasized, is responsible for morbidity and mortality in the vast majority of cancer cases, there is insufficient understanding of the factors that contribute to tumor dormancy and the involvement of stem cells in this phenomenon. However, based on the currently available literature, dormant tumors are likely to express stem cell characteristics with autophagy contributing to the capacity of tumor stem cells to survive in a prolonged state of dormancy.

References

Abedin, M.J., Wang, D., McDonnell, M.A., et al., 2007. Autophagy delays apoptotic death in breast cancer cells following DNA damage. Cell Death Differ. 14, 500–510.

Allan, A.L., Vantyghem, S.A., Tuck, A.B., et al., 2006–2007. Tumor dormancy and cancer stem cells: implications for the biology and treatment of breast cancer metastasis. Breast Dis. 26, 87–98 [Review].

Amaravadi, R.K., Yu, D., Lum, J.J., et al., 2007. Autophagy inhibition enhances therapy-induced apoptosis in a Myc-induced model of lymphoma. J. Clin. Invest. 117, 326–336.

Brackstone, M., Townson, J.L., Chambers, A.F., 2007. Tumour dormancy in breast cancer: an update. Breast Cancer Res. 9, 208–215.

Bristol, M.L., Di, X., Beckman, M.J., et al., 2012. Dual functions of autophagy in the response of breast tumor cells to radiation: cytoprotective autophagy with radiation alone and cytotoxic autophagy in radiosensitization by vitamin D3. Autophagy 8, 739–753.

Capparelli, C., Guido, C., Whitaker-Menezes, D., et al., 2012. Autophagy and senescence in cancer-associated fibroblasts metabolically supports tumor growth and metastasis via glycolysis and ketone production. Cell Cycle 11, 2285–2302.

Cufí, S., Vazquez-Martin, A., Oliveras-Ferraros, C., et al., 2011. Autophagy positively regulates the CD44(+) CD24(−/low) breast cancer stem-like phenotype. Cell Cycle 10, 3871–3885.

Dohi, E., Tanaka, S., Seki, T., et al., 2012. Hypoxic stress activates chaperone-mediated autophagy and modulates neuronal cell survival. Neurochem. Int. 60, 431–442.

Eisenberg-Lerner, A., Kimchi, A., 2009. The paradox of autophagy and its implication in cancer etiology and therapy. Apoptosis 14, 376–391 [Review].

Gewirtz, D.A., 2009. Autophagy, senescence and tumor dormancy in cancer. Autophagy 5, 1232–1234.

Gewirtz, D.A., Holt, S.E., Elmore, L.W., 2008. Accelerated senescence: an emerging role in tumor cell response to chemotherapy and radiation. Biochem. Pharmacol. 76, 947–957.

Goehe, R.W., Di, X., Sharma, K., et al., 2012. The autophagy-senescence connection in chemotherapy: must tumor cells (self) eat before they sleep? J. Pharmacol. Exp. Ther. 343, 763–778.

Gong, C., Bauvy, C., Tonelli, G., et al., 2013. Beclin 1 and autophagy are required for the tumorigenicity of breast cancer stem-like/progenitor cells. Oncogene 32, 2261–2272.

Hu, Y.L., Jahangiri, A., De Lay, M., et al., 2012. Hypoxia-induced tumor cell autophagy mediates resistance to anti-angiogenic therapy. Autophagy 8, 979–981.

Kim, K.W., Speirs, C.K., Jung, D.K., et al., 2011. The zinc ionophore PCI-5002 radiosensitizes non-small cell lung cancer cells by enhancing autophagic cell death. J. Thorac. Oncol. 6, 1542–1552.

Kundu, M., Thompson, C.B., 2008. Autophagy: basic principles and relevance to disease. Annu. Rev. Pathol. 3, 427–455 [Review].

Lin, C.I., Whang, E.E., Lorch, J.H., et al., 2012. Autophagic activation potentiates the antiproliferative effects of tyrosine kinase inhibitors in medullary thyroid cancer. Surgery 152, 1142–1149.

Liu, E.Y., Ryan, K.M., 2012. Autophagy and cancer – issues we need to digest. J. Cell Sci. 125, 2349–2358.

Lu, Z., Luo, R.Z., Lu, Y., et al., 2008. The tumor suppressor gene ARHI regulates autophagy and tumor dormancy in human ovarian cancer cells. J. Clin. Invest. 118, 3917–3929.

Michaud, M., Martins, I., Sukkurwala, A.Q., et al., 2011. Autophagy-dependent anticancer immune responses induced by chemotherapeutic agents in mice. Science 334, 1573–1577.

Mortensen, M., Soilleux, E.J., Djordjevic, G., et al., 2011. The autophagy protein Atg7 is essential for hematopoietic stem cell maintenance. J. Exp. Med. 208, 455–467.

Oliver, L., Hue, E., Priault, M., et al., 2012. Basal autophagy decreased during the differentiation of human adult mesenchymal stem cells. Stem Cells Dev. Jun 13.

Rausch, V., Liu, L., Apel, A., et al., 2012. Autophagy mediates survival of pancreatic tumour-initiating cells in a hypoxic microenvironment. J. Pathol. 227, 325–335.

Retsky, M.W., Demicheli, R., Hrushesky, W.J., et al., 2008. Dormancy and surgery-driven escape from dormancy help explain some clinical features of breast cancer. APMIS 116, 730–741 [Review].

Salemi, S., Yousefi, S., Constantinescu, M.A., et al., 2012. Autophagy is required for self-renewal and differentiation of adult human stem cells. Cell Res. 22, 432–435.

Schewe, D.M., Aguirre-Ghiso, J.A., 2008. ATF6alpha–Rheb–mTOR signaling promotes survival of dormant tumor cells *in vivo*. Proc. Natl. Acad. Sci. USA 105, 10519–10524.

Trumpp, A., Wiestler, O.D., 2008. Mechanisms of disease: cancer stem cells – targeting the evil twin. Nat. Clin. Pract. Oncol. 5, 337–347 [Review].

Wilson, E.N., Bristol, M.L., Di, X., et al., 2011. A switch between cytoprotective and cytotoxic autophagy in the radiosensitization of breast tumor cells by chloroquine and vitamin D. Horm. Cancer 2, 272–285.

Young, A.R., Narita, M., Ferreira, M., et al., 2009. Autophagy mediates the mitotic senescence transition. Genes Dev. 23, 798–803.

Yue, Z., Jin, S., Yang, C., et al., 2003. Beclin 1, an autophagy gene essential for early embryonic development, is a haploinsufficient tumor suppressor. Proc. Natl. Acad. Sci. USA 100, 15077–15082.

Death-Associated Protein Kinase 1 Suppresses Tumor Growth and Metastasis via Autophagy and Apoptosis

Padmaja Gade and Dhan V. Kalvakolanu

Abstract

Death associated protein kinase 1 (DAPK1) is a calcium- and calmodulin-dependent serine/threonine protein kinase that controls the cell cycle, apoptosis, autophagy, and tumor metastasis. Its expression is frequently suppressed in a wide variety of tumors. The tumor-suppressive function of DAPK1 is linked to its role in cell death via apoptosis and autophagy, as numerous cell death signals employ it. Importantly, several studies reveal a complex regulation of DAPK1 activity by various signaling pathways, thus modulating the balance between pro-apoptotic and prosurvival pathways. This chapter will describe the regulation of DAPK1 expression and the mechanisms of its function in apoptosis and autophagy.

© 2014 Elsevier Inc. All rights reserved.

INTRODUCTION

Aberrant growth promotion occurs owing to the inactivation of tumor suppressors and activation of oncogenes. The Hanahan–Weinberg model (Hanahan and Weinberg, 2000) suggests that at least 10 different genetic and physiologic alterations occur in a mammalian cell prior to reaching the full-blown malignant state. These include an acquisition of self sufficiency for perpetual growth, resistance to apoptosis, enhanced motility, development of neovasculature, activation of tumor-proliferating inflammation, and suppression of anti-tumor immunity. The blockade of cell division and/or an induction of programmed cell death are the primary innate tumor-suppressive mechanisms in mammals (Hanahan and Weinberg, 2000). The cell death nomenclature committee proposed 12 types of cell death modalities (4 typical and 8 atypical), depending on the morphology (Kroemer *et al.*, 2009). Among the typical ones, apoptosis, autophagy, necrosis, and cornification are the best characterized modes of cell death. Apoptotic cell death, once triggered, unfolds into a precisely choreographed series of proteolytic steps that dismantle organelles, and fragmentation of chromatin, culminating in self-elimination. While the contribution of loss in apoptotic machinery to tumor growth is well recognized, it is not the sole means by which a cell commits suicide. Autophagy, a process long known to play a protective role to alleviate the harmful effects of intracellular and environmental stress, also functions as a prodeath factor. Cornification, which represents terminal differentiation, is a special form of programmed cell death that primarily occurs in the epidermis. Although necrosis was considered an accidental uncontrolled form of cell death, accumulating data show that it is also mediated by specific set of signal transduction pathways and cell-degrading mechanisms involving the RIP family of serine/threonine kinases. In contrast to apoptosis and autophagy, in tumors necrosis is associated with inflammation, which further stimulates tumor cell survival and growth. Consistent with the morphological differences between autophagy, apoptosis, and necrosis, there are significant biochemical differences in these processes. While apoptosis is primarily a caspase-driven cell-dismantling process, necrosis is controlled by protein kinase-driven mitochondrial reactive oxygen species-dependent cellular explosion. Autophagy, on the other hand, occurs through protein kinases, ubiquitylation, and lysosome-mediated destruction of cellular contents. In general, apoptosis and autophagy do not cause inflammatory response.

The interferon (IFN) family of cytokines, originally identified as inhibitors of viral replication, influences cell survival through their effects on apoptosis and autophagy. IFNs induce these actions by regulating a number of genes (Stark *et al.*, 1998). The three main classes of IFNs, type I (IFN-α, β, ω, κ), type II (IFN-γ), and type III (IFN-λ1, λ2), use distinct receptors for inducing gene expression. Among these, IFN-γ is a potent immunomodulatory cytokine which regulates antiproliferative, anti-angiogenic, and adaptive immune responses (Stark *et al.*, 1998). IFN-γ causes tumor suppression by directly activating growth-suppressive genes and modulating cancer immunosurveillance.

Depending on the type and intensity of stimulus, cells execute different types of cell death programs that depend on various organelles. For example, apoptosis activated through the intrinsic pathway depends on mitochondria, whereas autophagy employs endoplasmic reticulum and lysosomes. Though suppression of tumorigenesis through a restoration of apoptosis is well known, the contribution of autophagy to suppression of tumorigenesis is still under exploration. Autophagy comes into the picture during at least three different phases in the development of a neoplastic cell (Eisenberg-Lerner *et al.*, 2009). Basal autophagy, which plays a housekeeping role, is essential for protein and organelle turnover and survival under stress or starvation. However, when autophagy exceeds minimal levels it promotes cell death. At the precancerous stage(s), autophagy eliminates cells bearing damaged DNA or organelles to maintain genomic integrity. If the damage or mutations are extensive and if the cells are transformed, elevated autophagy culminates in apoptosis and eliminates the transformed cells. Suppression of apoptosis and/or autophagy at this level will accelerate tumor development. Three different modes of interplay occur between apoptosis and autophagy, depending on the cellular microenvironment and stimulus. In the first form, both apoptosis and autophagy act as partners to induce cell death in a cooperative manner. In the second form, autophagy antagonizes apoptosis to promote cell survival. In the third form, autophagy acts as an enabler of apoptosis, thus promoting apoptotic cell death. Thus, both autophagy and apoptosis contribute to cell death from the front end in the first form, whereas in the third form autophagy indirectly promotes cell death through apoptosis. Such an interplay between apoptosis and autophagy has a major impact on tumor evolution (Eisenberg-Lerner *et al.*, 2009). Signifying the importance of these processes, several apoptosis- and/or autophagy-associated genes are downregulated in tumor cells. For example, many of the same regulators, such as *p53* and *p19^{ARF}* (regulatory genes), and also some basic cell death executive machinery like Atg5 and Bcl-2, participate in both processes (Eisenberg-Lerner *et al.*, 2009). Thus, it is of great interest to understand the molecular links between these two pathways and exploit them for the induction or inhibition of cell death.

DAPK1 activity is critical for apoptotic cell death induced by various signals, including hyperproliferation signals, death receptor activation, oncogene expression, ceramide, and TGF-β (Bialik and Kimchi, 2006). Importantly, DAPK1 activity is also critical for IFN-γ induced autophagic cell death in HeLa cells. Thus, DAPK1 is emerging as one protein that controls both autophagy and apoptosis. DAPK1 is a Ca^{2+}/calmodulin-regulated actin cytoskeleton-associated serine/threonine kinase (Bialik and Kimchi, 2006). It harbors an N-terminal kinase domain followed by a Ca^{2+}/calmodulin regulatory domain, ankyrin repeats, a cytoskeletal binding region, and a C-terminal death domain (Figure 19.1A). It is the founding member of a death-related kinase family which includes DAPK-related protein 2 (DAPK-2), Zipper interacting kinase (ZIPK or DAPK3), DAP kinase-related apoptosis-inducing protein kinase 1 (DRAK1), and DRAK2. These enzymes share a high degree of homology in their kinase domains but differ markedly in their non-catalytic domains and biological functions (Bialik and Kimchi, 2006). Although DAPK1 was originally identified as a regulator of IFN-γ-induced apoptotic death, it is also activated by disparate stimuli, such as TNF-α, Fas ligand, ceramide, TGF-β, arsenic trioxide, activated oncogenes, and DNA damage agents (Bialik and Kimchi, 2006) (Figure 19.1B). DAPK1 suppresses tumor cell metastasis. Consistent with this, DAPK1 expression is lost in a variety of tumor cell lines – in around 80% of primary B cell lymphoma and leukemia cell lines, and 30–40% of cell lines derived from bladder, breast, and renal carcinomas (Bialik and Kimchi, 2006).

DAPK1 AND APOPTOSIS

Apoptotic cell death is a homeostatic mechanism that maintains cell numbers in the body under different physiopathological conditions (Kroemer *et al.*, 2009). Aberrations in the

(A)

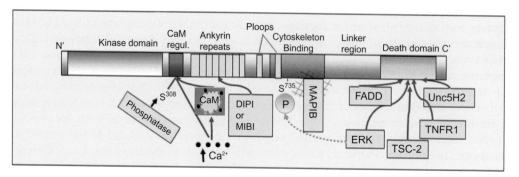

(B)

FIGURE 19.1   **(A) A modular representation of DAPK1 structure and its interactions promoting activation, autophagy and/or apoptosis.** DAPK1 protein harbors several domains with various functions, which accounts for its activation and/or participation in different pathways. In addition to the kinase domain, DAPK1 also harbors ankyrin repeats and death domains for mediating its interactions with other proteins as shown. The cytoskeletal binding domain facilitates DAPK1 localization to actin microfilaments in the cell. The Ca^{2+}/CaM binding regulatory domain (CaM regul.) facilitates activation of the kinase upon the election of cytosolic calcium levels. In addition to the CaM regulatory domain, autophosphorylation at S^{308} results in the inactive state of DAPK1, maintained in normal cells. ERK dependent phosphorylation at S^{735} of the cytoskeletal binding domain is known to regulate DAPK1 activity. See the text for more details. **(B) Upstream signals driving DAPK1 induction and activation, and cellular outcomes.** A wide variety of cell death stimuli regulate DAPK1. This results in p53-dependent or -independent activation of apoptosis and autophagy. Further, DAPK1-dependent phosphorylation of myosin light chain protein in association with weakening of the cortical actin network results in membrane blebbing, one of the hallmarks of programmed cell death.

regulation of apoptosis result in cell survival, and hence tumor cells gain selective advantage by hindering apoptosis. DAPK1 overexpression results in apoptotic morphological changes, including rounding and shrinkage of the cells. It participates in apoptotic pathways induced by TNF-α, TGF-β, and Fas (Bialik and Kimchi, 2006). The kinase activity of DAPK1 is required for the biological effects, whereas the death domain regulates its pro-apoptotic function by interacting with extracellular signal-regulated kinase (ERK), UNC5H2 (netrin-1 receptor), and members of the tumor necrosis factor receptor super family TNFR1 (TNF-α receptor) and Fas-associated protein with death domain (FADD) (Figure 19.1A) (Bialik and Kimchi, 2006).

ERK-dependent phosphorylation event at DAPK1 S^{735} (in the cytoskeletal binding domain) is known to be involved in the regulation of DAPK1 activity. Increased phosphorylation at S^{735} correlated well with increased phosphorylation of DAPK1 substrate, myosin- II regulatory light chain (MLC), and increased killing activity by the overexpressed DAPK1. In fact, the apoptotic effect of DAPK1 is the result of the bidirectional signals from ERK–DAPK1 interactions (Bialik and Kimchi, 2006) (Figure 19.2). Activated DAPK1 retains ERK in the cytoplasm and makes it unavailable for its growth-promoting activities.

In other models of apoptosis, DAPK1 is associated with tumor suppressor p53 (Figure 19.2). One of the mechanisms mediating the DAPK1-induced p53-dependent tumor suppression came from the study of malignant transformation in primary rodent embryonic fibroblasts (Martoriati et al., 2005). In this study, co-expression of Dapk1 with a combination of oncogenes, such as Myc/Ras or E1A/Ras, resulted in suppression of transformation by these pairs of oncogenes. Fibroblasts, expressing T antigen and Ras, were refractive to Dapk1-mediated tumor suppression and became susceptible to apoptosis only after deletion of the T antigen binding site of p53 (Martoriati et al., 2005). Further, studies using p53 knockout fibroblasts also showed that the transformation suppressive activity of DAPK1 was p53 dependent (Martoriati et al., 2005). In non-transformed cells, unscheduled activation of oncogenes induces activation of cell cycle check points and suppresses apoptosis to prevent uncontrolled division. One such oncogene-induced pathway involves Dapk1-dependent activation of p53 by $p19^{ARF}$, an inhibitor of Mdm2 (Martoriati et al., 2005). Dapk1 upregulated by hyperproliferative signals like E2F1 and c-myc activates an intrinsic p53-dependent apoptotic check point (Raveh et al., 2001). Dapk1 operates upstream of $p19^{ARF}$, activating p53 transcriptional activity. The upregulated Dapk1 and activated p53 suppress oncogenic transformation of cells (Raveh et al., 2001). Dapk1 overexpression induces p53 transcriptional activity in a $p19^{ARF}$-dependent manner in fibroblasts. Dapk1-induced cell death in fibroblasts requires both p53 and $p19^{ARF}$. DAPK1 is also a direct transcriptional target of p53 (Martoriati et al., 2005). Thus, an autoregulatory feedback loop exists between DAPK1 and p53, which controls apoptosis (Raveh et al., 2001). In the absence of DAPK1, p53 is only partially expressed.

Moreover, DAPK1 levels are inversely correlated with the metastatic potential of the tumors, and reintroduction of DAPK1 into the metastatic tumor cells suppresses their metastatic potential in vivo (Bialik and Kimchi, 2006). Overexpression of DAPK1 in carcinoma cell lines devoid of a functional p53 induces activation of autophagic cell death (Bialik and Kimchi, 2006). Thus, loss of DAPK1 expression in cancer cells may result in attenuation of p53-dependent apoptotic signals triggered by oncogenes. Occasionally DAPK1 is also linked to the apoptotic route in a p53-independent manner. For instance, TGF-β-induced DAPK1 activation and mitochondrion-dependent apoptosis is significantly blocked by expression of

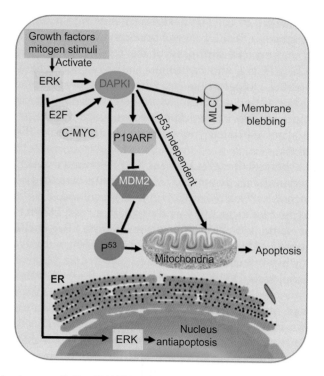

FIGURE 19.2 **Mechanisms mediating DAPK1 action in apoptosis.** Schematic representation of the mechanisms mediating the action of DAPK1 in apoptosis. ERK-dependent phosphorylation of DAPK1 is known to regulate DAPK1 activity. Increased DAPK1 activity leads to increased phosphorylation of myosin- II regulatory light chain (MLC) and increased membrane blebbing. The apoptotic effect of DAPK1 is the result of the bidirectional signals from ERK-DAPK1 interactions. Activated DAPK1 retains ERK in the cytoplasm and makes it unavailable for its growth promoting activities in the nucleus. Dapk1 is upregulated by hyperproliferative signals like E2F1 and c-myc which further activates an intrinsic p53 dependent apoptotic check point. DAPK1 operates upstream of p19ARF, activating p53 transcriptional activity. DAPK1 is also a direct transcriptional target of p53. Thus, an autoregulatory feedback loop exists between DAPK1 and p53, which controls apoptosis. Further, DAPK1 also induces apoptosis in a p53 independent manner. See the text for more details.

the dominant negative mutant of DAPK1 or by antisense inhibition of DAPK1 expression in p53-null hepatoma cells (Bialik and Kimchi, 2006). Thus, DAPK1 can also drive apoptosis in a p53-independent manner.

Interestingly, both ERK and UNC5H2 interact with the death domain of DAPK1 (Bialik and Kimchi, 2006). In the absence of Netrin1 (neuroimmune guidance cue), UNC5H2 (Netrin1 receptor) adopts an open confirmation and recruits PR65β/PP2A (a serine/threonine phosphatase) into the UNC5H2–DAPK1 complex. The recruitment of PR65β/PP2A led to dephosphorylation of DAPK1 at S^{308}, and activation of apoptosis. Interestingly, dephosphorylation of S^{308} opens the locked confirmation of the Ca^{2+}/calmodulin regulatory domain and increases its affinity for CaM, thus promoting DAPK1 catalytic activity. Further, the death domain of DAPK1 is known to interact with TNFR1 and FADD for inducing apoptosis. DAPK1, by interacting with TNFR1, regulates TNF-α-stimulated apoptosis. FADD, an intracellular apoptotic adaptor, recruits pro-caspase 8, which results in formation of the death inducing signaling complex (DISC). DAPK1 is known to be involved in the death receptor-induced apoptosis downstream of DISC formation and upstream of other caspases (Cohen *et al.*, 1999).

DAPK1 REGULATION

DAPK1 is subjected to regulation at many levels which shapes the outcome of its effects on cells. The loss of *DAPK1* expression is often linked to hypermethylation of its promoter region (Bialik and Kimchi, 2006). In some cancers, methylation level of specific genes will predict the clinical outcome. Initially, *DAPK1* was thought to be one of the genes whose expression levels correlated well with promoter hypermethylation. Further analysis of hypermethylation in primary cancer cells revealed that methylation at the *DAPK1* promoter is not the only reason for its loss of expression (Narayan *et al.*, 2003). Interestingly, a homozygous deletion in the CpG region of the *DAPK1* promoter and allelic loss of the *DAPK1* gene was found in a small number of pituitary adenomas and NSCLC cell lines, respectively. Indeed, restoration of DAPK1 expression in lung carcinoma cell lines attenuates their metastatic potential *in vivo*. A "CLL haplotype" was identified recently which resulted in an increased binding of the homeobox transcription factor HOXB7 to the *DAPK1* promoter, leading its suppression (Raval *et al.*, 2007). Further, an allelic variant of the *DAPK1* death domain ($N^{1347}S$) is known to attenuate ERK-dependent apoptosis in *vitro* and *in vivo* (Stevens *et al.*, 2007), by predominantly shifting the equilibrium towards autophagy. In renal cell carcinoma (RCC), although DAPK1 protein is present, its kinase activity is inactivated, although the mechanisms are not clear. Src kinase dependent phosphorylation of DAPK1 at Y^{491}/Y^{492} inhibited its activity, while ERK activation increased its activity by phosphorylation at S^{735} (Chen *et al.*, 2005; Wang *et al.*, 2007).

DAPK1 regulation through protein stabilization and turnover also appears to be critical in shaping its biological activities. DAPK1 degradation appears to be dependent on a ubiquitin–proteasome pathway (Lin *et al.*, 2009a). DIP-1, a ubiquitin ligase containing three ring fingers, binds directly to the ankyrin repeats of DAPK1 (Lin *et al.*, 2009a). Further studies demonstrated that DIP-1 is identical to mindbomb (MIB1) (Lin *et al.*, 2009b). Another E3 ubiquitin ligase, the carboxyl terminus of Hsc70-interacting protein (CHIP), indirectly binds to DAPK1 through Heat Shock Protein 90 (Hsp90) (Lin *et al.*, 2009a). Recently, KLHL20, a BTB-Kelch protein harboring potential dimerization domains, was found to bridge DAPK1 to Cullin3, thereby promoting DAPK1 ubiquitination and proteasomal degradation to control IFN responses (Lee *et al.*, 2010). Additionally, a DAPK1 isoform, s-DAPK1, undergoes destabilization in a proteasome-independent manner (Lin *et al.*, 2009b). All these findings suggest that DAPK1 levels are controlled only partly by promoter hypermethylation, and additional regulatory mechanisms as yet undefined do exist.

Under certain circumstances, DAPK1 might depend critically on transcriptional mechanisms for its activation. Indeed, TGF-β and p53 response elements responsible for *DAPK1* transcription were identified on the promoter (Bialik and Kimchi, 2006). Interestingly, in the Flt3ITD$^+$ subset of acute myeloid leukemias (AML), which rely on tyrosine kinase-dependent cell survival signals, *DAPK1* is repressed transcriptionally by mechanisms involving p52

NF-κB and histone deacetylases (HDACs) (Shanmugam *et al.*, 2011). HDACs cause deacetylation of histones, allowing them to wrap DNA more tightly and thus inhibit gene expression. In particular, the stimulus from the upstream signals drives p52 NF-κB and its partner relB to attract HDACs and possibly other repressors to the promoter, thus enforcing *DAPK1* repression in this subset of AMLs. Our studies showed that *DAPK1* is critically dependent on the transcription factor CCAAT/enhancer binding protein-β (C/EBP-β) for its IFN-induced expression (Gade *et al.*, 2008). Importantly, C/EBP-β-null MEFs do not mount IFN-γ-induced apoptosis and/or autophagy. C/EBP-β is a major transcriptional regulator of metabolism, pro- and anti-growth pathways, cell differentiation, immune responses, reproductive system development, and neoplastic growth (Li *et al.*, 2007). Such diverse functions of C/EBP-β suggest that it cooperates with different cellular factors in a gene- and signal-specific manner for regulating gene expression. C/EBP-β can associate with transcription factors outside its family, such as STAT3, Sp1, NF-κB, and retinoblastoma (pRb) tumor suppressor protein. Indeed, we have shown earlier that the MED1 (TRAP220/PBP/DRIP220/CRSP220) subunit of the transcriptional Mediator complex interacts with C/EBP-β in an IFN-induced manner and is required for IFN-induced C/EBP-β-dependent *DAPK1* expression. Interestingly, a decline in MED1 expression correlated with a loss of DAPK1 levels in a number of human lung carcinomas and cell lines (Gade *et al.*, 2009). More importantly, restoration of MED1 into cells strongly inhibited the metastatic potential of a lung cancer cell line through DAPK1 upregulation (Gade *et al.*, 2009). Similar to our studies, others also showed that downregulation of Med1 induces a strong tumorigenic phenotype (Ndong Jde *et al.*, 2009). Interestingly, in IFN-γ-stimulated pathways, C/EBP-β interacts with ATF6, a key ER stress activated transcription factor, for inducing *DAPK1* expression and autophagy (Gade *et al.*, 2012).

DAPK1 AND AUTOPHAGY

Autophagy, or "self-eating," is a catabolic process that involves degradation of nonfunctional cellular components through lysosomal machinery in budding yeast (Klionsky, 2007). Three types of autophagy are known to date, depending on the mode of delivery of target proteins for degradation and physiological functions: chaperone-mediated autophagy, microautophagy, and macroautophagy. Chaperone-mediated autophagy involves the recognition of damaged proteins with a specific heat shock cognate 70 (Hsc70)-recognition motif. Upon recognition, the substrate proteins are translocated to the lysosomes by Hsc70, where they undergo rapid degradation. Microautophagy involves the direct engulfment of cytoplasmic material through an invagination of the lysosomal membrane and subsequent degradation of the engulfed proteins. Macroautophagy, the major mechanism, involves the destruction of damaged cell organelles or protein aggregates, and involves the formation of a double-membrane structure, known as an autophagosome, around the target. Hereafter, macroautophagy will be referred to as autophagy. At basal levels, autophagy exerts homeostatic functions by eliminating long-lived or aggregated proteins and damaged organelles. Autophagy is induced by number of stresses, including starvation, growth factor depletion, accumulation of unfolded proteins in the ER, and invasion by pathogenic organisms, and is a central player in many diseases, including cancer. However, the biological regulators of these responses are not known fully.

The intimate link between tumor suppression and autophagy was initially unfolded by the identification of Beclin 1 (*BECN1*; an orthologue of yeast *Atg6*, the first identified mammalian autophagy gene) as an interactor of oncoprotein BCL2, whose overexpression suppressed tumor growth. Loss of its expression was found in many breast tumors. Deletion of *Becn1* causes embryonic lethality, indicating its importance to other biological processes. However, haplo-insufficiency of Beclin 1 resulted in the development of lymphomas, hepatocellular carcinomas, and lung adenocarcinomas, confirming its tumor-suppressive role (Zalckvar *et al.*, 2009). Recently, DAPK1 was identified as a novel regulator of autophagy (Harrison *et al.*, 2008) (Figure 19.1B). As mentioned above, overexpression of DAPK1 in the absence of p53 (carcinoma cell lines) exhibited hallmarks of autophagic cell death. Further, downregulation of DAPK1 by expressing antisense RNA attenuated IFN-γ-induced autophagy in HeLa cells. Peptide combinatorial libraries identified MAP1B, a major component of neuronal cytoskeleton, as a DAPK1 interacting protein (Figure 19.3) which functions as a positive cofactor in DAPK1 regulated autophagy (Harrison *et al.*, 2008). Further, MAP1B interacts with Atg8 (LC3), an autophagy marker which permits maturation of autophagosomes. DAPK1 induces autophagy in a *Beclin1*-dependent manner (Zalckvar *et al.*, 2009). DAPK1 phosphorylates Beclin 1 at T^{119} within its BH3 domain to promote its dissociation from Bcl-X_L and induction of autophagy (Zalckvar *et al.*, 2009). DAPK1 was recently shown to phosphorylate and activate protein kinase D (PKD), a known tumor suppressor that regulates trafficking from the trans-Golgi network (Eisenberg-Lerner and Kimchi, 2012). PKD functions in various cellular responses, including responses to oxidative stress. PKD functions downstream of DAPK1 and binds and phosphorylates Vps34, a major regulator of autophagy, during oxidative stress. This shows another mechanism by which DAPK1 regulates autophagy.

Autophagy has been linked to cell survival and also to cell death in a process termed type 2 or autophagic cell death (Klionsky, 2007). Perturbations in ER homeostasis lead to ER-dependent cell death. DAPK1 is an important component in ER-specific cell death types (Gozuacik *et al.*, 2008). Interestingly, *Dapk*$^{-/-}$ mouse embryonic fibroblasts (MEFs) showed protection against cell death induced by tunicamycin, an ER stress inducer, showing DAPK1's role in ER stress-mediated cell death (Gozuacik *et al.*, 2008). Indeed, *Dapk1*$^{-/-}$ mice showed protection against kidney damage caused by tunicamycin. Importantly, *Dapk1*$^{-/-}$ MEFs showed attenuation of autophagy induction, activated by ER stress, preceding cell death. However, how ER stress is coupled with autophagy was not explored. We recently reported a signaling cascade wherein IFN-γ stimulated proteolytic cleavage of ATF6 and an ERK1/2-dependent phosphorylation of C/EBP-β at T^{189} together control the expression of *DAPK1* and autophagy (Figure 19.3B) (Gade *et al.*, 2012). In steady state, ATF6 exists as an ER membrane-anchored precursor protein of 90 kDa and is held inactive by BiP, an inhibitory protein. ER stress induces dissociation of ATF6 from BiP and nuclear translocation of a 50-kDa active form for induction of gene expression via the Golgi apparatus, where it is cleaved by the enzymes S1P and S2P to generate an active DNA-binding form. We found defective autophagy in cells lacking either ATF6 or C/EBP-β (Gade *et al.*, 2012). Neither the C/EBP-β T^{189A} mutant, which is phosphorylation defective, nor the proteolysis-resistant ATF6 mutant induced autophagy. Only restoration of the corresponding wild-type gene products reinstated autophagy (Gade *et al.*, 2012). Further, *Atf6*$^{-/-}$ mice were relatively more sensitive to bacterial infections than the wild-type mice, and their macrophages are defective at

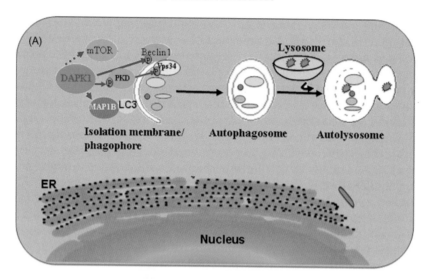

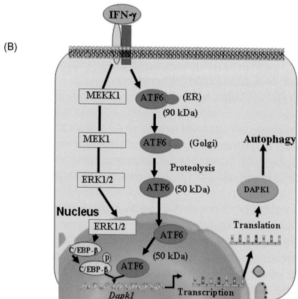

FIGURE 19.3   **(A) The role of DAPK1 in autophagy.** DAPK1 phosphorylates Beclin 1 and also interacts with MAP1B-LC3 for the induction of autophagy. DAPK1 phosphorylates PKD, which further phosphorylates Vps34 for induction of autophagy. DAPK1 indirectly activates mTOR activity, which is known to suppress autophagy. The double-membrane structures (isolation membrane or phagophore) formed upon induction of autophagy fuse around the damaged organelles and/ or protein aggregates, forming autophagosomes. Autophagosomes fuse with lysosomes to form autolysosomes, the degradative autophagic components. **(B) An IFN-γ stimulated ERK1/2 dependent phosphorylation of C/EBP-β at T^{189} through a MEKK1–MEK1–ERK1/2 axis.** A second arm involves IFN-γ stimulated translocation of ATF6 from the ER to the Golgi apparatus, wherein proteolytic processing of ATF6 releasing the transcriptionally active form (50 kDa) of ATF6 occurs prior to its nuclear entry. In the nucleus, ATF6 interacts with phosphorylated C/EBP-β for the induction of *Dapk1* expression and autophagy.

mounting autophagy upon infection (Gade *et al.*, 2012). Thus, our studies not only uncovered IFN-γ-stimulated *DAPK1* expression through transcription factors ATF6 and C/EBP-β and induction of autophagy, but also linked ER stress with autophagy through DAPK1 in driving antibacterial defense.

Autophagy is also activated through another pathway in which rapamycin binds to the mTORC1 complex and inactivates, leading to initiation of autophagy by the ULK1/Atg13/FIP200 complex (Klionsky, 2007). Tuberous sclerosis 2 (TSC-2), a major regulator of the mTORC1 pathway, was identified as a DAPK1 death-domain interacting partner by protein interaction screen (Stevens *et al.*, 2009). This interaction results in phosphorylation and inhibition of the TSC complex by DAPK1, which leads to the stimulation of mTORC1 activity and suppression of autophagy. Thus, DAPK1 acts as a suppressor and also promotes autophagy, depending on the upstream signals (Kang and Avery, 2010). Although DAPK1 is found to be necessary for IFN-γ-stimulated autophagy it seems not to be crucial for rapamycin- or starvation-induced autophagy, and thus probably explains these opposite functions (Kang and Avery, 2010). Further studies are needed to clarify the exact role of DAPK1 in these processes.

DAPK1 is connected to the regulation of endocytosis and can phosphorylate syntaxin-1A, a key component of the protein receptor complex required for docking and fusion of the synaptic vesicles that are required for autophagy (Lin *et al.*, 2009a). Further, syntaxin-1A, a major component of the exocytotic SNARE complex, is involved in NMDA receptor exocytosis. NMDA receptors (the major subtype of glutamate receptors) participate in rapid excitatory synaptic transmission. Importantly, in cerebral ischemia DAPK1 is recruited into the NMDA receptor complex, where it phosphorylates GRINB (NMDA receptor) at S^{1303}, inducing injurious Ca^{2+} influx through these channels and resulting in irreversible neuronal death (Tu *et al.*, 2010). Thus, DAPK1 acts as a signaling amplifier of NMDA receptors at extrasynaptic sites for mediating brain damage in stroke. Uncoupling of activated DAPK1 from the NMDA receptor complex protects the brain from damage in stroke. Indeed, the role of excitotoxins (NMDA) in mediating autophagy is known (Sadasivan *et al.*, 2010). Thus, it appears that DAPK1 has a critical role in mediating exocytotic vesicle-dependent autophagy in the central nervous system.

Tumor cells display an altered metabolic state known as the "Warburg effect," or aerobic glycolysis. In typical cells, pyruvate, the end product of glycolysis, is oxidized by the Krebs cycle (oxidative breakdown) in the mitochondrion to meet the cells' energy demands. However, in cancer cells much of the pyruvate generated by glycolysis is driven away from mitochondria to generate lactate (non-oxidative breakdown). Though lactate production is typically restricted to anaerobic conditions, in cancer cells glucose is channeled towards lactate production even in the presence of oxygen. The Warburg effect, or aerobic glycolysis, is critically dependent on a kinase known as PKM2 (pyruvate kinase M2). PKM2 acts at the level of generation of pyruvate, the end product of glycolysis from phosphoenol pyruvate (PEP), an intermediate product of glucose metabolism. Recently, a yeast two-hybrid screening identified PKM2 as a DAPK1 interacting protein (Mor *et al.*, 2012). There are two major isoforms of PK: M1 and M2. M1 is seen in most adult cells, while M2 is expressed mainly during embryogenesis. Expression of the PKM2 isoform was correlated with a shift towards increased glycolysis and a transformed state of cells. Ectopic expression of DAPK1$^{\Delta KD}$ increased the levels of cytoskeleton-bound PKM2 (insoluble PKM2), whereas depleting endogenous DAPK1 decreased cytoskeleton-bound PKM2 levels, thus connecting DAPK1 to metabolism

(Mor *et al.*, 2012). Additionally, PKM2 kinase activity causes dissociation of histone deacetylase 3 (HDAC3) from cyclin D1 promoter, allowing acetylation and expression of cyclin D1. Thus, PKM2 appears to have a role in cyclin D1-dependent cell cycle progression. Interestingly, IFN-γ and TNF-α induced DAPK1, downregulated cyclin D1 expression, and arrested cell cycle progression (Yoo *et al.*, 2012). Further substantiation is required to get a clear picture of DAPK1–PKM2 interactions with respect to cyclin D1 expression in the wider context of tumor growth, in a signal-dependent manner. Thus, a detailed characterization of the DAPK1 interacting proteins, its substrates, and their mechanisms of action in tumor growth and metastasis needs to be further defined.

DISCUSSION

DAPK1, located on human chromosome 9q21.33, is a well-known tumor suppressor (Bialik and Kimchi, 2006). It participates in a wide spectrum of cell death pathways, including IFN-γ-induced apoptotic and autophagic cell death. Recently, DAPK1 was demonstrated to be a critical modulator of cell fate decisions (Bialik and Kimchi, 2006). Although DAPK1 uses several cellular substrates to mediate its wide variety of functions, it is limited to higher-order organisms, given the absence of the DAPK1 family in yeast, where autophagy is known to occur.

Importantly, DAPK1 expression is downregulated in a wide variety of cancer types, including lung cancer, cervical carcinoma, lymphoma, nasopharyngeal carcinoma, and gastrointestinal tumors (Bialik and Kimchi, 2006). The mechanism for DAPK1 pro-apoptotic activity is not clear, although it is linked to its interaction with the cytoskeleton (Bialik and Kimchi, 2006). DAPK1 induction results in cytoskeletal reorganization and changes in the cell morphology, culminating in cell death (Bialik and Kimchi, 2006). Importantly, DAPK1 appears to play a critical nodal role directing signals towards apoptosis or autophagy. In ER-dependent pathways, DAPK1 could be activated by Ca^{2+} from the ER stores, while the formation of autophagophores (double-membrane vacuoles) is supported by the ER membrane (Harrison *et al.*, 2008). Further, DAPK1 has been shown to interact strongly with microtubules and MAP1B (an important protein for neuronal differentiation and its outgrowth), possibly promoting its interaction with MAP1LC3B (Harrison *et al.*, 2008). Both DAPK1 and MAP1B co-localized with α-tubulin and F-actin (Harrison *et al.*, 2008) may be involved in the sliding of the autophagosomes along the cytoskeletal structures and fusing with lysosomes, thus associating DAPK1 with autophagy.

Earlier, the existence of autophagic cell death was a matter of debate, as autophagy also functions to maintain cellular homeostasis. Autophagy, while providing an emergency nutrient supply during cell stress, and removing damaged proteins and organelles, can also lead to cell death when it fails to restore normal functions. Under these conditions, blocking autophagic cell death enhances the apoptotic cell death mode (Eisenberg-Lerner *et al.*, 2009). Both autophagy and apoptosis appear to be regulated by DAPK1. Indeed, DAPK1 is one of the first known proteins which directly connects autophagy to cell death mechanisms through Beclin 1. Beclin 1, a key intermediate in the unfolding of pro-autophagic signals to autophagosome formation, binds and regulates the properties of anti-apoptotic BCL2 family members, and *vice versa* (Zalckvar *et al.*, 2009). Importantly, Beclin 1 phosphorylation by

DAPK1 weakens its interaction with BCL-X$_L$ (an anti-apoptotic BCL2 family member), which explains a basis for the induction of autophagy (Zalckvar *et al.*, 2009). DAPK1 participates in oxidative stress-induced autophagy by phosphorylating PKD (Eisenberg-Lerner *et al.*, 2012). Autophagy acts as a double-edged sword in the evolution of tumors. Defective autophagy was demonstrated in many tumors, indicating autophagic cell death as a mechanism for tumor suppression. Although autophagy is a tumor-suppression mechanism, upon stress it enables tumor cell survival, particularly when apoptosis is defective (White and DiPaola, 2009). Only DAPK1-dependent phosphorylation of Beclin 1 and DAPK1 interaction with MAP1LC3B are known to date. Further analyses of the interactions of DAPK1 and its substrates with autophagic machinery need to be evaluated critically in the context of tumor growth. Understanding DAPK1 interactions with other autophagy products will provide the detailed mechanistic basis for autophagy induction during tumor suppression.

DAPK1 localizes to the cytoskeleton and can phosphorylate and/or regulate cytoskeletal proteins, thus influencing several cytoskeletal functions. Interestingly, phosphorylation of myosin II regulatory light chain (MLC) by DAPK1 is involved in membrane blebbing and formation of stress fibers, in addition to its role in the formation of autophagic vesicles (Bialik and Kimchi, 2006). Membrane blebbing is a common morphological feature of apoptotic cell death, resulting from weakening of the structural integrity of the cortical actin network owing to phosphorylation of MLC by DAPK1. Moreover, the enhanced contractility of myosin as a result of DAPK1 phosphorylation has a role in stress fiber formation. DAPK1 promoted stress fiber formation in serum-starved NIH3T3 cells, and is also necessary for serum-stimulated stress fiber formation in these cells (Bialik and Kimchi, 2006). Further, DAPK1 inhibits cell motility by blocking cell polarization in an integrin-mediated pathway (Bialik and Kimchi, 2006). In addition to the roles mentioned above, DAPK1 is also involved in the adhesion of cells to extracellular matrix (ECM) through its interaction with the cytoskeleton (Bialik and Kimchi, 2006). DAPK1 expression decreased adhesion of cells to the extracellular matrix by inhibiting integrin signaling by decreased Tyr phosphorylation of focal adhesion proteins FAK and paxillin (important components of integrin signaling) (Bialik and Kimchi, 2006). The combinational events of DAPK1, such as contractility, stress fiber formation, cell adhesion, and cell motility, can either accompany cell death or occur independently (Bialik and Kimchi, 2006). Importantly, these antimigratory effects of DAPK1 might explain a mechanism for the inhibition of tumor metastasis.

DAPK1 also antagonizes growth activation signals, as demonstrated by the negative cross-talk between DAPK1 and ERK, and specific inhibition of T cell receptor (TCR)-induced activation by DAPK1. Upon phosphorylation by ERK, DAPK1 retains ERK in the cytoplasm, making it unavailable for the nuclear substrates critical for cell survival. Thus, a negative cross-talk exists wherein ERK-activated DAPK1 promotes cell death by suppressing ERK-dependent survival (Bialik and Kimchi, 2006). TCR induces activation of NF-κB, a potent anti-apoptotic transcription factor, which further induces activation of downstream anti-apoptotic factors (Chuang *et al.*, 2012). Importantly, DAPK1 inhibits TCR-induced activation of NF-κB, which also explains a basis for DAPK1-mediated growth suppression. Further, DAPK1 is involved in an IFN-γ activated kinase cascade (a unique regulatory module), which initially facilitates translational repression; later, inhibition of DAPK1 permits inflammatory gene expression (Mukhopadhyay *et al.*, 2008). Thus, DAPK1 is a part of a negative feedback loop that is important for the regulation of inflammatory gene expression.

The role of DAPK1 in mediating cell death and also in antagonizing growth activation warrants understanding of DAPK1 regulation. A thorough understanding of DAPK1 regulation will help to develop drugs that can promote DAPK1 expression, since its expression is lost in many tumors. Interestingly, DAPK1 is regulated at transcriptional, post-transcriptional, and protein stability levels, affecting its expression. Our studies identified the transcriptional regulators of *DAPK1* in the IFN-γ-stimulated pathway (Gade *et al.*, 2012). Indeed, loss of C/EBP-β resulted in the inhibition of IFN-γ-induced apoptosis and autophagy. Thus, C/EBP-β is connected to the IFN-γ-induced autophagy through DAPK1. Further, C/EBP-β interacts with ATF6 upon IFN-γ stimulation for inducing DAPK1 dependent autophagy.

Autophagy, apart from tumor suppression, also has role in protection against microbial infections. Indeed, IFN-γ plays a critical role in mediating protection against infectious pathogens (Stark *et al.*, 1998). We recently demonstrated a connection between ER stress and autophagy in mediating antibacterial defenses through ATF6. Consistent with this, proteolytic activation of ATF6 and ER stress upon infection of cells with *Listeria monocytogenes* were recently reported (Pillich *et al.*, 2012). Interestingly, cells infected with *L. monocytogenes* mount autophagy as a defensive mechanism. Indeed, *Atf6$^{-/-}$* mice were prone to anthrax bacterial infection-induced mortality owing, in part, to defective autophagy (Gade *et al.*, 2012). Upon infection with *Bacillus anthracis*, macrophages from *Atf6$^{-/-}$* mice could not mount autophagy when compared to macrophages from wild-type mice. Additionally, *Atf6$^{-/-}$* macrophages also could not activate autophagy upon *Salmonella typhimurium* infection *in vitro*. Thus, ATF6 appears to have role in mediating protection against pathogens via autophagy (Gade *et al.*, 2012). Though autophagy limits intracellular microbial growth, intracellular microorganisms evolve strategies to evade this mechanism for their survival, which appears to be dependent on the actin cytoskeleton (Yoshikawa *et al.*, 2009). For example, ACTA of *L. monocytogenes*, a surface protein required for actin polymerization and actin-based bacterial motility, was found to play a pivotal role in evading autophagy (Yoshikawa *et al.*, 2009). ACTA protein was found to camouflage itself from host proteins and thus evades elimination by autophagy. Although the picture is incomplete, dynamic cross-interactions of various proteins at the actin cytoskeleton may be involved in evading autophagy.

Interestingly, other members of the DAPK family, ZIPK and DAPK2, are known to function in different settings of cell death, including autophagy (Gozuacik and Kimchi, 2006). DAPK2-induced cell death signals require DAPK1 function, as co-expression with a dominant negative mutant of DAPK1 resulted in attenuation of DAPK2-induced cell death. ZIPK interacts with DAPK1 at its kinase domain, and is phosphorylated by DAPK1 at different sites in the non-catalytic domain (Gozuacik and Kimchi, 2006). Phosphorylation of ZIPK by DAPK1 drives nuclear localization of ZIPK and increased cell death-inducing functions. Thus, the protein–protein interactions and kinase–substrate relationships among the DAPK family members suggest that the dynamic multiprotein complexes formed by these associations are capable of transmitting autophagic and/or apoptotic signals in response to various stress signals.

In sum, all these observations designate DAPK1 as stress-activated kinase which connects cellular stresses to apoptotic and/or autophagic pathways. Further, the widespread inactivation of DAPK1 in human tumors, and activation of apoptosis and/or autophagy upon reintroduction or activation of this kinase, elevates the possibility of using DAPK1-based therapeutic interventions against cancer. In the light of these roles played by DAPK1, it is very important to address how DAPK1 can modulate the critical balance between cell death and growth.

Acknowledgments

Studies are supported by the United States National Institutes of Health grant, CA78282, to DVK.

References

Bialik, S., Kimchi, A., 2006. The death-associated protein kinases: structure, function, and beyond. Annu. Rev. Biochem. 75, 189–210.

Chen, C.H., Wang, W.J., Kuo, J.C., et al., 2005. Bidirectional signals transduced by DAPK–ERK interaction promote the apoptotic effect of DAPK. EMBO J. 24, 294–304.

Chuang, Y.T., Lin, Y.C., Lin, K.H., et al., 2012. Tumor suppressor death-associated protein kinase is required for full IL-1beta production. Blood 117, 960–970.

Cohen, O., Inbal, B., Kissil, J.L., et al., 1999. DAP-kinase participates in TNF-alpha- and Fas-induced apoptosis and its function requires the death domain. J. Cell Biol. 146, 141–148.

Eisenberg-Lerner, A., Kimchi, A., 2012. PKD is a kinase of Vps34 that mediates ROS-induced autophagy downstream of DAPk. Cell Death Differ. 19, 788–797.

Eisenberg-Lerner, A., Bialik, S., Simon, H.U., et al., 2009. Life and death partners: apoptosis, autophagy and the cross-talk between them. Cell Death Differ. 16, 966–975.

Gade, P., Roy, S.K., Li, H., et al., 2008. Critical role for transcription factor C/EBP-beta in regulating the expression of death-associated protein kinase 1. Mol. Cell Biol. 28, 2528–2548.

Gade, P., Singh, A.K., Roy, S.K., et al., 2009. Down-regulation of the transcriptional mediator subunit Med1 contributes to the loss of expression of metastasis-associated dapk1 in human cancers and cancer cells. Intl. J. Cancer 125, 1566–1574.

Gade, P., Ramachandran, G., Maachani, U.B., et al., 2012. An IFN-gamma-stimulated ATF6-C/EBP-beta-signaling pathway critical for the expression of death associated protein kinase 1 and induction of autophagy. Proc. Natl. Acad. Sci. USA 109, 10316–10321.

Gozuacik, D., Kimchi, A., 2006. DAPk protein family and cancer. Autophagy 2, 74–79.

Gozuacik, D., Bialik, S., Raveh, T., et al., 2008. DAP-kinase is a mediator of endoplasmic reticulum stress-induced caspase activation and autophagic cell death. Cell Death Differ. 15, 1875–1886.

Hanahan, D., Weinberg, R.A., 2000. The hallmarks of cancer. Cell 100, 57–70.

Harrison, B., Kraus, M., Burch, L., et al., 2008. DAPK-1 binding to a linear peptide motif in MAP1B stimulates autophagy and membrane blebbing. J. Biol. Chem. 283, 9999–10014.

Kang, C., Avery, L., 2010. Death-associated protein kinase (DAPK) and signal transduction: fine-tuning of autophagy in Caenorhabditis elegans homeostasis. FEBS J. 277, 66–73.

Klionsky, D.J., 2007. Autophagy: from phenomenology to molecular understanding in less than a decade. Nat. Rev. Mol. Cell Biol. 8, 931–937.

Kroemer, G., Galluzzi, L., Vandenabeele, P., et al., 2009. Classification of cell death: recommendations of the nomenclature committee on cell death 2009. Cell Death Differ. 16, 3–11.

Lee, Y.R., Yuan, W.C., Ho, H.C., et al., 2010. The Cullin 3 substrate adaptor KLHL20 mediates DAPK ubiquitination to control interferon responses. EMBO J. 29, 1748–1761.

Li, H., Gade, P., Xiao, W., et al., 2007. The interferon signaling network and transcription factor C/EBP-beta. Cell Mol. Immunol. 4, 407–418.

Lin, Y., Hupp, T.R., Stevens, C., 2009a. Death-associated protein kinase (DAPK) and signal transduction: additional roles beyond cell death. Febs J. 277, 48–57.

Lin, Y., Stevens, C., Harrison, B., et al., 2009. The alternative splice variant of DAPK-1, s-DAPK-1, induces proteasome-independent DAPK-1 destabilization. Mol. Cell Biochem. 328, 101–107.

Martoriati, A., Doumont, G., Alcalay, M., et al., 2005. Dapk1, encoding an activator of a p19ARF-p53-mediated apoptotic checkpoint, is a transcription target of p53. Oncogene 24, 1461–1466.

Mor, I., Carlessi, R., Ast, T., et al., 2012. Death-associated protein kinase increases glycolytic rate through binding and activation of pyruvate kinase. Oncogene 31, 683–693.

Mukhopadhyay, R., Ray, P.S., Arif, A., et al., 2008. DAPK-ZIPK-L13a axis constitutes a negative-feedback module regulating inflammatory gene expression. Mol. Cell 32, 371–382.

Narayan, G., Arias-Pulido, H., Koul, S., et al., 2003. Frequent promoter methylation of CDH1, DAPK, RARB, and HIC1 genes in carcinoma of cervix uteri: its relationship to clinical outcome. Mol. Cancer 2, 24.

Ndong Jde, L., Jean, D., Rousselet, N., et al., 2009. Down-regulation of the expression of RB18A/MED1, a cofactor of transcription, triggers strong tumorigenic phenotype of human melanoma cells. Intl. J. Cancer 124, 2597–2606.

Pillich, H., Loose, M., Zimmer, K.P., et al., 2012. Activation of the unfolded protein response by *Listeria monocytogenes*. Cell Microbiol. 14, 949–964.

Raval, A., Tanner, S.M., Byrd, J.C., et al., 2007. Downregulation of death-associated protein kinase 1 (DAPK1) in chronic lymphocytic leukemia. Cell 129, 879–890.

Raveh, T., Droguett, G., Horwitz, M.S., et al., 2001. DAP kinase activates a p19ARF/p53-mediated apoptotic checkpoint to suppress oncogenic transformation. Nat. Cell Biol. 3, 1–7.

Sadasivan, S., Zhang, Z., Larner, S.F., et al., 2010. Acute NMDA toxicity in cultured rat cerebellar granule neurons is accompanied by autophagy induction and late onset autophagic cell death phenotype. BMC Neurosci. 11, 21.

Shanmugam, R., Gade, P., Wilson-Weekes, A., et al., 2011. A noncanonical Flt3ITD/NF-kappaB signaling pathway represses DAPK1 in acute myeloid leukemia. Clin. Cancer Res. 18, 360–369.

Stark, G.R., Kerr, I.M., Williams, B.R., et al., 1998. How cells respond to interferons. Annu. Rev. Biochem. 67, 227–264.

Stevens, C., Lin, Y., Sanchez, M., et al., 2007. A germ line mutation in the death domain of DAPK-1 inactivates ERK-induced apoptosis. J. Biol. Chem. 282, 13791–13803.

Stevens, C., Lin, Y., Harrison, B., et al., 2009. Peptide combinatorial libraries identify TSC2 as a death-associated protein kinase (DAPK) death domain-binding protein and reveal a stimulatory role for DAPK in mTORC1 signaling. J. Biol. Chem. 284, 334–344.

Tu, W., Xu, X., Peng, L., et al., 2010. DAPK1 interaction with NMDA receptor NR2B subunits mediates brain damage in stroke. Cell 140, 222–234.

Wang, W.J., Kuo, J.C., Ku, W., et al., 2007. The tumor suppressor DAPK is reciprocally regulated by tyrosine kinase Src and phosphatase LAR. Mol. Cell 27, 701–716.

White, E., DiPaola, R.S., 2009. The double-edged sword of autophagy modulation in cancer. Clin. Cancer Res. 15, 5308–5316.

Yoo, H.J., Byun, H.J., Kim, B.R., et al., 2012. DAPk1 inhibits NF-kappaB activation through TNF-alpha and INF-gamma-induced apoptosis. Cell Signal. 24, 1471–1477.

Yoshikawa, Y., Ogawa, M., Hain, T., et al., 2009. Listeria monocytogenes ActA is a key player in evading autophagic recognition. Autophagy 5, 1220–1221.

Zalckvar, E., Berissi, H., Eisenstein, M., et al., 2009. Phosphorylation of Beclin 1 by DAP-kinase promotes autophagy by weakening its interactions with Bcl-2 and Bcl-XL. Autophagy 5, 720–722.

TRIM13, Novel Tumor Suppressor: Regulator of Autophagy and Cell Death

Dhanendra Tomar and Rajesh Singh

Abstract

Ubiquitination is an important post-translational modification involved in regulation of a variety of cellular events by degradation, enzymatic activity, or signalosome regulation. Ubiquitin E3 ligases are critical regulators of ubiquitination, as they identify the target and determine the topology of ubiquitination. The TRIM family of ubiquitin E3 ligases belongs to RING family and is characterized by the presence of a tripartite motif (RING, B-Box, and coiled-coil domains). Some members of TRIM family proteins are known to degrade or modulate the activity of various oncogenes and tumor suppressors. TRIM13, an endoplasmic reticulum anchored protein also known as RFP2 and LEU5, is a tumor suppressor which is located at the 13q 14.3 chromosomal region and is deleted in multiple tumor types, especially in chronic lymphocytic leukemia (CLL) and multiple myeloma (MM). Various studies show that TRIM13 involved in both ERAD pathways (the autophagy–lysosome system and the proteasome system) regulates the cell death pathways and clonogenic ability of the cells. This protein regulates the autophagy pathway by interacting with the autophagy adaptors p62/SQSTM1 and DFCP1. Autophagy is involved in critical decisions regarding cell death and survival, and is thus a critical deciding factor in the process of tumorigenesis. This chapter reviews our work on TRIM13 and tumorigenesis, and gives a future perspective on the role of TRIM13 in tumorigenesis.

M.A. Hayat (ed): Autophagy, Volume 1
DOI: http://dx.doi.org/10.1016/B978-0-12-405530-8.00020-0

© 2014 Elsevier Inc. All rights reserved.

INTRODUCTION

Cancer is one of the leading causes of mortality worldwide. According to the latest report from the American Cancer Society, 1.64 million new cancer cases and 0.58 million deaths from cancer were projected to occur in the United States in the year 2012 alone (Siegel *et al.*, 2012). Cancer has been an intense focus of research for several decades due to the high cost to society. There are multiple factors involved in the onset of cancer, ranging from environmental to genetic. Tumorigenesis is characterized by uncontrolled proliferation and suppression of cell death pathways. During tumorigenesis, normal cells are transformed by acquiring features such as sustained proliferative signaling, activation of oncogenes, and disruption of tumor suppressors, the potential to invade surrounding or distant healthy tissues, stimulation of angiogenesis, and resistance to cell death induced by chemotherapeutic agents (Okada and Mak, 2004).

During tumorigenesis, numerous oncogenes disrupt the cell death pathways, leading to increased proliferation of the cells. Cell death is an essential part for the functioning of any biological system, ranging from development to immunity. The aberration in cell death leads to various pathological conditions such as cancer, neurodegeneration, inflammatory diseases, and autoimmunity (Fuchs and Steller, 2011). Multicellular organisms maintain cellular homeostasis by regulating cell proliferation and cell death to remove unwanted cells from the body (Fuchs and Steller, 2011). Programmed cell death (PCD) is characterized by removal of cells from the biological system in a programmed way (Fuchs and Steller, 2011). Programmed cell death is categorized in three major classes, namely apoptosis or type 1, autophagic or type 2, and, recently, necroptosis or type 3 cell death (Christofferson and Yuan, 2010). There are several other forms of cell death, including anoikis (which is almost identical to apoptosis except in its induction), cornification (a form of cell death exclusive to the eyes), excitotoxicity, and Wallerian degeneration. It has been observed that tumor suppressor genes trigger cell death in tumorigenic cells, while oncogenes inhibit cell death.

During the past two decades tremendous progress has been made in understanding the process of apoptosis (Type 1 PCD) (Fuchs and Steller, 2011), and this will not be discussed here in detail as excellent reviews are available. Autophagy (type 2 cell death) is another form of pro-/anti-cell death pathway, and plays a critical role in organ-specific tumorigenesis (Mizushima *et al.*, 2008). Autophagy is a lysosomal degradation pathway that plays a critical role in cell survival, differentiation, development, and homeostasis. This is one of the major mechanisms through which cells degrade misfolded protein, protein aggregates, and defective organelles during stress conditions and supply nutrients to help in cell survival (Figure 20.1). The autophagy pathway also leads to degradation of essential cellular components and induction of cell death in some specific conditions (Figure 20.1). Tumorigenesis involves the accumulation of dysfunctional organelles, which leads to accumulation of DNA damage in the genome of cells and in turn to either amplification/deletion of the critical genes, or aberration in signaling pathways, leading to tumorigenic conditions. Autophagy plays a crucial role in the maintenance of cellular homeostasis by removal of damaged organelles, and subsequently prevents genome damage and metabolic stress. It has been observed that autophagy is dysregulated in many cancers.

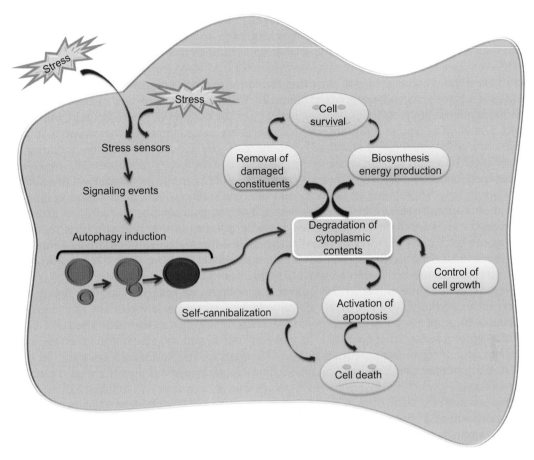

FIGURE 20.1 **Autophagy in cell death and survival.** Extra- or intracellular stress activates stress sensor proteins, which further activate the cascading signaling events that lead to the induction of autophagy. Autophagy induction results in degradation of cytoplasmic contents, which can be damaged organelles or cellular components. This results in production of new raw materials for biosynthesis, and in energy metabolism that leads to enhanced survival in stress conditions. Autophagy can also result in degradation of essential cellular components and activation of apoptosis by activating caspases, which results in the onset of cell death and suppression of cellular growth.

Autophagy is downregulated in brain cancer and liver cancer, while in breast cancer, colorectal cancer, gastric cancer, and pancreatic cancer high levels of autophagy have been observed.

Autophagy is primarily a survival mechanism, and provides protection to cells from cellular damage by different intra- or extracellular stimuli (Mizushima *et al.*, 2008). Autophagy is also known to be involved in the onset of cell death by caspase activation (Young *et al.*, 2012) or direct degradation of essential cellular components and subsequent cell death (Mizushima *et al.*, 2008). During tumorigenesis, initially autophagy inhibits oncogenic transformation by removing cellular organelles damaged by different cellular stresses, such as genotoxic molecules and ROS. Conversely, during later tumorigenic stages autophagy benefits tumor growth, as it provides an alternative energy source. It also acts as survival mechanism for the tumor cells that are in hypoxic areas of tumor growth.

Besides type 1 and type 2 programmed cell death pathways, necroptosis (type 3) is also involved in the regulation of various developmental and physiological processes (Wu *et al.*, 2012). Necroptosis is generally triggered in cells that have compromised caspase-dependent apoptosis. These two death pathways have intrinsic cross-talk and a mutual inhibitory effect. Details of necroptosis and its role in tumorigenesis are beginning to emerge.

Post-translational modifications of proteins play regulatory role in the initiation or termination of various cellular signaling pathways. The role of phosphorylation is well understood and has been the focus of intensive investigation for several decades. Post-translational modification of proteins by ubiquitin (a small 76 amino acid protein) plays a critical role in maintaining cellular homeostasis by regulating the turnover of proteins, protein–protein interactions, and activity. It has long been known that ubiquitin-mediated post-translational modification of proteins is involved in protein degradation (Komander and Rape, 2012), but recent experimental evidence clearly suggests it also has a role in the initiation and execution of various signaling processes (Komander and Rape, 2012).

The role of ubiquitination in the autophagy pathway is not well known. It has been observed that, during cellular stress conditions and many pathological conditions, there is accumulation of protein aggregates and dysfunctional organelles inside the cells. These protein aggregates and dysfunctional organelles are tagged by ubiquitin, which is recognized by adaptor proteins such as p62/SQSTM1, NBR1, Nix, and Optineurin and targeted to the autophagosomes for subsequent degradation in lysosomes (Johansen and Lamark, 2011).

The process of ubiquitination (conjugation of ubiquitin to target protein) involves the sequential action of three enzymes: E1 (ubiquitin activating enzyme), E2 (ubiquitin conjugating enzyme), and E3 (ubiquitin ligases). In the process of ubiquitination, E3 ligases are terminal enzymes which recognize the substrate and facilitate the conjugation of ubiquitin to the substrate (Komander and Rape, 2012). In the human genome, more than 700 ubiquitin E3 ligases have been predicted; however, their roles in different physiological and pathological processes are unclear.

The ubiquitin E3 ligases are broadly categorized into three classes: RING (Really Interesting New Gene), HECT (Homologous to the E6AP Carboxyl Terminus), and a poorly characterized U-Box E3 ligase family (Varshavsky, 2012). The Tripartite Motif (TRIM) or RBCC family proteins belong to the RING family of ubiquitin E3 ligases. These proteins are characterized by the presence of N-terminal RING finger (R) domain, one or two B-Boxes (B) and a coiled-coil (CC) domain, and C-terminal variable domains (Meroni and Diez-Roux, 2005). These proteins are known to play an important role in antiviral immune response, being involved in the TLR (Toll-like Receptor) and interferon pathways (Kawai and Akira, 2011). The innate immune response and interferon signaling play a critical role in the process of tumorigenesis and the maintenance of the tumor microenvironment. The role of TRIMs as ubiquitin ligases in the regulation of inflammation during tumorigenesis is not well studied, and only a few members are known to be involved in this process (Hatakeyama, 2011). In this chapter we describe the role of TRIM13 in the regulation of autophagy, and its novel role as a tumor suppressor.

TRIM13 (also termed LEU5, RFP2, DLEU5, or RNF77) is an endoplasmic reticulum-anchored ubiquitin E3 ligase involved in the regulation of ERAD pathways (Tomar *et al.*, 2012a). Recent studies suggest that TRIM13 is involved in the regulation of the autophagy pathway and plays critical role in cell death and survival during stress conditions (Joo *et al.*, 2011; Tomar *et al.*, 2012a). Its frequent deletion in cancer conditions, and some experimental evidence, suggests that TRIM13 is a candidate tumor suppressor gene. In the present chapter we summarize the various studies on TRIM13 and its role in autophagy and cell death, which are critical processes in the regulation of tumorigenesis.

TRIM FAMILY PROTEINS

TRIM/RBCC proteins are members of the RING family of E3 ligases and are characterized by the presence of tripartite motif consisting of the N terminus RING domain, B-Box, and coiled-coil (CC) domain variable C-terminal domain (Meroni and Diez-Roux, 2005). The RING (Really Interesting New Gene) family of ubiquitin E3 ligases is the largest group of E3 proteins, having more than 600 members (Deshaies and Joazeiro, 2009). Initially, RING domain proteins were postulated to play an important role in DNA functions as these proteins were shown to bind to DNA; later, these proteins were shown to be involved in transfer of ubiquitin to the target protein (Deshaies and Joazeiro, 2009). The RING domain is a characteristic zinc finger domain which has 40–60 residues. The RING domain has a cysteine-rich sequence motif, Cys–X2–Cys–X(9–39)–Cys–X(1–3)–His–X(2–3)–Cys–X2–Cys–X(4–48)–Cys–X2–Cys (where X is any amino acid), that binds to two zinc atoms in a cross-brace manner through seven cysteine and one histidine residues (Deshaies and Joazeiro, 2009).

The RING domain is present in many other proteins; however, in TRIM proteins it is generally followed by the B-Box domain. The RING domain of TRIM proteins is responsible for E3 ligase activity in the process of ubiquitination. The B-Box domain is also a zinc-binding motif, and there are two types of B-Box domains: type 1, where cysteine is the coordination residue, and type 2, where histidine is the coordination residue (Meroni and Diez-Roux, 2005). This domain is known to be involved in protein–protein and protein–DNA interactions (Meroni and Diez-Roux, 2005). The B-Box is followed by the CC domain, which is important for homo-/heterotypic interactions and results in complexes of higher molecular structures (Napolitano and Meroni, 2012). This domain may be significant in the formation of specific subcellular structures, and thus an orchestrator of specific functions of individual proteins (Napolitano and Meroni, 2012). The C-terminal region of TRIM proteins has varied domain architecture, such as COS (C-terminal subgroup one signature), FN3 (fibronectin type 3), PRY, SPRY, PHD (plant homeodomain), BROMO, FIL (filamin-type Ig), NHL (NCL-1, HT2A, and LIN-41), MATH (meprin and TRAF homology), ARF (ADP ribosylation factor-like), and transmembrane and Pyrin domains (Ozato *et al.*, 2008). The C-terminal region can harbor any of these distinct motifs alone or in combination. TRIM proteins were further classified in 11 subgroups based on these C-terminal motifs (Ozato *et al.*, 2008).

The TRIM proteins are found in all metazoans, ranging from flies to humans, but the number of TRIMs varies between species. In *Drosophila* there are less than 10 known members, whereas in humans more than 70 members are known, indicating that TRIM proteins have evolved extensively. There are several members of the TRIM proteins that are uniquely expressed in humans and are not present in any other species, suggesting that TRIM proteins may have unique functions in humans. The TRIM family proteins have multiple domains which have unique interactions in different cellular signaling conditions, and regulate developmental to innate immune processes. The TRIM proteins are extremely heterogeneous in tissue and organ expression, and they also form distinct multimeric protein structures targeted to different cellular compartments (Ozato *et al.*, 2008).

TRIMs: Different Roles in Varied Cellular Conditions

Ubiquitin E3 ligases are the most diverse proteins, and recognize the target protein and mediate the covalent linkage between target and ubiquitin moieties. They provide target specificity and uniqueness in the process of ubiquitination. The TRIM family proteins, having multiple domains, perform distinct functions depending upon their subcellular localization and translocation in different physiological and pathological conditions. Recent studies on TRIM family proteins showed that these proteins play an important role in vesicular trafficking. TRIM72 is involved in vesicular trafficking to the plasma membrane during membrane repair, thus regulating efficient cellular functions (Cai *et al.*, 2009). TRIM3 is also involved in regulation and trafficking of the EGF receptor to endosomal localization by ubiquitination (Mosesson *et al.*, 2009). TRIM32 protein plays important role in regulation of miRNA expression via c-Myc degradation, and their activity via directly interaction with the argonaute protein (Schwamborn *et al.*, 2009), which is directly involved in the regulation of various developmental and physiological processes.

Mutations in TRIM1 (MID2) and TRIM18 (MID1) lead to the onset of X-linked Opitz GBBB syndrome, which is characterized by various developmental defects (Short *et al.*, 2002). TRIM2 is highly expressed in the nervous system and regulates neuronal polarization; its deficiency leads to neurodegeneration (Khazaei *et al.*, 2011). TRIM9 is also expressed in the nervous system and repressed in Parkinson's disease (Tanji *et al.*, 2010). TRIM6 is involved in the maintenance of pluripotency in mouse embryonic stem cells (Sato *et al.*, 2012). Mutations in TRIM20, TRIM32, and TRIM37 are associated with familial Mediterranean fever, limb-girdle muscular dystrophy type 2H, and Mulibrey nanism, respectively (Avela *et al.*, 2000; Kudryashova *et al.*, 2005; Touitou, 2001).

Programmed cell death (PCD) is an evolutionarily conserved process which is observed in unicellular to multicellular organisms. This cellular process plays an important role in vital cellular processes, ranging from development to immunity. Ubiquitin-mediated posttranslational modification plays a critical role in the regulation of cell death pathways. As described in earlier sections, the TRIM family of ubiquitin E3 ligases has multiple domains, and each domain has a unique function. The role of TRIM family members in the regulation of cell death pathways is emerging, and to date only few are known to regulate apoptosis and autophagy. TRIM17 induces apoptosis in neuronal cells by degrading Mcl-1, which is an anti-apoptotic Bcl-2 family member (Magiera *et al.*, 2012). TRIM13 sensitizes cells to ionizing radiation-induced apoptosis by degrading AKT and MDM2 (Joo *et al.*, 2011). TRIM32 enhances tumor necrosis factor-induced apoptosis by inducing proteasomal degradation of the X-linked inhibitor of apoptosis (XIAP) (Ryu *et al.*, 2011). TRIM21 (Ro52) regulates death ligand-induced apoptosis by downregulating c-FLIP(L) (Zhang *et al.*, 2012), while TRIM28 and TRIM45 have antiproliferative activity (Chen *et al.*, 2012; Shibata *et al.*, 2012). These experimental evidences suggest that TRIMs have a critical role in regulation of apoptosis by modulating the levels of master regulators of apoptotic pathways.

Some experimental evidences suggest that E3 ligases may play a significant role in autophagy. Ubiquitin E3 ligases are known to regulate autophagy by regulating ubiquitination of the target protein, therefore playing an essential role in selective autophagy. The Atg family proteins, which are essential inducer and modulator proteins of autophagy, have a CC domain, and this domain has been shown to be involved in the induction and modulation of the autophagy pathway. TRIM family proteins also have a coiled-coil domain and form multimeric protein complexes or signalosomes. This evidence suggests that TRIM and Atg proteins may hetero-oligomerize and regulate autophagy. Two members of TRIM family (i.e., TRIM13 and TRIM21) are known to positively regulate autophagy during ER stress and regulation of the NF-κB pathway, respectively (Niida *et al.*, 2010; Tomar *et al.*, 2012a).

The TRIM family of ubiquitin E3 ligases is well known in antiretroviral signaling. TRIM5 was the first member to be characterized as an antiretroviral factor and pattern recognition receptor in the innate immune recognition of retroviruses. TRIM5 is involved in the antiretroviral response by interfering with the uncoating of viral particles during viral infection. TRIM11 and TRIM32 repress retroviral gene expression after integration of the viral genome and the host genome, while TRIM22 inhibits the viral assembly and transcription of the viral genome. These proteins also regulate the innate immune response and interferon pathways. TRIM25 is an important factor in RIG-I (Retinoic acid Inducible Gene-I)-mediated antiviral signaling, which regulates interferon production. TRIM25 ubiquitinates the caspase recruitment domain (CARD) of RIG-I and regulates its downstream signaling pathway (Gack *et al.*, 2008).

NF-κB and IFN pathways are also known to play a critical role in tumorigenesis. This has been an area of interest for a long time. The role of ubiquitination has also been of interest in regulation of these pathways. Ubiquitin E3 ligases, as mentioned above, recognize the substrate in these critical pathways and may regulate the process of oncogenesis. The NF-κB pathway is positively regulated by TRIM8, and acts as tumor inducer (Li *et al.*, 2011; Tomar *et al.*, 2012b). TRIM11 is highly expressed in gliomas, and positively regulates tumorigenesis. TRIM16 acts as a tumor suppressor in neuroblastoma cells and is repressed in squamous cell carcinoma (Cheung *et al.*, 2012). TRIM19, also known as promyelocytic leukemia protein (PML), is involved in promyelocytic leukemia and solid tumors (de The *et al.*, 1991). TRIM13 is deleted in various malignancies, regulates ERAD, autophagy, and cell death, and acts as a candidate tumor suppressor (Tomar *et al.*, 2012a). These studies clearly indicate that TRIM family protein members play a critical role in various cellular signaling pathways that lead to the onset of various pathological conditions. Here, we discuss further the recent studies demonstrating the role of TRIM13 in the regulation of autophagy and oncogenic transformation.

TRIM13: REGULATOR OF AUTOPHAGY AND TUMORIGENESIS

As discussed previously, members of the TRIM family proteins have been shown to be involved in different intracellular processes, such as cell signaling, trafficking, and apoptosis. TRIM13 is an endoplasmic reticulum-anchored ubiquitin E3 ligase involved in the regulation of ERAD pathways. TRIM13 regulates ERAD-I by targeting the ERAD substrate to proteasomal degradation with the help of valosin-containing protein (VCP), as well as in ERAD-II by inducing autophagy during ER stress conditions. Experimental evidence suggests that TRIM13 is involved in the regulation of the initiation step of autophagy and may form signaling complexes on the ER surface for regulation of autophagy. TRIM13 interacts with the autophagy adaptor protein p62/SQSTM1 and co-localizes with DFCP1, which is a marker for ER-induced autophagosomes, suggesting that TRIM13 is involved in the initiation and execution of autophagy during ER stress conditions.

TRIM13 is a multidomain protein, having N-terminal RING, B-Box, Coiled-Coil (CC) and C-terminal transmembrane (TM) domains. These different domains may perform discrete functions in different signaling pathways. Experimental evidence suggests that the RING domain of this protein is involved in ubiquitination of the ERAD substrate and its subsequent degradation by proteasomes, while the CC domain of this protein regulates autophagy. The RING domain of TRIM13 is also important for its auto-polyubiquitination and degradation during normal physiological conditions. During ER stress conditions, TRIM13 interacts with p62 through the CC domain and may help to assemble signalosomes through its partners, like p62 and DFCP1, for autophagy induction, which may be important in alleviating ER stress.

TRIM family proteins are known to form homo- or heteromeric protein complexes which regulate different cellular functions. Experimental evidence suggests that TRIM13 interacts with p62, which is a multidomain protein, having a UBA domain that binds to ubiquitinated proteins and determines their degradation fate through either UPS or autophagy. The turnover of TRIM13 is high in normal physiological conditions. TRIM13 is polyubiquitinated, recognized by p62, and degraded by autophagy and UPS pathways. During ER stress conditions, TRIM13 is stabilized, induces autophagy, is involved in ERAD pathways, and may play an important role in ER stress-related pathological conditions (Tomar *et al.*, 2012a). TRIM13 is also known to regulate apoptosis during exposure of cells to ionizing radiation. TRIM13 regulates the levels of pro- and anti-apoptotic proteins, increasing expression of pro-apoptotic proteins p53, p21, and Bax while strongly suppressing anti-apoptotic proteins MDM2, AKT, and Bcl-2 (Joo *et al.*, 2011). It induces the proteasomal degradation of anti-apoptotic proteins MDM2 and AKT to sensitize cells to ionizing radiation-induced apoptosis.

Experimental evidence suggests that TRIM13 regulates autophagy and apoptosis. Both of these processes play a critical role in the process of tumorigenesis. TRIM13 is present on chromosomal region 13q14.3, which has been found to be homozygously deleted in various malignancies, including B cell chronic lymphocytic leukemia (CLL) and multiple myeloma (MM). Due to its homozygous deletion in various malignancies, this gene has been assigned as a candidate tumor suppressor. TRIM13-mediated regulation of autophagy and apoptosis further strengthen this hypothesis. To prove this hypothesis, Tomar *et al.* have performed *in vitro* clonogenic assays to observe the effect of TRIM13 on the clonogenic ability of cells. Overexpression of TRIM13 decreased the colony-forming ability of the cells, while knockdown had the opposite effect (Figure 20.2); this further supports the earlier observation of its tumor suppressor activity.

Tomar and colleagues also monitored the role of TRIM13-induced autophagy in the regulation of the clonogenic ability of cells. The colony-forming assay suggest that

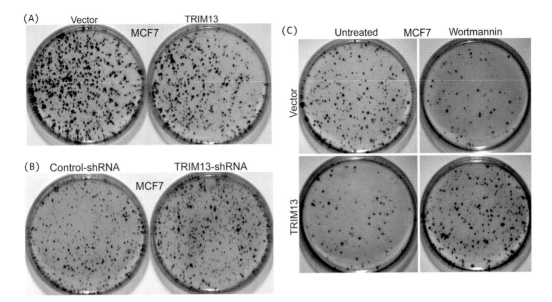

FIGURE 20.2 **TRIM13 regulates the clonogenic ability of cells.** To assess the role of TRIM13 in regulation of the clonogenic ability of cells, MCF7 cells were transfected with TRIM13 and TRIM13-shRNA along with empty vector and control shRNA. The overexpression of TRIM13 results in suppression of clonogenic ability (A), while knockdown of TRIM13 has the opposite effect (B). To elucidate the role of TRIM13-induced autophagy in regulation of the clonogenic ability of the cells, MCF7 cells were transfected with TRIM13 and treated with wortmannin (a chemical inhibitor of autophagy), and a colony-forming assay was done. Autophagy inhibition in TRIM13 overexpressing cells results in negation of TRIM13-mediated suppression of the clonogenic ability of the cells (C), which indicates that TRIM13-induced autophagy might be essential for its tumor suppressor activity.

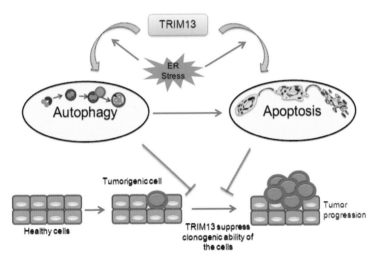

FIGURE 20.3 **TRIM13-mediated tumor suppression.** Experimental data suggest that TRIM13 induces autophagy and sensitizes cells to apoptosis. A number of tumor suppressors lead to induction of autophagy and apoptosis to suppress tumorigenesis. TRIM13-induced autophagy suppresses tumor progression by mitigating cellular stress though cellular damage is not controlled and stress condition is transcend this protein induces apoptosis to prevent its oncogenic transformation.

TRIM13-induced autophagy is essential for suppression of the clonogenic ability of cells, as the number of colonies was increased in TRIM13 overexpressing wortmannin-treated cells in comparison to untreated ones (Figure 20.2). Experimental evidence also suggests that the CC domain of TRIM13 is involved in regulation of the clonogenic ability of cells, which further strengthens the role of autophagy in tumor suppression, as this domain is involved in autophagy induction (Tomar et al., 2012a). TRIM13 and its cross-talk with p62 suggest that it may help to counteract cellular stress conditions and prevent the cells from acquiring a tumorigenic phenotype. This observation corroborate with that in an earlier study, which showed that selective elimination of p62 by autophagy is involved in the suppression of tumorigenic activity during the initial stages of tumorigenesis (Mathew et al., 2009).

DISCUSSION AND CONCLUSIONS

The role of autophagy in the process of tumorigenesis is complex and less well understood. Emerging reports suggest that this process plays both positive and negative roles in tumorigenesis. However, in established tumors, autophagy assists in the survival of tumor cells by protecting them from nutrient deprivation in hypoxic conditions, and also from chemotherapy-induced death. For the efficient management of tumor conditions, the molecular mechanism of the autophagy pathway and its regulation need to be studied. As discussed above, the post-translational modification of proteins regulates the activity, turnover, and signaling pathways during different physiological and pathological conditions. Ubiquitin-mediated post-translational modification plays critical role in the regulation of selective autophagy, as well as in the regulation of other signaling pathways. TRIMs are newly evolved proteins that help in the assembly of novel signaling complexes during many cellular stress conditions, such as genotoxicity, inflammation, and the innate immune response.

ER stress leads to the accumulation of unfolded proteins in the cellular environment which need to be cleared. Persistent accumulation of unfolded proteins in the cells leads to aberrations in the signaling pathways and transformation to a tumorigenic one. TRIM13 induces autophagy in response to ER stress, and can remove unfolded proteins and suppress the initial tumorigenic process. Such experimental evidences need to be further validated in animal models of tumorigenesis. The role of other TRIM family proteins in autophagy and tumorigenesis needs to be studied further to shed light on the molecular mechanism of tumorigenesis.

Acknowledgments

The research work in the authors' laboratories is funded by the Department of Biotechnology (DBT), Department of Science and Technology (DST), and Indian Council for Medical Research (ICMR), Government of India, and facilities developed under DBT program support to the Indian Institute of Advanced Research. Dhanendra Tomar received a Senior Research Fellowship from Council of Scientific and Industrial Research (CSIR), Government of India. We thank Sripada Lakshmi and Kritarth Singh for critical reading and helpful suggestions. This work constituted the PhD thesis work of Dhanendra Tomar.

References

Avela, K., Lipsanen-Nyman, M., Idanheimo, N., et al., 2000. Gene encoding a new RING-B-box–coiled-coil protein is mutated in Mulibrey nanism. Nat. Genet. 25, 298–301.

Cai, C., Masumiya, H., Weisleder, N., et al., 2009. MG53 nucleates assembly of cell membrane repair machinery. Nat. Cell Biol. 11, 56–64.

Chen, L., Chen, D.T., Kurtyka, C., et al., 2012. Tripartite motif containing 28 (Trim28) can regulate cell proliferation by bridging HDAC1/E2F interactions. J. Biol. Chem. 287, 40106–40118.

Cheung, B.B., Koach, J., Tan, O., et al., 2012. The retinoid signaling molecule, TRIM16, is repressed during squamous cell carcinoma skin carcinogenesis *in vivo* and reduces skin cancer cell migration *in vitro*. J. Pathol. 226, 451–462.

Christofferson, D.E., Yuan, J., 2010. Necroptosis as an alternative form of programmed cell death. Curr. Opin. Cell Biol. 22, 263–268.

Deshaies, R.J., Joazeiro, C.A., 2009. RING domain E3 ubiquitin ligases. Annu. Rev. Biochem. 78, 399–434.

de The, H., Lavau, C., Marchio, A., et al., 1991. The PML-RAR alpha fusion mRNA generated by the t(15;17) translocation in acute promyelocytic leukemia encodes a functionally altered RAR. Cell 66, 675–684.

Fuchs, Y., Steller, H., 2011. Programmed cell death in animal development and disease. Cell 147, 742–758.

Gack, M.U., Kirchhofer, A., Shin, Y.C., et al., 2008. Roles of RIG-I N-terminal tandem CARD and splice variant in TRIM25-mediated antiviral signal transduction. Proc. Natl. Acad. Sci. U.S.A. 105, 16743–16748.

Hatakeyama, S., 2011. TRIM proteins and cancer. Nat. Rev. Cancer 11, 792–804.

Johansen, T., Lamark, T., 2011. Selective autophagy mediated by autophagic adapter proteins. Autophagy 7, 279–296.

Joo, H.M., Kim, J.Y., Jeong, J.B., et al., 2011. Ret finger protein 2 enhances ionizing radiation-induced apoptosis via degradation of AKT and MDM2. Eur. J. Cell Biol. 90, 420–431.

Kawai, T., Akira, S., 2011. Regulation of innate immune signaling pathways by the tripartite motif (TRIM) family proteins. EMBO Mol. Med. 3, 513–527.

Khazaei, M.R., Bunk, E.C., Hillje, A.L., et al., 2011. The E3-ubiquitin ligase TRIM2 regulates neuronal polarization. J. Neurochem. 117, 29–37.

Komander, D., Rape, M., 2012. The ubiquitin code. Annu. Rev. Biochem. 81, 203–229.

Kudryashova, E., Kudryashov, D., Kramerova, I., et al., 2005. Trim32 is a ubiquitin ligase mutated in limb girdle muscular dystrophy type 2H that binds to skeletal muscle myosin and ubiquitinates actin. J. Mol. Biol. 354, 413–424.

Li, Q., Yan, J., Mao, A.P., et al., 2011. Tripartite motif 8 (TRIM8) modulates TNFalpha- and IL-1beta-triggered NF-kappaB activation by targeting TAK1 for K63-linked polyubiquitination. Proc. Natl. Acad. Sci. U.S.A. 108, 19341–19346.

Magiera, M.M., Mora, S., Mojsa, B., et al., 2013. Trim17-mediated ubiquitination and degradation of Mcl-1 initiate apoptosis in neurons. Cell Death Differ. 20, 281–292.

Mathew, R., Karp, C.M., Beaudoin, B., et al., 2009. Autophagy suppresses tumorigenesis through elimination of p62. Cell 137, 1062–1075.

Meroni, G., Diez-Roux, G., 2005. TRIM/RBCC, a novel class of "single protein RING finger" E3 ubiquitin ligases. Bioessays 27, 1147–1157.

Mizushima, N., Levine, B., Cuervo, A.M., et al., 2008. Autophagy fights disease through cellular self-digestion. Nature 451, 1069–1075.

Mosesson, Y., Chetrit, D., Schley, L., et al., 2009. Monoubiquitinylation regulates endosomal localization of Lst2, a negative regulator of EGF receptor signaling. Dev. Cell 16, 687–698.

Napolitano, L.M., Meroni, G., 2012. TRIM family: pleiotropy and diversification through homomultimer and heteromultimer formation. IUBMB Life 64, 64–71.

Niida, M., Tanaka, M., Kamitani, T., 2010. Downregulation of active IKK beta by Ro52-mediated autophagy. Mol. Immunol. 47, 2378–2387.

Okada, H., Mak, T.W., 2004. Pathways of apoptotic and non-apoptotic death in tumour cells. Nat. Rev. Cancer 4, 592–603.

Ozato, K., Shin, D.M., Chang, T.H., et al., 2008. TRIM family proteins and their emerging roles in innate immunity. Nat. Rev. Immunol. 8, 849–860.

Ryu, Y.S., Lee, Y., Lee, K.W., et al., 2011. TRIM32 protein sensitizes cells to tumor necrosis factor (TNFα)-induced apoptosis via its RING domain-dependent E3 ligase activity against X-linked inhibitor of apoptosis (XIAP). J. Biol. Chem. 286, 25729–25738.

Sato, T., Okumura, F., Ariga, T., et al., 2012. TRIM6 interacts with Myc and maintains the pluripotency of mouse embryonic stem cells. J. Cell Sci. 125, 1544–1555.

Schwamborn, J.C., Berezikov, E., Knoblich, J.A., 2009. The TRIM-NHL protein TRIM32 activates microRNAs and prevents self-renewal in mouse neural progenitors. Cell 136, 913–925.

Shibata, M., Sato, T., Nukiwa, R., et al., 2012. TRIM45 negatively regulates NF-kappaB-mediated transcription and suppresses cell proliferation. Biochem. Biophys. Res. Commun. 423, 104–109.

Short, K.M., Hopwood, B., Yi, Z., et al., 2002. MID1 and MID2 homo- and heterodimerise to tether the rapamycin-sensitive PP2A regulatory subunit, alpha 4, to microtubules: implications for the clinical variability of X-linked Opitz GBBB syndrome and other developmental disorders. BMC Cell Biol. 3, 1.

Siegel, R., Naishadham, D., Jemal, A., 2012. Cancer statistics, 2012. CA Cancer J. Clin. 62, 10–29.

Tanji, K., Kamitani, T., Mori, F., et al., 2010. TRIM9, a novel brain-specific E3 ubiquitin ligase, is repressed in the brain of Parkinson's disease and dementia with Lewy bodies. Neurobiol. Dis. 38, 210–218.

Tomar, D., Singh, R., Singh, A.K., et al., 2012a. TRIM13 regulates ER stress induced autophagy and clonogenic ability of the cells. Biochim. Biophys. Acta 1823, 316–326.

Tomar, D., Sripada, L., Prajapati, P., et al., 2012b. Nucleo-Cytoplasmic Trafficking of TRIM8, a Novel oncogene, is involved in positive regulation of TNF Induced NF-kappaB Pathway. PLoS One 7, e48662.

Touitou, I., 2001. The spectrum of Familial Mediterranean Fever (FMF) mutations. Eur. J. Hum. Genet. 9, 473–483.

Varshavsky, A., 2012. The ubiquitin system, an immense realm. Annu. Rev. Biochem. 81, 167–176.

Wu, W., Liu, P., Li, J., 2012. Necroptosis: an emerging form of programmed cell death. Crit. Rev. Oncol. Hematol. 82, 249–258.

Young, M.M., Takahashi, Y., Khan, O., et al., 2012. Autophagosomal membrane serves as platform for intracellular death-inducing signaling complex (iDISC)-mediated caspase-8 activation and apoptosis. J. Biol. Chem. 287, 12455–12468.

Zhang, J., Fang, L., Zhu, X., et al., 2012. Ro52/SSA sensitizes cells to death receptor-induced apoptosis by down-regulating c-FLIP(L). Cell Biol. Int. 36, 463–468.

21

Hypoxia-Induced Autophagy Promotes Tumor Cell Survival

Qipeng Zhang and Ke Zen

Abstract

Macroautophagy (hereafter referred to as autophagy) is a highly conserved biological process that degrades and recycles damaged, misfolded proteins or long-lived organelles. Previous studies show that hypoxia is common in solid tumors, and that hypoxia-induced autophagy is also found in these tumor cells. This chapter summarizes the recent literature on hypoxia-induced autophagy and reviews the prosurvival role of hypoxia-induced autophagy. We first review the mechanism of hypoxia-induced autophagy, and then analyze the several aspects of the protective role of this autophagic response for tumor cells: hypoxia-induced autophagy prolongs the lifespan of tumor cells, stimulates a more aggressive phenotype, and elevates the incidence of metastasis. Furthermore, hypoxia-induced autophagy enhances the resistance of tumor cells to cancer therapy. Potential autophagy inhibitors, including pharmacological inhibitors and siRNA or micro-RNA of autophagic genes, are reviewed and listed in the chapter. In summary, hypoxia-induced autophagy

© 2014 Elsevier Inc. All rights reserved.

promotes tumor cell survival. There is evidence of a tumor-suppressive role of autophagy in tumorigenesis, and the often observed autophagic cell death in extreme stress conditions is also discussed in this chapter. These phenomena can be attributed to the outcome of failed autophagic adaptation.

INTRODUCTION

Hypoxia in Normal and Tumor Cells

Oxygen (O_2) is an essential nutrient for all aerobic organisms. Oxygen serves as the terminal electron acceptor in the process of mitochondrial respiration that generates ATP. For this reason, oxygen deprivation impairs energy production and leads to an energy crisis in cells; even worse, accumulation of free radicals is a byproduct of impaired energy production that causes additional stress on proteins and DNA in the cell. When the oxygen tension in a cell, tissue, or organism is reduced, it experiences hypoxia. Hypoxia occurs under both physiologic and pathologic conditions, and has an effect on multiple aspects of an organism. For example, during early embryonic development, physiologic hypoxia stimulates development of the hematopoietic and circulatory systems to maintain the huge oxygen requirement for rapid cell proliferation (Covello and Simon, 2004). Therefore, humans develop complex respiratory and circulatory systems to ensure delivery of oxygen to meet the metabolic requirements of each of the 10^{14} cells of an adult organism. In many disease states, these systems fail and hypoxia becomes a major factor contributing to the pathophysiology of heart attack, stroke, and pulmonary hypertension, among others (Semenza, 1998). Importantly, rapidly growing tumors also experience hypoxia due to insufficient and defective vascularization. In fact, a major feature of solid tumors is hypoxia, which is supposed to promote tumor progression and increase treatment resistance (Brahimi-Horn et al., 2007). The role(s) of hypoxia in physiologic and pathologic conditions is a hot topic in current research.

Hypoxia-Inducible Factors (HIFs)

A major mechanism mediating adaptive responses to hypoxia is the regulation of transcription by hypoxia-inducible factors. HIF-1 is composed of HIF-1α and HIF-1β subunits; in particular cell types they may express HIF-2, which is composed of HIF-2α and HIF-1β subunits. This heterodimeric protein complex belongs to the basic helix–loop–helix (bHLH)/Per–Arnt–Sim (PAS) domain family of transcription factors (Gu et al., 2000). Under normal oxygen conditions, HIF-1α or HIF-2α is constantly and quickly hydroxylated on Pro^{402} and Pro^{564}, which is recognized by the von Hippel–Lindau protein (pVHL), leading to HIF-α ubiquitination and proteasomal degradation. Under hypoxic conditions, reduced oxygen slows down the activity of proly hydroxylase domain protein 2 (PDH2) and results in increased HIF stability. Under such conditions, the HIF-α subunits enter the nucleus and bind the stable β subunit, forming a functional transcriptional complex. All the HIF target genes have a cis-acting DNA sequence (5′–CGTG–3′) within their promoters or enhancers, called hypoxia response elements (HREs), which is the binding site for HIFs. HIF target

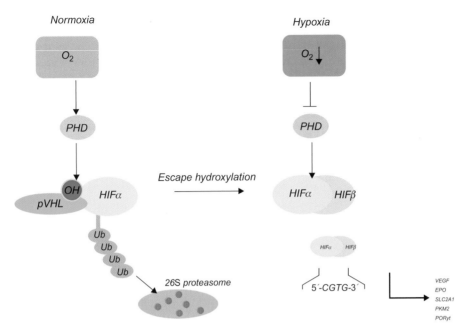

FIGURE 21.1 HIFs regulate the cell survival response to hypoxia. Under normal oxygen conditions, HIF-1α or HIF-2α is constantly and quickly hydroxylated by the proly hydroxylase domain protein (PHD), which is recognized by the von Hippel–Lindau protein (pVHL), leading to HIF-α ubiquitination and proteasomal degradation. In hypoxic conditions, reduced oxygen slows down the activity of PDH2 and results in increased HIF stability. Under such conditions, the HIF-α subunits enter the nucleus and bind the stable β subunit, forming a functional transcriptional complex. All the HIF target genes have a *cis*-acting DNA sequence (5′–CGTG–3′) within their promoters or enhancers, called the hypoxia response element (HRE), which is the binding site for HIF.

genes include the genes responsible for increasing oxygen delivery, such as erythropoietin (EPO), transferrin, vascular endothelial growth factor (VEGF), inducible nitric oxide synthase (NOS2), heme oxygenase 1 (HO1), and the genes responsible for decreased oxygen consumption, such as glucose transporters (GLUT1, GLUT3), hexokinase 1 and 2 (HK1, HK2), glucosephosphate isomerase (GPI), triosephosphate isomerase (TPI), glyceraldehydephosphate dehydrogenase (GAPDH), phosphoglycerate kinase 1 (PGKl), phosphoglucomutase (PGM), enolase 1 (ENOl), pyruvate kinase M (PKM), lactate dehydrogenase A (LDHA), etc. (Semenza, 1998). In summary, HIF in tissues is oxygen sensitive, and precisely regulates the delivery and consumption of oxygen (Figure 21.1).

HIF is also involved in many physiological and pathological situations. For example, during development, as normal cells proliferate, increased O_2 consumption results in hypoxia (reduced O_2 levels), which activates HIFs, leading to transcription of the VEGF gene, which encodes VEGF, a secreted protein that stimulates angiogenesis and thereby increases O_2 delivery. Since cancer cells are characterized as dysregulated cell proliferation, the blood vessels formed within solid tumors are often structurally and functionally abnormal, resulting in severe hypoxia. To adapt to the hypoxic microenvironment, cancer cells have to co-opt physiological responses to hypoxia that are mediated by HIFs (Semenza, 2012).

Hypoxia Induces Autophagy in Cells

Macroautophagy (hereafter referred to as autophagy) is a highly conserved biological process that degrades and recycles damaged, misfolded proteins or long-lived organelles. Autophagy can be induced by various stress factors, including nutrient starvation, growth factor withdrawal, hypoxia, etc. During this cellular "self-eating" process, selective or bulk portions of cytoplasm, including whole organelles, are sequestered in double-membrane vacuoles called autophagosomes. These structures fuse with lysosomes to form autophago-lysosomes, the site of degradation for the sequestered cargos. These "cargos" are degraded in lysosomes, thereby recycling energy and building blocks for the synthesis of new bio-molecules. The importance of autophagic signaling to homeostasis has been shown by the study of autophagy-defective systems. Autophagy primarily plays a prosurvival role in unfavorable growth conditions or under cellular stress. Autophagy is also constitutively active in cells, and plays an important role in quality control. Misfolded proteins and damaged organelles are degraded by this pathway. It is involved in many physiological and/or pathological processes, such as embryo development, cell differentiation, cell aging, and cell death. The initiation, elongation, and recycling of autophagosomes have been elegantly documented by numerous investigators, and are the subject of other chapters. Here, we focus on the activation and consequences of autophagy under hypoxic conditions (Figure 21.2).

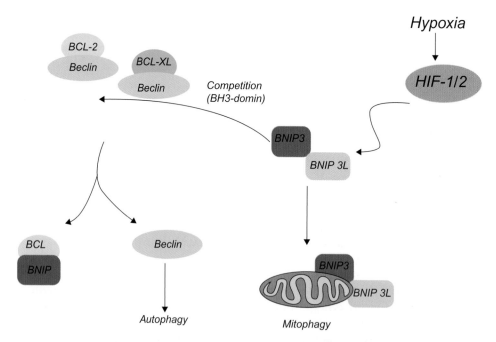

FIGURE 21.2 **The molecular mechanism of hypoxia-induced autophagy: hypoxia-induced expression of BNIP3 and/or BNIP3L proteins.** The BH3 domains of BNIP3 and BNIP3L displace Beclin 1 from the Bcl-2–Beclin 1 complex by competing with Bcl-2, and, because of the low affinity for Bcl-XL, BNIP3/BNIP3L is not capable of triggering cell death. Alternatively, BNIP3 and/or BNIP3L may be involved in mitophagy, the main clearance pathway of damaged mitochondria to prevent increased levels of ROS.

Hypoxia induces autophagy in various cells. Since autophagy is a stress-response and survival mechanism, it also contributes to the survival of established tumor cells under various stress conditions. In this chapter we focus on hypoxia-induced autophagy in tumor cells when tumors grow to a certain stage, and provide an overview of the autophagic signaling pathway, its role in tumor cell survival, and its connection to cancer migration and metastasis. In addition, we present a brief overview of the possible contribution of autophagic signaling to tumor-cell drug resistance.

HYPOXIA-INDUCED AUTOPHAGY PROMOTES TUMOR CELL SURVIVAL

Tumor Cells Employ Autophagy to Survive in a Hypoxic Microenvironment

A hypoxic microenvironment is very common in solid tumors. Although tumor tissues have increased angiogenesis, the rapid proliferation of tumor cells forms an increasing tumor size and the poorly functioning vascular network leads to an insufficient supply of nutrients and oxygen, especially in the center of the tumor. Gradients of oxygenation exist around individual perfused vessels, and range from normal values (~5%) near the vessel wall to anoxia in necrotic regions. Transient changes in blood flow also lead to strong temporal changes in oxygenation within specific tumor regions (Rouschop *et al.*, 2010). In such an extreme heterogeneous oxygen situation, the tumor cells and tumor stromal cells are under temporal and regional variable hypoxia. Therefore, tumor cells have to adapt to hypoxia. Autophagy is an important mechanism employed by tumor cells to survival in the hypoxic environment. It is reported that cells in the central region of a tumor tend to show higher levels of autophagy than do cells at tumor margins (Degenhardt *et al.*, 2006). Interestingly, in addition to inducing autophagy, hypoxia also leads to a physiological selective pressure in tumors for the expansion of variants that have lost their apoptotic potential, such as loss of the p53 tumor-suppressor gene or overexpression of the apoptosis-inhibitor protein Bcl-2 (Graeber *et al.*, 1996). In many tumor cells, apoptosis is inactivated. In these tumor cells with defects in apoptosis, survival of tumor cells under metabolic stress is dependent on autophagy. In fact, autophagy is essential for tumor cells to survive under metabolic stress. Genetic inactivation of autophagy will prevent tumor cell survival in response to metabolic stress when apoptosis is inactivated. Mathew and colleagues divided tumor cells under metabolic stress into to two stages: maintenance and preservation (Mathew *et al.*, 2007). During the maintenance phase, activities such as cell division and motility are sustained. Prolonged starvation and progressive autophagy cause cells gradually to shrink in size, but restoration of nutrients allows recovery. In the preservation phase, cell division and motility decrease, presumably as an energy conservation effort, creating the minimal cell that is capable of recovery (MCCR). Eventually, cells are defective in both apoptosis and autophagy; these cells undergo autophagic cell death after failure of restoration of nutrients to allow recovery. Even in tumor cells with normal activity of apoptosis, inhibition of autophagy enhances apoptotic cell death under metabolic stress. As for the tumor cells with a double defect in apoptosis and autophagy, these fail to tolerate metabolic stress, undergo metabolic catastrophe, and die by necrosis (Figure 21.3).

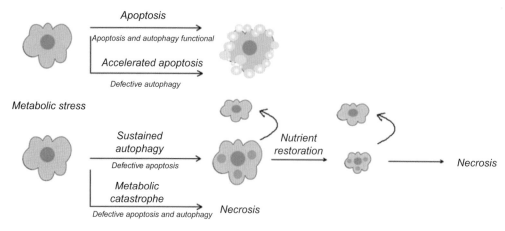

FIGURE 21.3 **Autophagy plays a prosurvival role in established tumor cells.** Mathew and colleagues have reviewed tumor cell death under metabolic stress. (1) In tumor cells with normal apoptotic activity, excessive metabolic stress may trigger cell apoptosis; inhibition of autophagy will enhance apoptotic cell death under metabolic stress conditions. (2) In tumor cells with defective apoptotic activity, the cells will endure two different stages (the maintenance and preservation stages). During the maintenance phase, activities such as cell division and motility are sustained. Prolonged starvation and progressive autophagy cause cells to gradually shrink in size, but restoration of nutrients allows recovery. In the preservation phase, cell division and motility decrease, presumably as an energy conservation effort, creating the minimal cell that is capable of recovery (MCCR). These cells undergo an autophagic cell death after failure of restoration of nutrients to allow recovery. Tumor cells with a double defect, in both apoptosis and autophagy, fail to tolerate metabolic stress, undergo metabolic catastrophe, and die by necrosis.

Molecular Mechanism of Hypoxia-Induced Autophagy

HIF is a key transcription factor that regulates hundreds of genes expressions, allowing cells to adapt rapidly to a large range of reduced oxygen concentrations and survive. It was demonstrated that a BH3-only protein, the bnip3 gene, emerged as one of the HIF-regulated genes that was induced during hypoxia (Bellot et al., 2009). Rapid and full induction of BNIP3 could protect cells from death through an autophagic process. HIF-1 and HIF-2 appear to be evenly matched in their capacity to induce BNIP3-dependent autophagy. In agreement with these studies, HIF-1-dependent expression of BNIP3 was described to be essential in mitochondrial autophagy (also called mitophagy), as described in MEFs (Zhang et al., 2008) and later in mole rat heart tissue (Band et al., 2009). Hypoxia impairs mitochondrial respiration, eventually leads to more damaged mitochondria, and causes production of reactive oxygen species (ROS) in tumor cells. Mitophagy (specific mitochondrial autophagy) is the main clearance pathway for damaged mitochondria. In fact, mitophagy is necessary to prevent increased levels of ROS (Rouschop et al., 2009).

BNIP3L is a homolog of BNIP3; BNIP3L shares 56% sequence similarity with BNIP3. Interestingly, BNIP3L is also induced by hypoxia, and is shown to trigger mitophagy and to be essential in the final steps of erythroid differentiation (Sandoval et al., 2008). Simple knockdown of BNIP3 or BNIP3L was sufficient to partially suppress autophagy. However, the strength of the response is enhanced when dual ablation of BNIP3 and BNIP3L is performed. These results reveal that expression of BNIP3 and BNIP3L is required for hypoxia-induced autophagy. Furthermore, they found that knockdown of BNIP3 and BNIP3L increased cell death in hypoxia, as did ablation of Beclin 1 or Atg5 in the same cells.

Regarding the mechanism by which BNIP3 and BNIP3L are capable of triggering autophagy, there is a proposed possible working model (Mazure and Pouyssegur, 2009). In this model, BNIP3 and BNIP3L compete with Beclin 1 for its interaction with Bcl-2. Bcl-2-bound Beclin 1 is then replaced and released, thus initiating autophagy. In detail, as a novel atypical BH3-only protein, Beclin 1 interacts with Bcl-2 or Bcl-XL and thus controls the balance between apoptosis and autophagy. BNIP3 and BNIP3L, both overexpressed in hypoxia, possess the atypical BH3 domains, which are the determinants in displacing Beclin 1 from Bcl-2/Beclin 1 or Bcl-XL/Beclin 1 complexes. Free Beclin 1 can thus induce autophagy.

There are some other molecules involved in hypoxia-induced autophagy, such as SQSTM1/p62 (Pursiheimo *et al.*, 2009) and DJ-1/PARK7 (Vasseur *et al.*, 2009). These molecules may act as an upstream activator or a downstream independent effector of HIF1 function in cancer cells. It is important to note that in anoxia (<0.1% oxygen) a HIF-independent autophagic response is induced, generated via AMPK–mTOR and unfolded protein-response (UPR) pathways. The autophagic cell death that is often observed in these extreme stress conditions should be seen as the outcome of failed adaptation (Mazure and Pouyssegur, 2010).

Hypoxia-Induced Autophagy is Associated with an Aggressive Tumor Phenotype and Elevated Incidence of Metastasis

The hypoxic core of tumors can induce autophagy and promote survival of these more aggressive cells. Hypoxia is implicated in the loss of E-cadherin expression during epithelial–mesenchymal transition (EMT), which is essential for cancer cell invasion and metastasis. This loss in E-cadherin maintains the mesenchymal migratory state enhanced by HIF induction of the c-MET receptor of hepatocyte growth factor and matrix metalloproteases, a set of conditions that magnifies migration of cells in search of nutrients (Semenza, 2010). During such migration, cancer cells detach from the original nest and move to a new place. This process of cancer metastasis necessarily requires that tumor cells survive in an isolated environment that is without nutrient support from the primary tumor. This metastasis-prone state may be particularly dependent on autophagy, as cells in isolation are expected to be more reliant on autophagy (Mathew *et al.*, 2007). The expression of LC3 (autophagy marker) has been reported to be strongly associated with the metastasis and poor clinical prognosis of human melanoma (Han *et al.*, 2011). Furthermore, the hypoxia-induced autophagic response is reported to be associated with an aggressive phenotype and elevated incidence of metastasis of head and neck squamous cell carcinomas (Vigneswaran *et al.*, 2011). In their study, two different murine squamous cell carcinoma cells (B4B8 and LY-2 cells) were injected into mice to establish the immunocompetent murine HNSCC models. The non-aggressive B4B8 cancer cells exhibited a slow growth rate and lack of metastatic spread, while aggressive LY2 tumors demonstrated a rapid growth rate with regional and distant metastasis. They found that the intratumoral hypoxia fraction in B4B8 tumors was significantly lower than in LY2 tumors, and that the hypoxic areas in B4B8 tumors exhibited an increased apoptosis rate compared with that of LY2 tumors. In contrast, autophagy was evident in the hypoxic areas in LY2 tumors. Furthermore, induction of hypoxia *in vitro* elicited autophagy but not apoptosis in LY2 cancer cells. The extremely aggressive pancreatic ductal adenocarcinoma (PDA) is characterized by a small population of highly therapy-resistant cancer stem cells capable of self-renewal and migration. Similarly, it is reported that markers for hypoxia, CSCs, and autophagy are co-expressed in patient-derived tissue of PDA (Rausch et al., 2012). Hypoxia starvation (H/S) enhanced clonogenic survival and migration of established pancreatic cancer cells with stem-like properties, while pancreatic tumor cells with fewer stem cell markers did not survive these conditions. Clinically, the autophagy marker protein LC3A was correlated with hypoxia and may be used as a poor prognostic marker for patient survival in human clear cell ovarian cancer (Spowart et al., 2012).

Hypoxia-Induced Autophagy Enhances the Resistance of Tumor Cells to Cancer Therapy

Current cancer therapies, such as angiogenesis inhibitors, inhibit the strong demand for angiogenesis in order to suppress or kill tumor cells; inhibition of angiogenesis will reduce the bloodstream in tumor tissues, which inflicts metabolic stress and hypoxia. Furthermore, conventional surgery, radiation, and chemotherapy disrupt tumor architecture and vascularization, leaving any remaining tumor cells potentially susceptible to metabolic stress. The treated tumor cells are particularly vulnerable because of their high metabolic demand and reliance on glycolysis (Mathew et al., 2007). In such a situation, autophagy is critical for a cancer cell's viability, as a stress-relieving and prosurvival function. Specifically, although the tumor cells decrease their oxygen demands by using an anaerobic pathway, they also sense the reduced oxygen tension and begin a hypoxic response, which leads to sustained hypoxia-induced autophagy. Therefore, genetic or pharmacologic autophagy inhibition preferentially sensitizes cancer cells to treatment. Literature regarding these studies has been reviewed (Morselli et al., 2009), including both pharmacological inhibitors of autophagy (e.g., 3-methyladenine, hydroxychloroquine, bafilomycin A1, monensin) and siRNAs that target essential modulators of the autophagic machinery (e.g., Atg3, Atg4b, Atg4c, Bec-1/Atg6, Atg10, and Atg12) and then sensitize cancer cells to a various of stress conditions (e.g., glucose and amino acid deprivation, growth factor withdrawal, detachment from the extracellular matrix (i.e., anoikis), estrogen receptor antagonism with tamoxifen, androgen deprivation, radiation therapy, and DNA alkylation damage with cyclophosphamide). Inhibition of autophagy with either chloroquine or Atg5-targeted short hairpin RNAs (shRNAs) facilitated tumor regression induced by p53 reactivation and DNA damage. These studies provide evidence that autophagy serves as a survival pathway in tumor cells treated with apoptosis activators, and a rationale for the use of autophagy inhibitors such as chloroquine in combination with therapies designed to induce apoptosis in human cancers.

Currently, several clinical investigations are examining whether pharmacologic inhibition of autophagy, using an autophagy inhibitor, can augment the efficacy of standard anticancer regimens. For example, it is reported that HIF-1α/AMPK-dependent hypoxia-induced autophagy is triggered by the devascularization in anti-angiogenic therapy. Hu et al. (2012) reported that, when compared with pretreatment specimens from the same glioblastoma patients, increased regions of hypoxia and higher levels of autophagy-mediating

BNIP3 were found in specimens from patients which are clinically resistant to the VEGF-neutralizing antibody bevacizumab. They demonstrated that when treated with bevacizumab alone, human glioblastoma xenografts showed increased BNIP3 expression and hypoxia-associated growth, which could be prevented by addition of the autophagy inhibitor chloroquine. *In vivo* targeting of the essential autophagy gene Atg7 would disrupt tumor growth when combined with bevacizumab treatment (Hu *et al.*, 2012).

Potential Autophagy Inhibitors

To enhance the antitumor effect, autophagy inhibitors may be combinative when used with antitumor therapies. Pharmacological inhibitors of autophagy (e.g., chloroquine, 3-methyladenine) and siRNAs or microRNAs that target essential modulators of the autophagic genes (e.g., siRNAs targeting Atg5, miR-30a targeting Bec-1) have been shown to sensitize cancer cells to a wide spectrum of stress conditions caused by antitumor therapies. Here, we have divided the autophagy inhibitors into two groups: small molecular inhibitors, and siRNAs or microRNA inhibitors.

Pharmacological Inhibitors of Autophagy

Currently, only chloroquine and its derivative hydroxychloroquine are FDA-approved agents able to inhibit autophagy; these affect the degradation stage of autophagy through preventing acidification of lysosomes. 3-Methyladenine (3-MA) and wortmannin repress the formation of autophagosomes by restraining the recruitment of class III PI3K to the membrane. Bafilomycin A1 (BafA) is a direct inhibitor of vacuolar ATPase, and interferes with the fusion of autophagosomes with lysosomes (Zhou *et al.*, 2012).

siRNA or microRNA of Autophagic Genes

Recently, inhibition of autophagy by exogenous siRNA or endogenous microRNA has been reported. For example, using the siRNA approach, by targeting Atg5, Atg6, and Atg7, in combination with tamoxifen in MCF7 cells can result in decreased cell viability concomitant with increased mitochondrial-mediated apoptosis. In a similar fashion, the combination of autophagy knockdown and tamoxifen treatment resulted in reduced cell viability in the estrogen receptor-positive T-47D and tamoxifen-resistant MCF7-HER2 breast cancer cell lines (Qadir *et al.*, 2008). MiR-30a is supposed to be able to sensitize the tumor cells to chemotherapy through suppressing the key autophagic genes Beclin 1 and Atg5 (Zou *et al.*, 2012). These findings indicate that dysregulation of miR-30a may interfere with the effectiveness of antitumor drugs' induced apoptosis by an autophagy-dependent pathway, thus representing a novel potential therapeutic target in tumor therapy.

DISCUSSION

This chapter has reviewed the adaptive response role of hypoxia-induced autophagy, which is supposed to be promoting the survival of tumor cells. However, autophagy is a double-edged sword for tumors (Long and Ryan, 2012): autophagy is potentially tumor-suppressive at the initial stages of cancer development. For example, accumulating evidence shows the inactivation of autophagy genes in certain human cancers (Liang et al., 1999), and in autophagy-compromised mice (Beclin 1+/−) a tumor is more likely to occur (Qu et al., 2003). These results indicate that autophagy is potentially tumor-suppressive before cells change into tumor cells. In this sense, autophagy, as an intracellular quality control mechanism, prevents malignant transformation and cancer progression. Nevertheless, if healthy cells have transformed into cancer cells, during progression of the tumor autophagy may subsequently switch to confer a tumor-promoting role by supplementing the metabolic needs of growing tumors in nutrient- and oxygen-deprived conditions. Besides the above roles, autophagy has many other facets and plays multifunctional roles in healthy or tumor cells. Furthermore, the role of autophagy in tumorigenesis is likely dependent on different tumor stages, such as initiation, progression, metastasis, and/or development of treatment resistance. It is important to decide when, where, and how to suppress autophagy during tumor therapy.

The detailed mechanism of hypoxia-induced autophagy still needs further study. During hypoxia, BNIP3 and BNIP3L are upregulated by stabilized HIFs, but the specific molecular mechanisms of BNIP3 and BNIP3L involved in autophagy are still uncertain. It has been proposed that the BH3 domains of BNIP3 and BNIP3L expressed in hypoxia displace Beclin 1 from the Bcl-2– Beclin 1 complex, while, because their low affinity for Bcl-XL, BNIP3/BNIP3L are not capable of triggering cell death. It is important that BNIP3/BNIP3L's affinity for Bcl-XL is measured. The intimate mechanism by which BNIP dimers and/or heterodimer complexes disrupt the Beclin 1–Bcl complexes also needs further investigation (Mazure and Pouyssegur, 2009, 2010). In addition, it has been demonstrated that mTOR inhibition by hypoxia does not require AMPK or LKB1; HIF-1 also has the ability to suppress the mTOR pathway through its activation of REDD1, which represses mTORC1, resulting in stimulation of autophagy (Brugarolas et al., 2004). There may be different pathways involved in the mechanism of hypoxia-induced autophagy; Papandreou et al. (2008) found that extreme hypoxia is able to activate a HIF-1-independent process, and the hypoxia-induced autophagic response is Atg5- and AMPK-activity dependent but is independent of the activities of BNIP3 and BNIP3L (Papandreou et al., 2008). Rouschop et al. (2010) reported that hypoxia stimulates autophagy in a ROS- and HIF-1-independent mechanism involving PERK activation in response to unfolded protein stress, resulting in the transcriptional upregulation of the autophagy genes Atg5 and LC3 (Rouschop et al., 2010). These reports, however, are still controversial; further study is needed with replication of the experimental conditions to draw a clear conclusion. Understanding the molecular mechanism of hypoxia-induced autophagy is helpful for selecting the target protein and designing autophagy inhibitors.

In tumor cells, hypoxia often occurs combined with other stresses, such as nutrient deprivation and DNA damage. All the above stresses could induce autophagy in tumors; it is hard to discriminate hypoxia-induced autophagy from other stresses. Unlike nutritional materials, oxygen is a material that cannot be stored and is not reusable; what is worse, lack of oxygen will lead mitochondria to produce more ROS and oxidative stress occurs, which is detrimental to the cell. In fact, hypoxic conditions are indispensable for cancer growth and progression; hypoxia leads to a vicious circle in cells. Prosurvival autophagy is employed to maintain homeostasis and help cells to overcome the stresses. Autophagy is an effective and important survival response of tumor cells; therefore, inhibition of autophagy is effective in killing tumor cells. Importantly, inhibition of autophagy can be applied under any circumstances; as mentioned above, if the apoptosis pathway is still uncompromised, inhibition of autophagy will lead to apoptotic cell death of the tumor cells, while if the apoptosis pathway is inactivated, inhibition of autophagy will lead the tumor cells susceptible to the stresses to die in a necrotic manner.

It is worth noting that the role(s) of autophagy occur in the tumor stromal microenvironment. Cancer cells are not pure homogeneous populations *in vivo*; instead, they are embedded in "cancer cell nests" that are surrounded by stromal cells. Furthermore, cancer cells show a broad spectrum of bioenergetic states, with some cells using aerobic glycolysis while others rely on oxidative phosphorylation as their main source of energy. In addition, there is mounting evidence that metabolic coupling occurs in aggressive tumors, between epithelial cancer cells and the stromal compartment, and between well-oxygenated and hypoxic compartments. As discussed above, the roles of autophagy in tumors are very complex. In recent years, attention to autophagy in the tumor stroma, which is referred to as "autophagic tumor stroma," has created a new paradigm to understand the role of autophagy in cancer. The Lisanti group has proposed a hypothesis. This group demonstrated that epithelial cancer cells use oxidative stress to induce autophagy in the tumor microenvironment (Salem *et al.*, 2012). As a consequence, the autophagic tumor stroma generates recycled nutrients that can then be used as chemical building blocks by anabolic epithelial cancer cells. Similarly, Zhao *et al.* (2012) proposed that the autophagic tumor stroma is a phenomenon of adaptation at a certain stage of tumor development, and has a prominent role in tumor growth and progression, and the spread of tumors (Zhao *et al.*, 2012).

Tumor cells are more active metabolically, and the poor vascularization of tumors causes hypoxia and nutrient deprivation. Antitumor therapy also puts stresses on tumor cells, and these natural and artificial stresses lead to a stronger demand for autophagy of tumor cells, and therefore autophagy may be a useful target for tumor therapy. Better understanding of the mechanism of hypoxia-induced autophagy and carefully choice of the target for autophagy, in combination with traditional antitumor treatments, will bring a benefit for tumor therapies.

Acknowledgments

This work was supported by grants obtained from the National Natural Science Foundation of China (31100777, 31000478, 81250044, and 90608010) and the National Basic Research Program of China (973 Program No. 2011CB504803). We thank Dr Jie Xu for producing the figures.

References

Band, M., Joel, A., Hernandez, A., et al., 2009. Hypoxia-induced BNIP3 expression and mitophagy: *in vivo* comparison of the rat and the hypoxia-tolerant mole rat, *Spalax ehrenbergi*. FASEB J. 23, 2327–2335.

Bellot, G., Garcia-Medina, R., Gounon, P., et al., 2009. Hypoxia-induced autophagy is mediated through hypoxia-inducible factor induction of BNIP3 and BNIP3L via their BH3 domains. Mol. Cell Biol. 29, 2570–2581.

Brahimi-Horn, M.C., Chiche, J., Pouyssegur, J., 2007. Hypoxia and cancer. *J. Mol. Med.* (Berl.) 85, 1301–1307.

Brugarolas, J., Lei, K., Hurley, R.L., et al., 2004. Regulation of mTOR function in response to hypoxia by REDD1 and the TSC1/TSC2 tumor suppressor complex. Genes Dev. 18, 2893–2904.

Covello, K.L., Simon, M.C., 2004. HIFs, hypoxia, and vascular development. Curr. Top. Dev. Biol. 62, 37–54.

Degenhardt, K., Mathew, R., Beaudoin, B., et al., 2006. Autophagy promotes tumor cell survival and restricts necrosis, inflammation, and tumorigenesis. Cancer Cell. 10, 51–64.

Graeber, T.G., Osmanian, C., Jacks, T., et al., 1996. Hypoxia-mediated selection of cells with diminished apoptotic potential in solid tumors. Nature 379, 88–91.

Gu, Y.Z., Hogenesch, J.B., Bradfield, C.A., 2000. The PAS superfamily: sensors of environmental and developmental signals. Annu. Rev. Pharmacol. Toxicol. 40, 519–561.

Han, C., Sun, B., Wang, W., et al., 2011. Overexpression of microtubule-associated protein-1 light chain 3 is associated with melanoma metastasis and vasculogenic mimicry. Tohoku J. Exp. Med. 223, 243–251.

Hu, Y.L., DeLay, M., Jahangiri, A., et al., 2012. Hypoxia-induced autophagy promotes tumor cell survival and adaptation to antiangiogenic treatment in glioblastoma. Cancer Res. 72, 1773–1783.

Liang, X.H., Jackson, S., Seaman, M., et al., 1999. Induction of autophagy and inhibition of tumorigenesis by beclin 1. Nature 402, 672–676.

Long, J.S., Ryan, K.M., 2012. New frontiers in promoting tumor cell death: targeting apoptosis, necroptosis and autophagy. Oncogene 31, 5045–5060.

Mathew, R., Karantza-Wadsworth, V., White, E., 2007. Role of autophagy in cancer. Nat. Rev. Cancer. 7, 961–967.

Mazure, N.M., Pouyssegur, J., 2009. Atypical BH3-domains of BNIP3 and BNIP3L lead to autophagy in hypoxia. Autophagy 5, 868–869.

Mazure, N.M., Pouyssegur, J., 2010. Hypoxia-induced autophagy: cell death or cell survival? Curr. Opin. Cell Biol. 22, 177–180.

Morselli, E., Galluzzi, L., Kepp, O., et al., 2009. Anti- and pro-tumor functions of autophagy. Biochim. Biophys. Acta 1793, 1524–1532.

Papandreou, I., Lim, A.L., Laderoute, K., et al., 2008. Hypoxia signals autophagy in tumor cells via AMPK activity, independent of HIF-1, BNIP3, and BNIP3L. Cell Death Differ. 15, 1572–1581.

Pursiheimo, J.P., Rantanen, K., Heikkinen, P.T., et al., 2009. Hypoxia-activated autophagy accelerates degradation of SQSTM1/p62. Oncogene 28, 334–344.

Qadir, M.A., Kwok, B., Dragowska, W.H., et al., 2008. Macroautophagy inhibition sensitizes tamoxifen-resistant breast cancer cells and enhances mitochondrial depolarization. Breast Cancer Res. Treat. 112, 389–403.

Qu, X., Yu, J., Bhagat, G., et al., 2003. Promotion of tumorigenesis by heterozygous disruption of the beclin 1 autophagy gene. J. Clin. Invest. 112, 1809–1820.

Rausch, V., Liu, L., Apel, A., et al., 2012. Autophagy mediates survival of pancreatic tumor-initiating cells in a hypoxic microenvironment. J. Pathol. 227, 325–335.

Rouschop, K.M., Ramaekers, C.H., Schaaf, M.B., et al., 2009. Autophagy is required during cycling hypoxia to lower production of reactive oxygen species. Radiother. Oncol. 92, 411–416.

Rouschop, K.M., van den Beucken, T., Dubois, L., et al., 2010. The unfolded protein response protects human tumor cells during hypoxia through regulation of the autophagy genes MAP1LC3B and ATG5. J. Clin. Invest. 120, 127–141.

Salem, A.F., Whitaker-Menezes, D., Lin, Z., et al., 2012. Two-compartment tumor metabolism: autophagy in the tumor microenvironment and oxidative mitochondrial metabolism (OXPHOS) in cancer cells. Cell Cycle 11, 2545–2556.

Sandoval, H., Thiagarajan, P., Dasgupta, S.K., et al., 2008. Essential role for Nix in autophagic maturation of erythroid cells. Nature 454, 232–235.

Semenza, G.L., 1998. Hypoxia-inducible factor 1: master regulator of O2 homeostasis. Curr. Opin. Genet. Dev. 8, 588–594.

Semenza, G.L., 2010. Defining the role of hypoxia-inducible factor 1 in cancer biology and therapeutics. Oncogene 29, 625–634.

Semenza, G.L., 2012. Hypoxia-inducible factors: mediators of cancer progression and targets for cancer therapy. Trends Pharmacol. Sci. 33, 207–214.

Spowart, J.E., Townsend, K.N., Huwait, H., et al., 2012. The autophagy protein LC3A correlates with hypoxia and is a prognostic marker of patient survival in clear cell ovarian cancer. J. Pathol. 228, 437–447.

Vasseur, S., Afzal, S., Tardivel-Lacombe, J., et al., 2009. DJ-1/PARK7 is an important mediator of hypoxia-induced cellular responses. Proc. Natl. Acad. Sci. USA 106, 1111–1116.

Vigneswaran, N., Wu, J., Song, A., et al., 2011. Hypoxia-induced autophagic response is associated with aggressive phenotype and elevated incidence of metastasis in orthotopic immunocompetent murine models of head and neck squamous cell carcinomas (HNSCC). Exp. Mol. Pathol. 90, 215–225.

Zhang, H., Bosch-Marce, M., Shimoda, L.A., et al., 2008. Mitochondrial autophagy is an HIF-1-dependent adaptive metabolic response to hypoxia. J. Biol. Chem. 283, 10892–10903.

Zhao, X., He, Y., Chen, H., 2012. Autophagic tumor stroma: mechanisms and roles in tumor growth and progression. Int. J. Cancer. 132, 1–8.

Zhou, S., Zhao, L., Kuang, M., et al., 2012. Autophagy in tumorigenesis and cancer therapy: Dr Jekyll or Mr. Hyde? Cancer Lett. 323, 115–127.

Zou, Z., Wu, L., Ding, H., et al., 2012. MicroRNA-30a sensitizes tumor cells to cis-platinum via suppressing beclin 1-mediated autophagy. J. Biol. Chem. 287, 4148–4156.

Index

Note: Page numbers followed by "*f*" and "*t*" refers to figures and tables, respectively.